HANDBOOK of BREAST IMAGING

Handbooks of Diagnostic Imaging

Series Editor
RONALD L. EISENBERG, M.D.
Professor and Chairman
Department of Radiology
Louisiana State University Medical Center
Shreveport, Louisiana

Volumes Already Published

Handbook of Gastrointestinal Imaging, edited by R. Kristina Gedgaudas-McClees, M.D.

Handbook of Head and Neck Imaging, edited by June M. Unger, M.D.

Forthcoming Volumes

Handbook of Neurologic Imaging, by J. Robert Kirkwood, M.D.

Handbook of Pediatric Imaging, by Lori L. Barr, M.D., and Susan D. Stansberry, M.D.

HANDBOOK of BREAST IMAGING

Edited by

Mary Ellen Peters, M.D.

Professor
Department of Radiology
University of Wisconsin Medical School
Madison, Wisconsin

Dawn R. Voegeli, M.D.

Staff Radiologist
Patuxent Medical Group
Howard County General Hospital
Columbia, Maryland

Kathleen A. Scanlan, M.D.

Assistant Professor
Department of Radiology
University of Wisconsin Medical School
Madison, Wisconsin

Churchill Livingstone
New York, Edinburgh, London, Melbourne

Library of Congress Cataloging-in-Publication Data

Handbook of breast imaging / edited by Mary Ellen Peters, Dawn R. Voegeli,
   Kathleen A. Scanlan.
      p.   cm. — (Handbooks of diagnostic imaging)
   Includes bibliographies and index.
   ISBN 0-443-08620-6
   1. Breast — radiography.   2. Breast — Diseases — Diagnosis.
3. Breast — Tumors — Diagnosis.   I. Peters, Mary Ellen.   II. Voegeli, Dawn R.
III. Scanlan, Kathleen A.   IV. Series.
   [DNLM: 1. Breast Neoplasms — radiography.   2. Mammography.   WP 815
H236]
RG493.5.R33H36   1989
618.1'907572 — dc20
DNLM/DLC
for Library of Congress   89-15760
                                                                   CIP

© **Churchill Livingstone Inc. 1989**

Distributed in the United Kingdom by Churchill Livingstone, Robert Stevenson House, 1 – 3 Baxter's Place, Leith Walk, Edinburgh EH1 3AF, and by associated companies, branches, and representatives throughout the world.

Accurate indications, adverse reactions, and dosage schedules for drugs are provided in this book, but it is possible that they may change. The reader is urged to review the package information data of the manufacturers of the medications mentioned.

The Publishers have made every effort to trace the copyright holders for borrowed material. If they have inadvertently overlooked any, they will be pleased to make the necessary arrangements at the first opportunity.

Acquisitions Editor: *Robert A. Hurley*
Assistant Editor: *Nancy Terry*
Production Designer: *Charlie Lebeda*
Production Supervisor: *Jocelyn Eckstein*

Printed in the United States of America

First published in 1989

Contributors

Margaret I. Fagerholm, M.D.
Assistant Professor, Department of Radiology, University of Wisconsin Medical School, Madison, Wisconsin

Enid F. Gilbert-Barness, M.D.
Professor, Department of Pathology, University of Wisconsin Medical School, Madison, Wisconsin

Mary Ellen Peters, M.D.
Professor, Department of Radiology, University of Wisconsin Medical School, Madison, Wisconsin

Lucinda K. Prue, R.T.R.
Radiology Technician, Department of Radiology, University of Wisconsin Medical School, Madison, Wisconsin

Frank Ranallo, Ph.D.
Director of Radiological Physics Services, Department of Medical Physics, University of Wisconsin Medical School, Madison, Wisconsin

Kathleen A. Scanlan, M.D.
Assistant Professor, Department of Radiology, University of Wisconsin Medical School, Madison, Wisconsin

Dawn R. Voegeli, M.D.
Staff Radiologist, Patuxent Medical Group, Howard County General Hospital, Columbia, Maryland

William H. Wolberg, M.D.
Professor of Surgery and Human Oncology, University of Wisconsin Medical School, Madison, Wisconsin

Preface

We have often been asked by our residents for an introductory book to mammography and a study guide for boards. We wrote *Handbook of Breast Imaging* to fulfill this need. It is our hope that other radiology residents as well as general radiologists interested in learning mammography will find it valuable.

The text is organized to reflect the information and procedures required at various stages of the mammographic examination. Anatomy and physiology of the breast, common clinical problems from a surgeon's perspective, pathology of breast carcinoma, physics of screen-film mammography, and positioning for the mammogram are discussed initially. The radiology of the normal breast is described prior to the discussion of the abnormal mammogram. Subsequent chapters address the mammographic findings in benign and malignant processes and in the postoperative and irradiated breast. Separate chapters review galactography, ultrasound, preoperative localization, and the mammographic report.

As in any other radiographic study, one's ability to read a mammogram is often dependent on mammographic presentations one has seen previously. We have, therefore, chosen to present the material through the use of numerous illustrations and a short but comprehensive text.

We are grateful to Mrs. Sally Jeglum for her patience in typing the manuscript, to Mr. Max Westrich for the preparation of the line drawings, and to our contributors — Drs. Margaret Fagerholm, Enid Gilbert-Barness, Frank Ranallo, and William Wolberg and Mrs. Lucinda Prue — for lending their expertise.

Mary Ellen Peters, M.D.
Dawn R. Voegeli, M.D.
Kathleen A. Scanlan, M.D.

Contents

1

Anatomy and Physiology of the Breast

Mary Ellen Peters

A working knowledge of the anatomy and physiology of the breast is required to understand its pathologic conditions as well as for interpretation of the mammogram.

ANATOMY

The mammary gland is enclosed between the superficial and deep layers of the superficial fascia. Approximately one-half of the gland overlies the fascia of the pectoralis major, with the remainder overlying the axillary and serratus anterior fascia laterally and the obliquus externus and rectus abdominis fascia inferiorly. Between the deep layer of the superficial fascia and the pectoralis fascia is the "retromammary space," which is filled with loose areolar tissue. Through this space traverse the posterior suspensory ligaments, projections of the deep layer of the superficial fascia, which fuse with the pectoralis fascia. The mammary gland is attached to the overlying skin by bands of connective tissue originating between the glandular fat lobules. These bands are called Cooper's ligaments (Fig. 1-1).

The long axis of the mammary gland is directed toward the axilla. The portion that extends into the axilla is termed the axillary tail, or the tail of Spence. In some women accessory glandular tissue, separate from the main gland, develops in the axilla. This may occur unilaterally or bilaterally. Knowledge of this normal variant is important to the radiologist, since carcinoma as well as benign masses can arise within it. One could also mistake the accessory axillary tissue for an abnormal mass if this variant is not known.

The glandular portion of the breast is composed of fibrous, adipose, and epithelial tissues and is divided into 15 to 20 lobes, arranged in a radial pattern. Each lobe drains separately via a duct; just beneath the surface of the nipple, however, some of the ducts join. Usually there are no more than 5 to 10 openings (papillae) on the surface of the nipple. Proceeding distally from the nipple, the collecting ducts branch, ending in the terminal ductal lobular unit (TDLU), which is comprised of an extralobular terminal duct, intralobular terminal duct, and ductules. The ductules are the most distal structures and have a saclike appearance (Fig. 1-2). (Ductules are also known as acini in the lactating breast.)

The lobule is the smallest structural unit of the gland and is composed of an intralobular terminal duct, ductules, and a surrounding vascular connective tissue that comprises the bulk of the lobule (Fig. 1-2). In the sexually mature woman, the lobule measures approximately 500 μm in diameter, and it is here that milk is secreted.

1

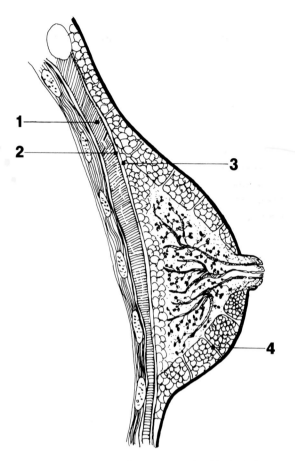

Fig. 1-1 Sagittal section of the breast. 1, pectoralis major; 2, pectoralis fascia; 3, superficial fascia; 4, Cooper's ligaments.

The ducts are surrounded by a specialized connective tissue that is more cellular and vascular than ordinary connective tissue. Lymphatic vessels are present within the connective tissues. Elastic tissue also invests the ducts but does not extend into the lobules. In the lobules the connective tissue is more cellular and vascular than that surrounding the ducts.

The epithelium of the ductal-lobular system comprises two layers. The superficial cell layer adjacent to the lumen is composed of true epithelial cells, which are cuboidal in the lobule and columnar in the extralobular ductal system. The deep cell layer throughout the entire system is composed of myoepithelial cells.

Although the large ducts can be involved with carcinoma, the smaller ducts are most often affected. Well-

ings[12,13] has demonstrated that ductal and lobular carcinoma in situ and invasive ductal and lobular carcinoma arise in the TDLU. Fibrocystic changes and fibroadenoma also develop in the TDLU.

LYMPHATICS

The lymphatic vessels arise in the periductal spaces. More than 75 percent of the total lymphatic drainage is into the ipsilateral axillary nodes, with the remainder draining into the ipsilateral internal mammary chain. Both groups of nodes receive lymph from all four quadrants. In a very small percentage of patients, lymph is received by the posterior intercostal nodes.

The axillary nodes are usually the first to be involved with metastatic disease, although other groups may be affected. Contralateral nodal involvement is only seen in the presence of ipsilateral lymphatic obstruction. The subcutaneous lymphatics are also an important route for spread of breast carcinoma. They anastomose with the deep lymphatics of the ipsilateral breast and the subcutaneous lymphatics over the contralateral breast and the abdominal wall.

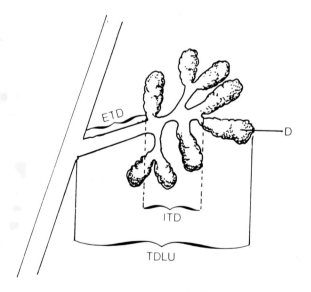

Fig. 1-2. Terminal ductal lobular unit (TDLU). *ETD*, extralobular terminal duct; *ITD*, intralobular terminal duct; *D*, ductule. The lobule consists of the intralobular terminal duct, ductules, and surrounding connective tissue. (From Wellings and Wolfe,[13] with permission.)

Lymph nodes are commonly found within the fibroglandular tissues of the breast. They are almost always located superiorly and laterally.

PHYSIOLOGY

Stimulation of breast growth at puberty is primarily under the influence of the ovaries, but the anterior pituitary gland and hypothalmus are also involved. Estrogen causes elongation and branching of the ducts, deposition of adipose tissue, an increase in the volume and elasticity of the connective tissues, and an increase in the vascularity. With the onset of ovulation and the production of progesterone, lobules are formed.

During the menstrual cycle, histologic changes occur that are dependent on the varying amounts of estrogen and progesterone. Vogel et al.[11] have studied these changes on specimens from reduction mammoplasty and subcutaneous mastectomy obtained for reasons other than cancer. They found, as have others, that different lobules in the same breast can vary in morphologic appearance. The morphology most consistent in serial sections formed the basis of their analysis.

From day 3 to day 7 of the menstrual cycle, and corresponding to a rise in estrogen, Vogel et al.[11] observed epithelial proliferation characterized by an irregular increase in cell layers. On days 8 to 14, stratified differentiation of epithelial cells occurred. The lumen of the acini and ducts grew larger on days 15 to 20, an effect thought to be the result of a rise in progesterone. During days 21 to 27, the luminal epithelial cells produced secretions, which also appeared to be a progestational effect. During this same time period, intralobular stromal edema and venous congestion occurred, changes Vogel thought were secondary to a sex steroid-induced histamine effect on the microcirculation. It has been theorized that the edema and congestion account for the "fullness" women experience just prior to menses. During days 28 to 2, when secretion ceased, there was loss of stromal edema and a decrease in luminal size.

During pregnancy and lactation, the lobules, as well as the acini within each lobule, proliferate, and the cells begin to secrete. Involution of the lobules occurs following cessation of lactation.

Menopausal involution of the lobule affects both the epithelium and its surrounding stroma. The epithelium flattens, loses secretory activity, and finally disappears completely. The loose connective tissue of the lobules transform into dense, hyalinized connective tissue. In this manner, the lobule is converted into ordinary stroma, which in the process of involution is replaced by fat.

SUGGESTED READINGS

1. Azzopardi J: Problems in Breast Pathology. WB Saunders, Philadelphia, 1979
2. Dewhurst J: Breast disorders in children and adolescents. Pediatr Clin North Am 28:287, 1981
3. Egan RL: Breast Imaging: Diagnosis and Morphology of Breast Diseases. WB Saunders, Philadelphia, 1988
4. Gray H: Edited by Goss CM, Gray's Anatomy. 29th Ed. Lea & Febiger, Philadelphia, 1973
5. Haagensen CD: Diseases of the Breast. 3rd Ed. WB Saunders, Philadelphia, 1986
6. Lanyi M: Diagnosis and differential Diagnosis of Breast Calcifications. Springer-Verlag, New York, 1986
7. Millis RR: Atlas of Breast Pathology. MTP Press Limited, Lancaster, England, 1984
8. Tabar L, Dean PB: Teaching Atlas of Mammography. Thieme-Stratton, New York, 1983
9. Townsend CM: Breast lumps. Clin Symp 32:3, 1980
10. Turner-Warwick RT: The lymphatics of the breast. Br J Surg 46:574, 1959
11. Vogel PM, Georgiade NG, Fetter BF et al: The correlation of histologic changes in the human breast with the menstrual cycle. Am J Pathol 104:23, 1981
12. Wellings SR: Developments of human breast cancer. Adv Cancer Res 31:287, 1980
13. Wellings SR, Wolfe JN: Correlative studies of the histological and radiographic appearance of the breast parenchyma. Radiology 129:299, 1978

TDIU = ETD + ITD + Tem.durhige
(remory) Scalps I I tragemin + Siah

2

Pathology of the Breast

Enid F. Gilbert-Barness

Breast carcinoma occurs in approximately 6 percent of the American female population and accounts for approximately 30,000 deaths annually in the United States. Mammary carcinoma is rare under 25 years of age and has a peak incidence at or around the menopause.

Many breast carcinomas are hormone-dependent. The demonstration of estrogen and progesterone receptors by radioimmunoassay and by immunocytochemistry using the immunoperoxidase technique on the tissue specimen has been important in directing hormonal therapy in such patients. Receptors have been found to be predictive of hormonal responsiveness, as indicated in Table 2-1.

Biopsy of a minimal nonpalpable mammographic lesion requires a mammogram of the biopsy specimen to identify the focus and to ensure that the lesion is selected for microscopic examination by the pathologist.

Epithelial tumors of the breast have their origin in the terminal ductal lobular units (TDLU). TDLU consists of the extralobular terminal duct, the intralobular terminal duct, and the terminal ductules (Fig. 2-1). The mammary lobule is composed of the intralobular terminal duct and the terminal ductules, within a loose connective tissue stroma. Benign lesions such as fibroadenoma and the full spectrum of "fibrocystic changes" have their origin in the TDLU. Fibrocystic changes may exhibit epitheliosis, epithelial hyperplasia, and preneoplastic atypical hyperplasia. In situ carcinomas (intraductal carcinoma and lobular in situ carcinoma)

appear to arise from pre-existing epithelial intraductal or intralobular hyperplasias. It has been estimated that in the human the time required for progression from normal to preneoplasia to neoplasia is 10 to 20 years; however, there may be regression or disappearance of the preneoplastic lesion.

The relative risk of invasive breast carcinoma based on the pathologic examination of the benign breast lesion has been defined in the summary consensus of the American College of Pathologists. Lesions diagnosed pathologically as adenosis, sclerosing or florid, apocrine metaplasia, macro- and/or microcysts, duct ectasia, fibroadenoma, fibrosis, mild hyperplasia (more than two but no greater than four epithelial cells in depth) mastitis, periductal mastitis, and squamous metaplasia have no increased risk for the development of breast carcinoma. Those lesions that are related to a slightly increased risk for invasive carcinoma (1.5 to 2 times) include hyperplasia of moderate or florid degree or with a solid or papillary pattern. Lesions with a moderately increased risk (5 times) include atypical hyperplasia (borderline lesion), either ductal or lobular.

A classification of primary breast carcinoma is shown in Table 2-2.

IN SITU LOBULAR CARCINOMA

Lobular carcinoma in situ tends to occur in younger women and produces no gross morphologic changes; it

Table 2-1 Receptors Predictive of Hormonal Responsiveness in Breast Carcinoma

Estrogen Receptors	Progesterone	Percent of Breast Carcinomas	Percent Hormonally Responsive
+	+	35	75
+	−	30	30
−	+	5	40
−	−	30	10

is a histologic diagnosis. About 10 percent of breast carcinomas arise within the terminal ductules of the lobules. Lobular carcinomas are usually multicentric and frequently bilateral. The likelihood of carcinoma being present in the contralateral breast in in situ lesions is 20 percent. The lesion is most often found in the upper-outer or upper-inner quadrants, within 5 cm of the nipple.

Microscopically the terminal ductules of the lobules are enlarged and filled with small, dark cells with few mitotic figures and usually no necrosis. The tumor cells are uniform, and the nuclei are round and uniform. The lesion may be difficult to differentiate from lobular hyperplasia. In the latter, the lesions are in normal-sized lobules, and the terminal ductules preserve the central lumen.

INFILTRATING LOBULAR CARCINOMA

Infiltrating lobular carcinoma is characterized by infiltration of the stroma by cells that are arranged in an "Indian file" arrangement in a dense fibrous stroma. The cells are small, round, and fairly uniform in size and shape, with hyperchromatic nuclei (Fig. 2-2). In approximately 80 percent of infiltrating lobular carcinomas there are foci of lobular carcinoma in situ.

INTRADUCTAL CARCINOMA

The noninfiltrating intraductal carcinoma (comedo carcinoma) tends to be multicentric but confined to the

Table 2-2 Classification of Primary Breast Carcinoma

I. Lobular carcinoma
  A. In situ (LCIS)
  B. Invasive (ILC)
II. Ductal carcinoma
  A. In situ (intraductal, comedo carcinoma)
  B. Invasive (infiltrating) adenocarcinoma, adenocarcinoma with productive fibrosis
    1. Not otherwise specified (NOS), usual
    2. Medullary carcinoma with lymphoid infiltration, atypical medullary carcinoma
    3. Mucinious or colloid carcinoma
    4. Papillary carcinoma
    5. Tubular carcinoma
    6. Inflammatory (ductal adenocarcinoma with dermal lymphatic invasion)
    7. Paget's disease
III. Stromal tumors — fibrosarcoma, liposarcoma, angiosarcoma
IV. Cystosarcoma phyllodes
 V. Rare tumors — adenoid cystic, apocrine, glycogen rich, metaplastic squamous, carcinosarcoma

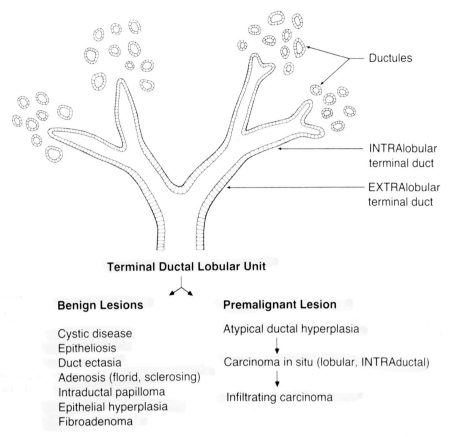

Ductules

INTRAlobular
terminal duct

EXTRAlobular
terminal duct

Terminal Ductal Lobular Unit

Benign Lesions

Cystic disease
Epitheliosis
Duct ectasia
Adenosis (florid, sclerosing)
Intraductal papilloma
Epithelial hyperplasia
Fibroadenoma

Premalignant Lesion

Atypical ductal hyperplasia

↓

Carcinoma in situ (lobular, INTRAductal)

↓

Infiltrating carcinoma

Fig. 2-1. Diagrammatic representation of the terminal duct lobular unit (TDLU) of the breast.

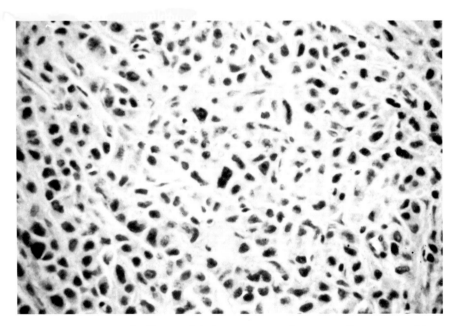

Fig. 2-2. Microscopic appearance of infiltrating lobular carcinoma. The tumor cells are arranged in an "Indian file" pattern. (H & E, ×100.)

medium-sized ducts. Proliferation of tumor cells within the ducts eventually fills and plugs the ducts. The centers of these distended ducts undergo necrosis. Cheesy material can be readily excreted upon pressure, hence the term comedo carcinoma. Microscopically there are dilated ducts filled with neoplastic cells with central necrosis (Fig. 2-3). If the tumor progresses, it may extend through the basement membrane and infiltrate the stroma, thus becoming an infiltrating ductal carcinoma.

INFILTRATING
DUCTAL CARCINOMA

The not otherwise specified (usual) infiltrating ductal carcinoma is the most common form of carcinoma of the breast and accounts for 70 to 80 percent of mammary carcinomas. On gross examination an infiltrating ductal carcinoma usually appears hard, averages 2 cm in diameter, and rarely exceeds 4 to 5 cm. The tumor may appear to be discrete, but more commonly is ill-defined and extends imperceptibly into the surrounding breast parenchyma (Fig. 2-4). On section, when there is a dense fibrous stroma (scirrhous carcinoma),

the tumor cuts with the consistency of an "unripe pear," producing a grating sound.

Microscopically the tumor usually has a dense collagenous hylanized stroma, with nests and clusters of neoplastic cells sometimes arranged in an acinar formation (Fig. 2-5). The cells are round to polygonol or compressed, with considerable pleomorphism. They contain hyperchromatic nuclei but are usually fairly uniform in size and shape. There are few mitoses, and the cytoplasm of the cells is amphophilic or clear. The tumor cells infiltrate surrounding fibrofatty tissue and frequently invade perivascular and perineural spaces.

MEDULLARY CARCINOMA

Approximately 4 percent of all mammary carcinomas are medullary in type. These tumors are usually deeply situated in the breast parenchyma; they tend to be large, fleshy masses up to 5 to 10 cm in diameter that are circumscribed and movable. The dense fibrous stroma seen in ductal carcinomas is not present; therefore they do not retract on the cut surface. The lesion has a soft, fleshy, brainlike consistency that is soft, par-

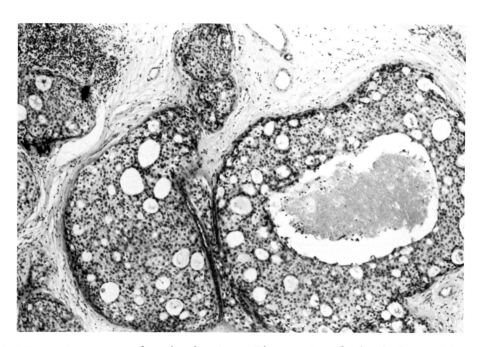

Fig. 2-3. Microscopic appearance of intraductal carcinoma. The tumor is confined to the ducts, and there is central necrosis. (H & E, ×100.)

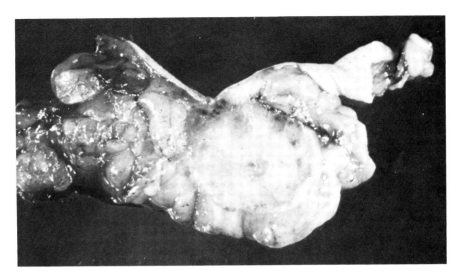

Fig. 2-4. Gross appearance of adenocarcinoma of breast. The tumor is poorly delimited and extends to the overlying skin surface.

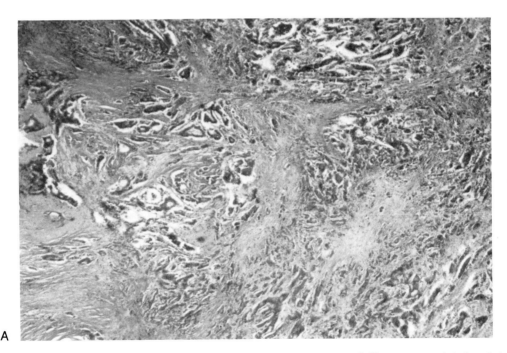

A

Fig. 2-5. **(A)** Microscopic appearance of infiltrating ductal adenocarcinoma with fibrotic stroma (scirrhous). (H & E, ×40.) *(Figure continues.)*

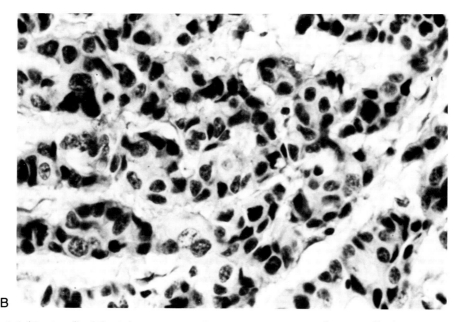

B

Fig. 2-5 *(Continued).* **(B)** High-power view showing acinar pattern of tumor cells. (H & E, ×100.)

tially cystic, bulky, and opaque and tends to resemble lymphoid tissue. Histologically, medullary carcinoma is highly cellular, with scant stroma. It is composed of large masses and sheets of polygonol cells with slightly basophilic cytoplasm, vesicular nuclei, and prominent nucleoli. A striking lymphocytic infiltration is usually prominent (Fig. 2-6). Mitoses are usually frequent; the presence or absence of the lymphoid infiltration appears to be of no prognostic significance.

MUCINOUS CARCINOMA (COLLOID OR GELATINOUS CARCINOMA)

This tumor comprises approximately 3 percent of all mammary carcinomas and has a considerably better prognosis than infiltrating ductal carcinoma. It has a slow growth pattern, frequently over many years, and is characterized by a large, bulky, well-demarcated, but unencapsulated mass (Fig. 2-7). The tumor has a soft gelatinous consistency and a slimy cut surface. Central cystic softening is frequently present.

Microscopically the tumor may form large lakes and pools of basophilic mucin, with small islands of neoplastic cells (Fig. 2-8). The tumor cells form an acinar arrangement and sometimes have a signet-ring pattern caused by cytoplasmic distention with intracellular mucin. There may be significant pleomorphism and invasive characteristics.

PAPILLARY LESIONS OF THE BREAST

Papillary lesions of the breast may develop within ducts or within cysts. Such lesions are usually not palpable and present with a serous or bloody discharge from the nipple. Distinguishing the benign papillary lesion from the frankly malignant tumor may be difficult. Invasion is considered the best evidence of malignancy. Papillary tumors most often occur in women just prior to, or during, menopause. Papillary carcinomas are usually 5 cm or more in diameter and represent about 1 percent of all mammary carcinomas.

Microscopic examination shows papillary fronds, with frank evidence of invasion of the surrounding ducts (Fig. 2-9). Mitoses are usually frequent. Lymphoid cells marginating the tumor may be seen. Frequently the lesion is borderline; however, most borderline lesions behave in a benign fashion and are usually cured by local excision.

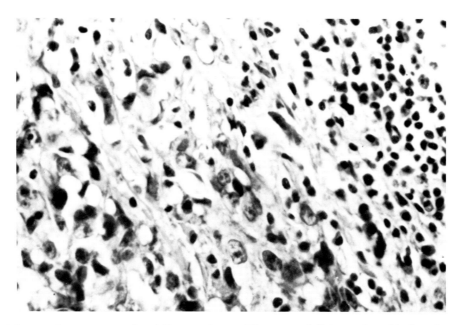

Fig. 2-6. Microscopic appearance of medullary carcinoma. The tumor *(left)* is marginated by lymphocytes *(right)*. (H & E, ×100.)

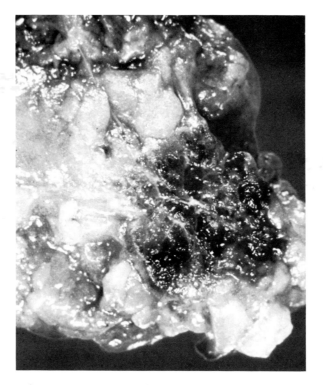

Fig. 2-7. Gross appearance of mucinous carcinoma of breast. The cut surface has a glistening mucoid appearance.

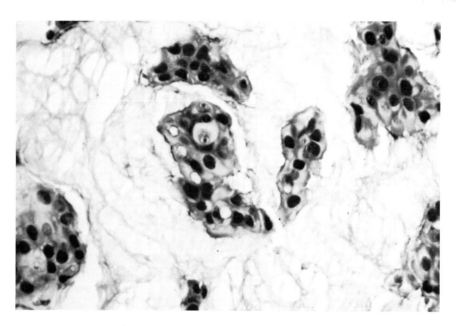

Fig. 2-8. Microscopic appearance of mucinous carcinoma of breast. The tumor cells are in small clusters within a sea of mucus. (H & E, ×100.)

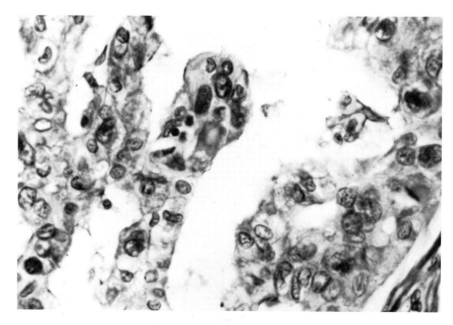

Fig. 2-9. Microscopic appearance of papillary carcinoma of breast. The tumor has a distinct papillary pattern with pleomorphism of the cells and high mitotic index with bridging and a cribriform pattern. (H & E, ×250.)

Papillary carcinoma has a better prognosis than ductal carcinoma, with a slower growth rate. Axillary lymph node metastases are not prominent.

TUBULAR CARCINOMA

Tubular carcinoma is a distinctive, well-differentiated type of mammary carcinoma. This tumor is usually no more than 1 to 2 cm in diameter. Microscopically it is composed of single-layered tubules in a fibrous stroma arranged in a uniform pattern. Sheets, papillary formations, and necrosis are absent, and mitoses are rare. Tubular and infiltrating ductal carcinoma patterns may coexist. Pure tubular carcinoma has a considerably better prognosis, with axillary lymph node metastases present in less than 25 percent of cases.

INFLAMMATORY CARCINOMA

Inflammatory carcinoma comprises less than 1 percent of all breast carcinomas. The entire breast is red, with brawny induration and widespread edema of the skin, simulating an inflammatory process. The nipple is usually crusted and retracted. The term, however, is a misnomer; the tumor is an infiltrating ductal carcinoma with widespread dermal lymphatic invasion. The presence of dermal lymphatic infiltration denotes a grave prognosis.

PAGET'S DISEASE

Paget's disease of the breast is a lesion of the nipple caused by infiltration of the epidermis by ductal carcinoma. It is an eczematoid lesion of the nipple that extends to involve the areola and surrounding skin. It is a manifestation of an underlying carcinoma of the breast with a malignant intraductal component. It occurs in an older age group and comprises less than 5 percent of mammary carcinomas.

A connection between the underlying carcinoma, within a duct, and the epidermis of the overlying skin of the nipple can usually be demonstrated if sufficient histologic sections are made. The tumor cells are large, pale, and vacuolated, lie within the epidermis (Fig. 2-10), and are similar to the underlying carcinoma. The

tumor can easily be confused with malignant melanoma and Bowen's disease, an intraepidermal squamous cell carcinoma. The prognosis is somewhat less favorable than the simple noninvasive ductal carcinoma. About 30 to 40 percent of patients have metastases at the time of diagnosis. The overall 10-year survival postmastectomy is approximately 60 percent.

STROMAL TUMORS

Cystosarcoma Phyllodes

Cystosarcoma phyllodes is a stromal breast tumor that is usually benign. It occurs in the same age group as breast carcinoma. Although the tumor may reach a large size, more than one-half measure less than 5 cm in diameter. Microscopically, this tumor resembles a giant fibroadenoma. Cystosarcomas are usually well circumscribed, firm, and gray-white in color; necrosis, cystic degeneration, and hemorrhage are seen only in large tumors. It has been suggested that the term cystosarcoma phyllodes be reserved for the malignant lesion and that the less aggressive form, which pursues a benign course, should be called giant fibroadenoma. The clinical presentation is similar to that of a fibroadenoma. The tumor tends to be totally or partially encapsulated and may be very large at the time of initial presentation, sometimes occupying most of the breast. When excessively large, it may ulcerate the overlying skin and become fixed to the underlying chest wall. Microscopically, cystosarcoma phyllodes has a highly cellular stroma and pleomorphism with an increased mitotic rate of the stromal cells. The epithelial portion of the tumor is benign and is similar to that seen in fibroadenoma. Those tumors that appear malignant histologically are characterized by stromal cells that simulate a fibrosarcoma with eight or more mitotic figures per high-power field. Some borderline lesions have less pleomorphism, are less cellular, and have lower mitotic rates. The capacity for a malignant cystosarcoma to metastasize is dependent upon the size of the tumor. Approximately 10 percent of malignant cystosarcomas metastasize, usually first to the lungs, although bone and visceral metastases may also occur. Axillary lymph node metastases usually occur relatively late, after pulmonary metastases. The metastatic lesions show only the sarcomatous pattern without the epithelial component. Cystosarcomas of borderline histo-

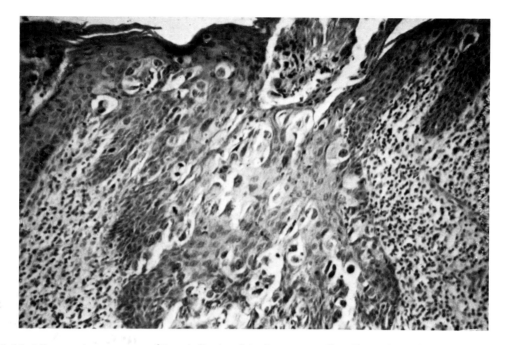

Fig. 2-10. Microscopic appearance of Paget's disease of nipple. Tumor cells infiltrate the epidermis. (H & E, ×100.)

logic malignancy rarely metastasize and usually only after local recurrence. A simple mastectomy appears to be the treatment of choice.

BENIGN LESIONS OF THE BREAST THAT MAY BE CONFUSED WITH CARCINOMA

A number of benign breast lesions may be confused either grossly or microscopically with carcinoma.

Acute Mastitis and Breast Abscess

Acute mastitis and breast abscess usually occur during lactation and may present as a localized area of induration. However, the lesion is usually painful. When the inflammation undergoes healing, fibrous scar tissue remains, and the localized area of firmness, often with retraction of the overlying skin, may simulate carcinoma.

Fat Necrosis

Patients with fat necrosis have a history of trauma in about 50 percent of cases. The lesion may present as a more or less well-defined nodule of firm consistency that may later become densely fibrotic and calcified. These lesions rarely exceed 2 cm in diameter and may resemble mammary carcinoma.

Fibrocystic Changes

The term *fibrocystic changes* encompasses the spectrum of cystic hyperplasia, chronic cystic mastitis, fibrosis, adenosis, sclerosing adenosis, epitheliosis, and atypical epithelial hyperplasia. One or more of these histologic lesions may coexist and/or be characterized by some degree of fibrosis of the stroma and epithelial hyperplastic lesions that may simulate breast carcinoma. Only atypical hyperplasia, mentioned previously, appears to predispose to a progression into breast carcinoma.

Fibroadenoma

Fibroadenoma may occur at any age but is more common before 30 years, at an earlier age than most patients with breast carcinoma. It is usually a small, movable, palpable nodule, 2 to 3 cm in diameter, rarely exceeding 5 cm. It occasionally contains areas of calcification.

Although it usually presents characteristic clinical features, surgical enucleation and pathologic examination are required to confirm its benign nature.

METASTASES FROM BREAST CARCINOMA

About two-thirds of all patients presenting with breast carcinoma have metastases to lymph nodes (Fig. 2-11) at the time of initial diagnosis. Axillary lymph node metastases are divided into three levels by the border of the pectoralis minor muscle (Fig. 2-12). The pattern of nodal spread is influenced by the location of the cancer in the breast. Tumors arising in the outer quadrants involve the axillary nodes alone in about 50 percent of cases; in an additional 15 percent, both internal mammary and axillary lymph nodes are involved. Cancers arising in the inner quadrants and center of the breast affect the axillary nodes alone in about 25 percent of cases while in another 40 percent internal mammary nodes are involved. Distant metastases via vascular spread may involve any organ, and widespread dissemination may be encountered. Frequent sites for metastases (Fig. 2-13) are the lungs, bones, liver, and adrenals. Some usual sites for metastatic involvement, such as the pituitary gland, eyes, and skin, are not infrequent in mammary carcinoma.

PROGNOSIS OF BREAST CARCINOMA

The prognosis of breast cancer has been determined and recommended by the American Joint Committee for Cancer and employs TNM (tumor size, nodal involvement, and metastases) as shown in Table 2-3.

The prognosis as determined by nodal involvement alone is shown in Table 2-4. The level of lymph node metastasis (Fig. 2-12, Table 2-5) and the histologic type of carcinoma also affects the prognosis (Tables 2-6 and 2-7). Poor prognostic signs include satellite nodules in the skin over the breast, extensive skin ulcerations, extensive edema of the skin, edema of the arm, extension to the chest wall, fixation of axillary nodes, spread to internal mammary or supraclavicular nodes, intradermal lymphatic invasion, and distant metastases.

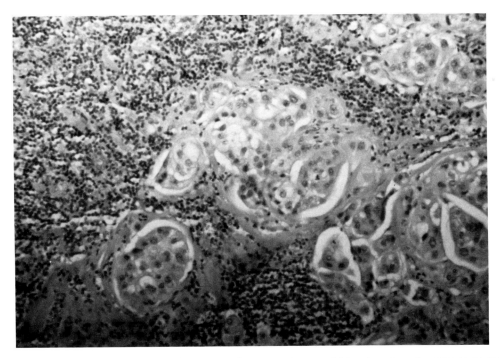

Fig. 2-11. Microscopic appearance of metastatic breast carcinoma within a lymph node. (H & E, ×100.)

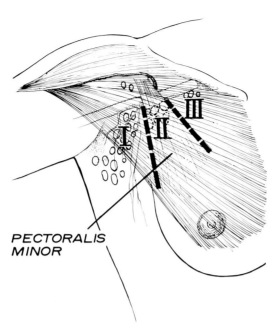

PECTORALIS MINOR

Fig. 2-12. Axillary lymph nodes divided into three levels by the borders of the pectoralis minor muscle. *Level 1,* nodes below the muscle; *level 2,* nodes beneath the muscle; *level 3,* nodes above the muscle. Level 3 is a key to prognosis (see Table 2-3) and a mark of the thoroughness of the axillary dissection. (From McDivitt et al.,[17] with permission.)

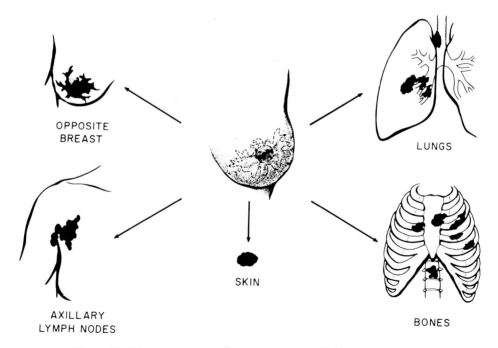

OPPOSITE BREAST

LUNGS

AXILLARY LYMPH NODES

SKIN

BONES

Fig. 2-13. The common sites for metastatic spread of breast carcinoma.

Table 2-3 Prognosis of Breast Carcinoma

PRIMARY TUMOR (T)

TX   Tumor cannot be assessed

T0   No evidence of primary tumor

Tis   In situ ductal carcinoma (intraductal); in situ lobular carcinoma; Paget's disease of nipple with or without intraductal carcinoma

Note: Paget's disease with a demonstrable tumor is classified according to the size of the tumor

T1   Tumor 2 cm or less in greatest dimension
  - T1a   No fixation to underlying pectoral fascia or muscle
  - T1b   Fixation to underlying pectoral fascia and/or muscle
    - i.   Tumor < 0.5 cm
    - ii.   Tumor > 0.5 < 1.0 cm
    - iii.   Tumor > 1.0 < 2.0 cm

T2   Tumor more than 2 cm but not more than 5 cm in its greatest dimension
  - T2a   No fixation to underlying pectoral fascia or muscle
  - T2b   Fixation to underlying pectoral fascia and/or muscle

T3   Tumor of any size with direct extension to chest wall or skin
  - T3a   No fixation to underlying pectoral fascia or muscle
  - T3b   Fixation to underlying pectoral fascia and/or muscle

T4   Tumor of any size with direct extension to chest wall or skin
  Note: Chest wall includes ribs, intercostal muscles, and serratus anterior muscle, but not pectoral muscle
  - T4a   Fixation to chest wall
  - T4b   Edema (including peau d'orange), ulceration of the skin of the breast, or satellite skin nodules confined to the same breast
  - T4c   Both of the above

Dimpling of the skin, nipple retraction, or any other skin changes except those in T4b may occur in T1, T2, or T3 without affecting the classification

Note: Causes of inflammatory carcinoma should be reported separately

LYMPH NODES (N)

NX   Regional lymph nodes cannot be assessed (not removed for study or previously removed)

N0   No evidence of homolateral axillary lymph nodes not fixed to one another or to other structures
  - N1a   Micrometastasis < 0.2 cm in lymph node(s)
  - N1b   Gross metastasis in lymph node(s)
    - i.   Metastasis more than 0.2 cm but less than 2.0 cm in one to three lymph nodes
    - ii.   Metastasis more than 0.2 cm but less than 2.0 cm in four or more lymph nodes
    - iii.   Extension of metastasis beyond the lymph node capsule (less than 2.0 cm in dimension)
    - iv.   Metastasis in lymph nodes more than 2.0 cm in dimension

N2   Metastases to homolateral axillary lymph nodes that are fixed to one another or to other structures

N3   Metastasis to homolateral supraclavicular or intraclavicular lymph node(s)

DISTANT METASTASES (M)

MX   Not assessed

M0   No (known) distant metastasis

M1   Distant metastasis present

(Data from Copeland.[6])

The overall 5-year survival of breast carcinoma is 35 to 40 percent. The 5-year survival rate for all patients treated by radical mastectomy is on the order of 50 percent.

The American Joint Committee on Cancer Staging of Breast Cancer can be summarized as follows:

Stage I: Relatively small cancers (up to 2 cm), localized to the breast

Stage II: Larger cancers (including those up to 5 cm) and/or those with regional freely movable axillary metastases

Stage III: Cancers with extensive local and/or regional spread

Stage IV: Distant metastases

Table 2-4 Nodal Involvement in Breast Carcinoma

Nodes Involved	Percent
All nodes negative	44
Internal mammary nodes only	9
Axillary nodes only	22
Both internal mammary and axillary nodes	25

Table 2-5 Effect of the Level of Axillary Metastases on Prognosis

Levels Involved	Crude 5-Year Survival (%)	Relative 5-Year Survival (%)	Relative 20-Year Survival (%)
None	75	83	65
I	56	62	38
II	41	47	31
III	28	31	11

(From McDivitt et al.,[17] with permission.)

Table 2-6 Cancer of Breast

Histologic Type	Percent of Cases	Percent 5-Year Survival	Percent 10-Year Survival
Ductal	78	54	38
Lobular	8	50	32
Medullary	4	63	50
Colloid	3	73	59
Comedo	5	73	58
Papillary	2	83	56

Table 2-7 Comparison of Special Histologic Types of Infiltrating Breast Carcinoma with Ordinary Infiltrating Duct Carcinoma (Infiltrating Duct Carcinoma with Productive Fibrosis)

Histologic Type	Infiltrating Duct Carcinomas with Productive Fibrosis	Infiltrating Lobular Carcinoma	Medullary (Infiltrating)	Colloid (Infiltrating)	Comedo-carcinomas (Infiltrating)	Papillary (Infiltrating)
Percent of total[a]	78.1	8.7	4.3	2.6	4.6	1.2
Average age (years)	50.7	53.8	49.0	49.7	48.6	51.9
Location		Standard	More in upper half of breast	Standard	Mostly subareolar	More in lower half of breast
Average delay time in seeking treatment (months)	5.6	5.1	4.1	5.4	5.9	5.8
Average size (cm)	3.1	3.5	3.4	3.8 (Not confirmed in Melamed et al's series[b])	3.9 (Either very small or very large)	3.4
Node involvement (%)	60	60	44	32	32	17
Median survival of treatment failures (years)	3.75	3.25	2.25	4.3	2.7	5
Crude survival (%)						
5 years	54	50	63	73	73	83
10 years	38	32	50	59	58	56
Actuarial survival (%)						
5 years	59	57	69	76	84	89
10 years	47	42	68	72	77	65
20 years	38	34	62	62	74	65

[a] Eight cancers of miscellaneous type excluded from tabulation.
[b] Melamed MR, Robbins GF, and Foote FW, Jr.: Prognostic significance of gelatinous mammary carcinoma. Cancer 14:699–704 1961.
(From McDivitt et al.,[17] with permission.)

SUGGESTED READINGS

1. Adair FE, Munzer JT: Fat necrosis of the female breast: a report of 110 cases. Am J Surg 74:117, 1947
2. Arthes FG: The pill, estrogens and the breast. Epidemiologic aspects. Cancer 28:1391, 1971
3. Azzopardi JG: Problems in Breast Pathology. In: Major Problems in Pathology. Vol. II WB Saunders, Philadelphia, 1979
4. Beahrs O, Myers MH (ed): American Joint Commission on Cancer. Manual for Staging of Cancer. 2nd Ed. JB Lippincott, Philadelphia, 1983
5. Commission on Clinical Oncology of the Union Internationale Contre le Cancrum (International Union Against Cancer—UICC): TNM Classification of Malignant Tumors. International Union Against Cancer, Geneva, 1968
6. Copeland M: Clinical Staging System for Carcinoma of

the Breast. American Joint Committee for Cancer Staging and End Result Reporting. June, 1962

7. Cutler SJ, Christine B, Barclay TH: Increasing incidence and decreasing mortality rates for breast cancer. Cancer 28:1376, 1971

8. Editorial: Steroid hormones and breast cancer. Lancet 2:521, 1972

9. Ellis DL, Teitelbaum SL: Inflammatory carcinoma of the breast. A pathologic definition. Cancer 33:1045, 1974

10. Fechner RE: Histologic variants of infiltrating lobular carcinoma of the breast. Hum Pathol 6:373, 1875

11. Fisher ER, Gregoria RM, Fisher B: THe pathology of invasive breast cancer. Cancer 6:1, 1975

12. Foote FW Jr., Stewart FW: Lobular carcinoma in situ. A rare form of mammary cancer. Am J Pathol 17:491, 1941

13. Haagensen CD: Diseases of the Breast. 2nd Ed. WB Saunders, Philadelphia, 1971

14. Haagensen CD, Stout AP, Phillips JS: Papillary neoplasms. Ann Surg 113:18, 1951

15. Korenman SG, Dukes BA: Specific estrogen binding by the cytoplasm of human breast carcinoma. J Clin Endocrinol Metab 30:639, 1970

16. McDivitt RW, Oberman HA, Ozzello L, Kaufman N (eds): The Breast. International Academy of Pathology Monograph. Williams & Wilkins, Baltimore, 1984

17. McDivitt RW, Stewart FW, Berg JW: Tumors of the Breast. Atlas of Tumor Pathology 2nd Series, Fascicle 2. Armed Forces Institute of Pathology, Washington, DC, 1967

18. Norris HJ, Taylor HB: Relationship of the histologic features to behavior of cystosarcoma phyllodes. Cancer 20:2090, 1967

19. Ridolfi RL, Rosen PP, Port A, et al: Medullary carcinoma of the breast. A clinicopathologic study with 10 year follow-up. Cancer 40:1365, 1977

20. Robbins GF, Berg JW: Bilateral primary breast cancer: a prospective clinicopathological study. Cancer 17:1501, 1964

21. Shapiro S, Strax P, Venet L, Fink R: The search for risk factors in breast cancer. Am J Public Health 58:820, 1968

22. van Bogaert LJ, Maldague P: Histologic classification of pure primary epithelial breast cancer. Hum Pathol 9:175, 1978

23. Wellings SR: Development of Human Breast Cancer. p. 287. In: Advances in Cancer Research. Vol. 31. Academic Press, Orlando, FL, 1980

24. Wheeler JE, Enterline HT: Lobular carcinoma of the breast in situ and infiltrating. In: Pathology Annual. Vol. II. New York, 1976

3

Clinical Diagnosis of Breast Masses

William H. Wolberg

The major clinical challenge of breast disease management is accurate diagnosis. Accurate diagnosis requires an understanding of breast disease and the modalities available to diagnose it. Equally as important as recognizing the diagnostic tools is understanding their limitations. The clinical dilemma is how to avoid benign biopsies and still minimize the number of nondiagnosed cancers. Even defining what constitutes a breast mass can be difficult at times. Both breast cancer and benign conditions cause nonpalpable mammographically identified abnormalities. How does one distinguish between what is benign and what is malignant? More importantly, what are the sensitivity and specificity of the diagnostic tests in the hands of each individual user? In this chapter, several benign conditions and how they are distinguished from cancer are discussed.

BENIGN CONDITIONS

Fibroadenoma are benign growths that may develop any time after puberty and are overwhelmingly the most common breast tumors in women under the age of 25 years. Fibroadenomata are usually single, firm, discrete, and freely movable. Skin changes and nipple retraction do not occur, and a correct clinical diagnosis can be made in the vast majority of instances. Fibroadenoma is rarely associated with breast cancer. Carcinoma developing in a fibroadenoma was found in 2 of my

series of 300 breast cancers. Cystosarcoma phyllodes is similar to a giant fibroadenoma and may be either benign or malignant. Accurate histologic diagnosis of malignant and benign cystosarcoma is sometimes difficult. When malignant, cystosarcoma rarely spreads to axillary lymph nodes.

Fibrocystic breast disease is the most common cause of breast masses. This diagnosis can be made histologically in over one-half of premenopausal women and includes so many conditions as to be a virtually useless term. However, it is useful to distinguish the following major pathologic types: epitheliosis (papillomatosis), adenosis, and macrocystic disease. Epitheliosis is a common, benign proliferation of the epithelial cells that line the distal ducts. These cells frequently form protuberances into the duct, hence the inaccurate term "papillomatosis." These ductal protuberances are not true papilloma and to refer to this condition as papillomatosis is confusing. Adenosis is a comprehensive term including all the non-neoplastic glandular hyperplasias that clinically produce the benign fibrous, lumpy breasts found commonly in premenopausal women. The term macrocystic disease covers the aspect of fibrocystic disease that produces gross cysts.

Breast cysts can usually be tentatively diagnosed by palpation, but sometimes they feel like cancer. Fine-needle aspiration without cytologic examination is used to establish a definitive diagnosis. Prerequisites for the diagnosis of a cyst by fine-needle aspiration are (1) nonbloody fluid is obtained, (2) the lump disappears, and (3) the breast examination is normal 6 weeks later. Cytologic examination of nonbloody aspirated fluid is usually unnecessary. Two series demonstrated positive cytology in only 3 of 10,000 cyst aspirates (McCarty KS Jr. and Kline TS, personal communication).

The common benign epithelial abnormalities included under the term of fibrocystic disease are found almost exclusively prior to menopause. Breast epithelial elements undergo atrophy at menopause. Postmenopausal estrogen replacement reverses menopausal breast epithelial atrophy, simulates benign breast disease, and thereby increases the complexity of breast diagnosis. When dealing with problems in premenopausal women, tactile breast examination is best performed 7 to 10 days after the onset of menses, when the breast glandular elements are least prominent.

Sterile benign inflammatory conditions of the breast include mammary duct ectasia and squamous metaplasia of the lactiferous duct, both of which present most commonly as periareolar fistulae in nonlactating women. Extensive mammary duct ectasia is unusual but may involve the entire breast and require a simple mastectomy for management. Squamous metaplasia of the lactiferous duct produces an epithelial plug of the duct at the nipple and causes a comedonelike process in the terminal duct. In contrast to duct ectasia, the lobules are not involved. Fat necrosis is a sterile inflammatory breast condition that follows trauma to the breast. Clinical presentation often resembles that of cancer, and bizarre cells are sometimes seen in fine-needle aspiration cytology.

Both benign and malignant breast disease may be associated with nipple discharge. Fibrocystic disease and intraductal papilloma are the most frequent causes of nipple discharge. Galactorrhea and galactocele are conditions due to faulty milk production. Milk can be distinguished from other nipple discharge by the presence of fat globules. The likelihood that nipple discharge is associated with cancer depends on the age of the patient and the character of the discharge. The following data provide useful guidelines for managing patients with nipple discharge. Devitt reported 1.6 percent cancers associated with nipple discharge in women younger than age 55 and 13.3 percent cancers associated with nipple discharge in women age 55 and older.[2] Ciatto et al. reported that cytologically suspicious cases were always associated with a bloody discharge, except for an occasional case with a purulent discharge.[1] In the absence of a mass, young women with nonbloody discharge, particularly from both breasts and/or multiple ducts, can be clinically followed. In older women and in selected younger ones, mammography may be a useful diagnostic adjunct. Bloody nipple discharge should be examined cytologically.

CARCINOMA

Breast cancer includes noninvasive and invasive types. The noninvasive types rarely metastasize and, if they do, one should question whether invasion was missed on the original pathologic examination. The two types of noninvasive cancer are lobular carcinoma in situ and intraductal carcinoma. Both are associated with an increased risk for subsequently developing breast cancer; lobular carcinoma in situ is associated with a bilateral risk, whereas the risk with intraductal is unilateral.

The major pathologic types of invasive carcinoma, lobular and ductal, have similar clinical behaviors. Less frequently encountered types with peculiar clinical characteristics are medullary, tubular, and adenoid cystic carcinomas and Paget's disease. Medullary carcinoma comprises about 5 percent of breast cancers and is characterized by a large local tumor appearing before metastases occur. Central necrosis is common and may appear cystic on ultrasound. Tubular and adenoid cystic carcinomas constitute about 1 percent of breast cancers and are characterized by their benign behavior. Paget's disease constitutes about 2 percent of breast cancers and is characterized by eczematoid nipple changes produced by nipple invasion from either invasive or noninvasive cancers.

DIAGNOSIS

Fine-needle aspiration biopsy for the cytologic diagnosis of breast masses is becoming more popular in this country, and its use is discussed in detail. For purposes of cytologic diagnosis, solid breast masses can be divided into those of epithelial and those of nonepithelial origin. The former include fibrocystic breast disease, fibroadenoma, and cancer. Nonepithelial masses include fat necrosis, post-traumatic damage, mammary duct ectasia, and lipoma. In premenopausal women, when epithelial cells are obtained fine-needle aspiration has been successful; the rule in postmenopausal women is that a positive diagnosis of a benign condition be made. Otherwise open surgical biopsy is essential.

Palpable masses are accessible for initial and for frequent follow-up tactile examination and are amenable to cytologic diagnosis based on fine-needle aspiration. In the presence of a discrete mass, fine-needle aspiration may precede either mammography or ultrasound for diagnosing breast masses. However, mammograms should be obtained before nondiscrete lesions are aspirated because aspiration may cause hemorrhagic distortion and the loss of valuable mammographic diagnostic information. On the other hand, mammography is superfluous for diagnosing a palpably accessible lesion.

Clinical application of fine-needle aspiration requires definition of the purpose of the cytologic diagnoses and knowledge of one's performance parameters. If the cytologic diagnosis is the definitive diagnosis prior to mastectomy, false positives must be minimized at the expense of a reciprocal increase in the false negatives. If the cytologic diagnosis avoids surgical biopsy of benign breast masses, false negatives must be minimized, and a reciprocal increase in the false positives must be accepted. I use fine-needle aspiration cytology to avoid biopsying benign masses. An intraoperative frozen section is done to determine whether the cytologically diagnosed cancer is invasive or noninvasive. Invasive and noninvasive cancers cannot be distinguished cytologically, and an axillary lymph node dissection is done

only for invasive cancers. With the same frozen section, the cytologic diagnosis is confirmed. Therefore, I use aspiration cytology to minimize the number of surgical biopsies needed to diagnose breast masses. In this context, an occasional false positive is acceptable, but a false negative is devastating. Our algorithm[4] has been skewed to avoid false negatives, and our false-positive rate is slightly higher than that reported by some. Test results based on 293 fine-needle aspirates (153 benign, 127 malignant, and 13 inadequate specimens, 8 of which were benign and 5 malignant) compare favorably with those reported in the literature. With our data set, exclusive of the 13 inadequate samples that were automatically biopsied, there were 147 true negatives, 6 false positives, 125 true positives, and 2 false negatives. The test performance statistics are sensitivity 0.984, specificity 0.954, and predictability of a positive 0.954. Lesions diagnosed cytologically as benign are followed clinically. A decision not to biopsy based on negative cytology requires complete assurance that the aspirate includes material from the clinically demonstrated mass. Astute clinical judgement must be exercised in cases with benign cytology to distinguish lesions that are suitable for clinical follow-up from those that require biopsy. However, with documented satisfactory test parameters, only clinical follow-up is necessary for most breast masses diagnosed cytologically as benign.

Nonpalpable breast masses that are identified only mammographically are more difficult to diagnose than are palpable masses. Deciding which nonpalpable, mammographically identified "abnormalities" require biopsy is a major problem in dealing with breast disease. In this context, I find the Moskowitz data on nonpalpable abnormalities very helpful.[3] Table 3-1 shows the incidence of cancer (both invasive and in situ) asso-

Table 3-1 Incidence of Cancer for Different Mammographic Patterns

Mammographic Pattern	Predictive Value for Cancer	Percent of Total Cancers Diagnosed with this Pattern
Punctate calcification	11.5	20.5
Mass		
Possibly malignant	5.4	7.3
Definitely malignant	73.7	6.8
Benign	2.2	2.9

(Data from Moskowitz.[3])

ciated with such abnormal mammographic patterns, based on biopsy of all calcifications and densities found in the Cincinnati Breast Cancer Detection Demonstration Project (BCDDP). These data provide a useful starting point for discussing biopsy indications with the patient.

Breast diagnosis can be difficult at times, and the best interests of patient and physician are not served by inflated claims of diagnostic accuracy. Diagnostic test users must know their personal test-performance parameters. Unfortunately, there is a trade-off between diagnostic sensitivity and diagnostic specificity. Diagnostic specificity suffers with improved sensitivity, and diagnostic sensitivity suffers with improved diagnostic specificity. The price for missing the diagnosis of breast cancer is so great that the tendency is to de-emphasize specificity and to biopsy anything that might be a cancer. Despite liberal biopsy, many cancers will not be diagnosed until after they have metastasized. Ultimately, an acceptable rate for benign biopsies to diagnose breast cancer must be determined and the information generated, in order to further a general understanding of the limits of breast cancer diagnosis.

SUGGESTED READINGS

1. Ciatto S, Bravetti P, Cariaggi P: Significance of nipple discharge clinical patterns in the selection of cases for cytologic examination. Acta Cytol 30:17, 1986
2. Devitt JE: Benign disorders of the breast in older women. Surg Gynecol Obstet 162:340, 1986
3. Moskowitz M: Minimal breast cancer redux. Radiol Clin North Am 21:93, 1983
4. Wolberg WH, Tanner MA, Loh WY, Vanichsetakul N: Application of a statistical approach to fine needle aspiration diagnosis of breast masses. Acta Cytol, 31:737, 1987

4
Physics of Screen-Film Mammography

Frank N. Ranallo

As with any medical imaging method, the objective of mammography is to provide optimal image quality for visualizing pathology, at the minimum possible risk to the patient. The mammographic examination places exceptionally high demands on image quality because of the small size and radiographic subtlety of the lesions that must be detected. Thus mammography requires substantially greater sharpness and contrast detectability than does general radiographic imaging.

The risk to the patient in mammographic examination is essentially the carcinogenic risk from the radiation delivered to the radiosensitive glandular tissue of the breast. In common with the vast majority of radiographic examinations, the carcinogenic risk to the individual patient from a mammographic examination is exceedingly small. The risk that a properly performed mammographic examination of a 40-year-old patient will induce cancer during the lifetime of that patient is most probably less than 1 in 10,000, perhaps substantially less. With older patients, the risk is even further reduced. This risk is not totally negligible, especially when considering the risk vs. benefit of screening large numbers of asymptomatic women under age 50. Responsibly, the clinician should try to limit any risk to the patient to as low a level as possible, consistent with a satisfactory result in the examination. Thus the reduction of radiation dose is a valid consideration in mammography. However, it is important not to overreact to the very small level of radiation risk in mammography. The image quality needed to make accurate diagnoses must not be seriously compromised in an attempt to reduce patient dose to unrealistically low levels. In such cases the risk to the patient due to a missed diagnosis may be much greater than any risk from radiation exposure. With the proper equipment selection, optimized exposure and development techniques, and a suitable program of quality assurance testing, it is possible to obtain very high quality mammograms at radiation doses that are *reasonably* low.

Because of the technical difficulties of providing a sufficiently high level of image quality at an acceptably low radiation dose, mammography has evolved into the use of dedicated imaging systems that can be optimized for this specific type of examination. Two distinct types of imaging methods are currently used in breast imaging: xeroradiography and screen-film imaging. The basic difference between them lies in the type of image receptor employed—the xeroradiographic plate vs. the screen-film cassette—and the resultant differences in image characteristics. These two types of image receptors have significant differences in patient dose, exposure latitude, and the x-ray energy spectrum required for optimum exposure.

Though xeroradiographic imaging requires the use of a specialized image receptor in place of the screen-film cassette, it is possible to utilize a conventional x-ray system to produce the x-rays. However, significantly better imaging results can be achieved by the use of totally dedicated xeroradiographic systems for mammography. In these units the tubes and generators are optimized to provide the appropriate x-ray energies and image sharpness; also proper patient positioning and compression is facilitated.

While dedicated units are *recommended* for xeromammography, dedicated units in mammographic screen-film imaging are *absolutely essential,* due to the even lower x-ray beam energies required and the need for vigorous uniform compression of the breast. It is simply not possible to produce a quality screen-film mammogram using conventional x-ray equipment, and the use of such equipment in screen-film mammography is strongly discouraged. In the remainder of this chapter, as we discuss the technical requirements of the various components of the screen-film mammographic system, the need for a carefully designed, dedicated system will become obvious.

Why should the radiologists and radiographers involved in mammography become familiar with the technical aspects of mammographic imaging? One reason is the need to make an informed decision in the purchase of a mammographic system. Some features such as ease of use, patient positioning and compression are relatively easy to investigate. However, the dedicated screen-film mammographic systems currently available vary substantially in their image quality and dosimetry characteristics. Discerning the differences between units in these areas is a much more difficult task. Much of the information supplied by the manufacturers can lead to erroneous conclusions unless one has an adequate understanding of the equipment characteristics that affect image quality and dose and a knowledge of the methods by which technical data on equipment performance are reported. For example, the dose for mammographic imaging can be expressed in many different ways. In order to compare patient doses from two different units, one must specify the exact type of dose measure used, the phantom thickness and composition, and the film density obtained, along with other imaging factors such as kVp and processing parameters (chemistry, time, and temperature).

A second reason is to provide for the optimal use of the mammographic system. Proper selection of imaging techniques and options, such as kVp, phototimer adjustments, developer temperature, and grid selection, can strongly affect the image quality and patient dose. A final related reason is the need for proper quality assurance to ensure the maintenance of optimal equipment performance. Once a facility for mammographic imaging is set up, proper imaging techniques must be established and means implemented for maintaining image quality and low patient dose. The questions of the methods and frequencies of checking equipment performance and the selection of personnel to perform these tests must be addressed. These activities are vitally important to the proper functioning of the mammographic facility.

The involvement of a physicist with expertise in diagnostic radiology in equipment acquisition, technique selection, and quality assurance can be very beneficial. Even when a physicist is associated with the clinical team, the physicians and technologists should acquaint themselves with the important technical aspects of mammographic imaging. This will allow them to better interact with the physicist and utilize the information he or she provides them. The clinicians need to make important decisions affecting the functioning of the mammographic facility. An ability to access and understand basic technical information is a great aid to this decision-making.

The remainder of this chapter discusses the basic concepts of image quality and patient dose and looks at how they are affected by the various components of a mammographic screen-film imaging system. The chapter concludes with a discussion of quality assurance methods.

IMAGE QUALITY

The subject of image quality in screen-film imaging is more easily understood by considering the two major aspects of image quality: *Image sharpness* and *low contrast detectability.* Although for clarity these two topics are discussed separately, in the end they need to be combined: the ability to visualize much of the important pathology in mammography, such as minute calcifications, is dependent on both the image sharpness and the low contrast detectability of the imaging system.

Image Sharpness

Image sharpness relates to the ability of the imaging system to discern fine detail in relatively high contrast objects. Image sharpness can be measured by the use of a lead foil resolution pattern. An x-ray image of several types of resolution patterns is shown in Figure 4-1. Typically, this device contains several groups of line patterns covering a range of sizes. The lines of lead foil in each group are separated by a distance equal to their width. One can make a quick and simple evaluation of image sharpness by a visual determination of the finest line pattern that can be resolved in an image of the resolution pattern. A more complete evaluation looks at the contrast level of each size pattern in the image and reports the contrast as a function of the number of line pairs per millimeter (lp/mm) in the pattern (also referred to as "cycles per millimeter"). This function is essentially what is referred to as the modulation transfer function, or MTF, of the imaging system.

The resultant image sharpness of the total imaging system is the sum of the sharpness characteristics of the various components of the system. The components critical to image sharpness include the x-ray tube and the screen-film cassette. The x-ray tube affects image sharpness by virtue of its focal spot size and the amount of off-focus radiation it emits. The effect of the focal spot size is influenced by the imaging geometry: the

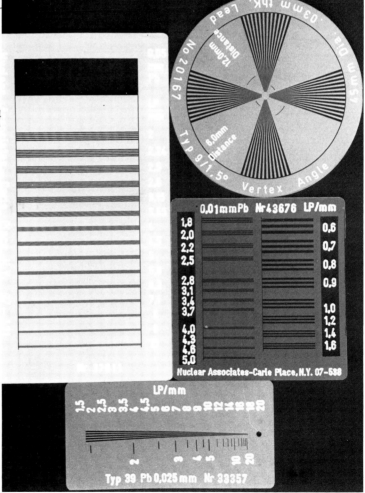

Fig. 4-1. An x-ray image of four different types of resolution patterns.

distance from the focal spot to the film and the distance between the breast and the film. Image sharpness is also affected by the characteristics of both the intensifying screen(s) and film and by whether close contact between them is maintained by the cassette. An additional very important contributor to image sharpness — or rather the lack of image sharpness — is patient motion. Equipment characteristics can contribute to this problem. If long exposure times are required, blurring due to patient motion is more likely. If the assembly containing the x-ray tube and image receptor is not mechanically stable, motion blurring may occur. Magnification imaging in mammography can make extreme demands on image quality factors. It requires both a very small focal spot size and an absolute minimum of patient motion.

Low Contrast Detectability

Low contrast detectability describes how well an imaging system is able to detect relatively large low contrast objects. It is affected by the combination of two image properties: image contrast and image noise. Consider a very simplified imaging situation in which the following manufactured object is imaged: a uniform "tumor" embedded in a volume of uniform "tissue." In the image you would expect to see a small area of raised or lowered density surrounded by a uniform background. The difference in density between the image of the tumor and the background tissue is the *image contrast* for the tumor. If you look closely at the film, however, you will notice that the images of both the tumor and the background are not perfectly uniform, even though the objects themselves were manufactured to be perfectly uniform. These fluctuations in density over the image, which are inherent limitations of the imaging process and do not reflect actual textures in the objects being imaged, are called *image noise*. Since these artificial or "artifactual" density fluctuations compete with the real density fluctuations produced by subtle features in the objects, the image noise interferes with our detection of subtle object features. In simple terms, to be able to recognize that an area in an image with a density different from the background density is a "real" feature, the eye must judge that it is unlikely that this area of different density could have resulted simply from the noise in the image. In other words, the image contrast must exceed the image noise. The visibility of a low contrast object can be obscured by either a loss in image contrast or an increase in image noise.

Low contrast detectability can be measured by imaging a phantom containing suitable low contrast objects. Several types of mammographic test phantoms contain "masses" that serve this purpose.

The image contrast of an object is affected in part by the difference in x-ray attenuation in the object compared with the x-ray attenuation of the material around it. That difference in attenuation can be increased by lowering the energy of the x-ray photons used to form the image; this can be accomplished by lowering the kVp technique or by using k-edge filters (such as molybdenum). The use of an antiscatter grid can increase image contrast by removing much of the scatter radiation in the x-ray beam exiting the patient. These methods all increase contrast without increasing image noise.

Image contrast can also be increased by selecting a film with higher contrast or by modifying film processing methods. This increase in contrast, however, is also accompanied by an increase in image noise, so that the increase in low contrast detectability may be minimal. It is important to increase film contrast to a level at which the visibility of low contrast objects actually is limited by image noise rather than simply by the fact of the contrast of the objects being too low for the eye to detect. However, increasing film contrast beyond that level simply reduces the exposure latitude of the image without significantly increasing the detectability of low contrast objects.

↑ # photons ↓ quant mottle

Image noise is of three types: quantum mottle, film graininess, and structure noise. *Quantum mottle* exists because the image is formed by the absorption of a finite number of individual x-ray photons. The larger the number of photons absorbed to form the image, the smaller the quantum mottle. Suppose you wanted to reduce the patient dose by one-half and could do so either by using a new film that was twice as sensitive as your current film or by using a new intensifying screen that could absorb twice the percentage of x-ray photons as your current screen. In either case you could cut your mAs technique (and patient dose) in half. If you chose the new film, you would find a significant increase in quantum mottle since you would now be forming an image with only one-half the number of x-ray photons. If, instead, you chose the new screen you could reduce patient dose without increasing quantum mottle. Again, only one-half the number of x-ray photons would strike the screen, compared with your original technique, but the screen would absorb twice as many of the photons that hit it. The net result is that the same number of x-ray photons are absorbed to form the image as with the original screen. Of course, unless the new screen obtained its greater absorbing powers from a newer technology, it would have to be thicker and thus have less image sharpness.

Film graininess exists because the film emulsion is composed of discrete grains of silver halide crystals. It produces a noise with a much finer structure than quantum mottle. While graininess is not a significant noise factor in most areas of radiology, in mammography its effect on image noise is not negligible, since it can interfere with the detection of very fine structures such as microcalcifications.

Structure noise can come from any object within the x-ray beam. While some amount of quantum mottle and film graininess is unavoidable, structure noise is due to imperfections in the imaging system. If the intensifying screens or antiscatter grid is improperly manufactured or damaged, it may produce a mottle or artifact in the image that is reproduced on all films. Textures in the materials used as the x-ray filter, breast support, or compression device may show up in the images. Great care must be taken in the selection and fabrication of these materials. Because of the great sensitivity of the mammographic imaging system it can visualize even minor defects.

Visibility of Pathologies

The concepts of image sharpness and low contrast detectability are to some extent idealized to simplify the understanding and actual testing of image quality. Image sharpness describes the visibility of small objects of high contrast, while low contrast detectability describes the visibility of large objects of low contrast. In some cases the visibility of specific pathology is determined almost solely by either the image sharpness or the low contrast detectability properties of the imaging system. For example, in computed tomography (CT) imaging, bone detail depends principally on image sharpness, while the imaging of soft tissue tumors depends on low contrast detectability. In many cases, though, the visibility of pathology is dependent on *both* image sharpness and low contrast detectability. The visibility of microcalcifications in mammography is such a case. Here the objects to be visualized are both

very small and also of low contrast, since their small size does not allow much additional attenuation of the x-ray beam. Hence the visibility of microcalcifications can be diminished if either the image sharpness or low contrast detectability of the imaging system is degraded.

Mammography phantoms that contain specks and fibrils produce images that are very useful in evaluating the total image quality of mammographic systems in a way that is clinically relevant. The imaging of the specks and fibrils depends on both the image sharpness and low contrast detectability of the imaging systems.

PATIENT DOSE

The radiation dose received by the breast is affected by many different components of the imaging system. The factors that influence dose include: the generator type, the actual kVp used, the x-ray tube anode material, the x-ray filter, the use and type of antiscatter grid, the type of film and intensifying screen, the processing technique, and the film density. The effect of each of these factors on image quality and dose will be discussed in the next section of this chapter. At this point the discussion will focus on the ways of expressing patient dose.

First let's review the meaning of the three types of quantities and units encountered in radiation dosimetry. One quantity, called "exposure" and given in units of *roentgens (R)*, measures the ionizing strength of the radiation in air: 1 R will cause the production of 2.58×10^{-4} coulombs of ionization per kilogram of air. This measurement of exposure is performed using an air-filled ion chamber. Another quantity, called "absorbed dose," is given in units of *rads* — 1 rad corresponds to the absorption of 100 ergs of energy per gram of tissue. For soft tissue (or water), an exposure of 1 R at the surface of the tissue will produce an absorbed dose of about 0.8 to 0.9 rad in the surface tissue. A third quantity, called "dose equivalent," is given in units of *rems* and is simply the product of absorbed dose times a "quality factor" that reflects the relative biological damage caused by different forms of ionizing radiation (x-rays, beta particles, alpha particles, neutrons). Since the quality factor for x-rays is 1.0, the expression of radiation dose in either *rads* or *rems* will be numerically equal in diagnostic radiology.

The three types of radiation quantities described above can also be expressed using the newer, preferred SI units. In the SI system, exposure is directly expressed in units of coulombs per kilogram ($C\ Kg^{-1}$), with 1 R equaling $2.58 \times 10^{-4}C\ kg^{-1}$. The unit of absorbed dose in the SI system is the *gray (Gy)* — 1 Gy equals 100 rad and corresponds to the absorption of 1 joule of energy per kilogram of tissue. Often the unit centigray (cGy) is used; this is 1/100 of a gray and is equal to 1 rad. The SI unit of dose equivalent is the *sievert (Sv)*, with 1 Sv equaling 100 rem.

Table 4-1 lists the various ways that patient dosimetry has been expressed in the literature. Since the resultant numbers can vary by more than a factor of 10, it is very important that one understand which method of dose description is being used when one looks at dose figures.

Surface exposure — free in air — without backscatter is the direct measurement obtained when an ion chamber is placed at the point in space where the surface of the breast would normally be in the imaging process. Here no phantom is used. If instead the measurement is made with a breast equivalent material placed where the breast would normally be and with the ion chamber placed on top of the phantom, the exposure meter will now read *surface exposure — including backscatter,* a slightly higher number. (When radiation impinges on an object, some fraction of the radiation that enters the object is scattered back out; this is called *backscatter*.) This exposure reading directly above the surface of the breast can be numerically converted to the dose received by the surface tissue of the breast, the *surface dose*. Since the amount of backscatter in mammography is generally less than 10 percent, and the conversion from surface exposure (in R) to surface dose (in rads) changes the number by only 10 to 20 percent, the numerical differences among the first three dosimetry measurements are not very significant.

The above measurements of surface exposure and dose can also be obtained using thermoluminescent dosimeter (TLD) chips that can be placed on the surface of the breast or phantom instead of using an ion chamber. TLDs are small chips typically composed of lithium fluoride. If these chips are exposed to radiation and later heated, they will give off a light glow during heating that is proportional to the radiation dose they absorbed. There are several organizations in the United States that offer TLD dosimetry services. These services will send you TLDs that can be placed on patients or phantoms during an x-ray exposure. You then return the TLDs for analysis and a report of the radiation doses. These services provide clinical institutions with an easy, accurate method of monitoring radiation exposures in clinical examinations, without the need for purchasing expensive radiation measurement equipment.

The next three dosimetry measurements all refer to the absorbed dose at a point of the breast other than the surface or to some average dose over the breast tissue. These measurements all give numbers substantially less than the first three types because of the attenuation of the radiation as it passes through the breast. These measurements can be made directly by placing TLDs within a breast equivalent phantom. In practice, they are usually calculated from the surface exposure using published tables that were derived from actual depth dose experiments.

The *midbreast dose* is simply the dose to the breast tissue at a depth equal to one-half the compressed thickness of the breast. It is a somewhat better measure of the radiation risk to the breast than surface dose, but it still falls substantially short of accurately representing the true risk to the entire breast. This is especially the case in screen-film mammography, in which the midbreast dose may significantly underestimate the radiation risk.

There is a problem with the reporting of midbreast dose that occurs with some TLD services. In some cases the dose to the breast is reported as midbreast dose, but the number given is actually the dose at a 3 cm depth in the

Table 4-1 Dosimetry Specifications Used in Mammography

Specification	Units
Surface exposure — free in air (without backscatter)	R
Surface exposure — including backscatter	R
Surface dose (includes backscatter)	rad
Midbreast dose	rad
Mean absorbed dose	rad
Mean glandular dose	rad

breast. This is the true midbreast dose only for a 6 cm compressed breast. For a more typical 4 to 5 cm compressed breast, the dose figure given is much lower than the true midbreast dose.

A much better way to report patient dose is the *mean absorbed dose* to the breast. This is the dose averaged over the entire breast. The best measure of patient dose is the *mean glandular dose.* Here the dose is given as an average over the glandular tissue of the entire breast. The rationale for using the mean glandular dose is that it gives the average radiation dose to the tissue at greatest risk and thus best represents the true radiation risk to the patient.

Table 4-2 gives some typical values for the surface exposure and for the mean glandular dose for both screen-film and xeroradiographic systems. (For screen-film systems the midbreast dose is about 60 percent of the mean glandular dose; for xeroradiographic systems the midbreast dose is about 80 to 90 percent of the mean glandular dose.) Note that while the surface exposures for screen-film and xeroradiography are similar, the mean glandular doses are not: The mean glandular doses for screen-film systems are significantly lower than for xeroradiography. Each of the three screen-film systems listed utilizes single screen and single emulsion films. Kodak (Rochester, NY) has recently introduced a new screen-film system that utilizes double screens and double emulsion films. Kodak claims that this new

system can cut radiation exposure in half. Likewise, Xerox (Pasadena, CA) has introduced a new imaging system (Xerox 175) that it also claims will cut patient doses in half compared with conventional xeroradiography, while providing improved image quality.

COMPONENTS OF A MAMMOGRAPHIC SCREEN-FILM IMAGING SYSTEM

In order to better understand how the performance of the screen-film mammography system is affected by the characteristics of its various components, it is helpful to look at each of these components individually. Figure 4-2 shows a schematic diagram of a screen-film mammographic system, indicating many of its major components.

The X-Ray Generator and the Production of X-Rays

The x-ray generator is the device that produces the high voltage (or "potential") that is applied across the x-ray tube. Ideally, at the start of an x-ray exposure this voltage would instantaneously jump to the selected value. The voltage would remain constant at the selected level until the end of the exposure, at which time the tube voltage would drop instantaneously back to zero. This, of course, is an idealization; no generator

Table 4-2 Typical Values of Surface Exposure and Mean Glandular Dose for Screen-Film, Xeroradiographic, and Film Systems[a]

Imaging System	Surface Exposure (R)	Mean Glandular Dose (rad)
Screen-film		
Min-R screen/Min-R film/no grid	0.8	0.12
Min-R screen/OM-1 film/no grid	0.4	0.06
Min-R screen/OM-1 film/grid	1.0	0.15
Xeroradiography		
Positive mode	1.0	0.40
Negative mode	0.8	0.30
Film	2–20	0.6–3

[a] The figures given are for a single view of an "average" breast.

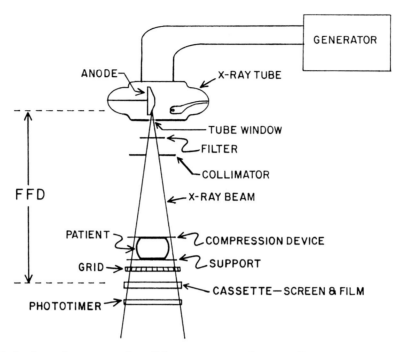

Fig. 4-2 A schematic representation of the components of a screen-film mammographic system.

can actually provide this perfect performance. The generator types that come closest are called *constant potential generators*; they provide tube potentials that are very nearly constant during the exposure time. Other generator types produce tube potentials that vary during the exposure time. A plot of tube potential versus time is referred to as the *kV waveform*. The value of tube potential that occurs at the peaks of the kV waveform is called the *kVp*. The variation of the kV waveform during the exposure is described by the term *kV ripple*. The kV ripple is normally given as a percent of the kVp. For example, if the kVp is 30 kVp and the kV waveform varies between 27 and 30 kV, the kV ripple would be 10 percent. Constant potential units usually have kV ripple of only a few percent. In mammography, *three-phase* units normally have a generator type referred to as *three-phase, six-pulse*, which yields a kV ripple of 10 to 25 percent. *Single-phase* generators produce kV waveforms that approach 100 percent ripple. Although this kV ripple is reduced somewhat by the capacitance of the high-voltage cables between the generator and the tube (the cables are able to "hold" the voltage as it drops and prevent it from going down to zero between the voltage peaks), the kV ripple of single-phase units is still substantially greater than that of three-phase units.

When an x-ray exposure is initiated, the generator places a high voltage across the x-ray tube. Electrons, evaporated from the hot cathode filament in the tube, are accelerated across the tube by this high voltage until they hit the tube's anode and are stopped. At this point some of the energy of the electrons is converted into x-ray photons, which then leave the x-ray tube to form the x-ray beam. As an example, if a constant potential of 30 kV is placed across the x-ray tube, the individual electrons will each attain an energy of 30,000 electron volts, or 30 keV, just before hitting the anode. In hitting the anode, any individual electron may convert anywhere from 0 to 100 percent of its energy into an x-ray photon. Thus the x-ray photons produced will have a range or spectrum of energies from 0 to 30 keV. This spectrum of x-ray photons is modified by the addition of filtration at the exit port of the x-ray tube. While filters like aluminum predominately remove the low energy photons, a *k-edge filter* like molybdenum removes both the very low energy photons and also most of the photons with energies above its k-edge (20 keV for molybdenum). If a molybdenum filter is added to the exit port, most of the x-ray photons with energies below 15 kev and above 20 keV are removed from the x-ray beam. The remaining photons, predominately between 15 and 20 keV, have close to the optimum energy for screen-film mammographic imaging.

The energy spectrum of the photons leaving the x-ray tube and filter can be described by a graph that plots the number of photons produced versus the energy of the photons. This energy spectrum is affected by the material of the anode surface. A tungsten anode will produce an x-ray spectrum that is smooth or continuous. A molybdenum anode will also produce a continuous spectrum of x-ray photons but in addition will produce a large number of extra x-ray photons between 17 and 20 kev; these additional photons are the "characteristic" radiation of molybdenum. Since this photon energy is near optimum for screen-film mammography, tubes with molybdenum anodes and molybdenum filters are most commonly used in screen-film mammography.

An example of a typical x-ray spectrum for screen-film mammography is given in Figure 4-3. Note the great attenuation of the x-ray photons above 20 keV by the molybdenum filter. Also note the two peaks of characteristic x-radiation produced by the molybdenum anode. Figure 4-4 shows the x-ray spectrum of this same x-ray beam after it has passed through 5 cm of tissue. The vertical scale has been amplified by a factor

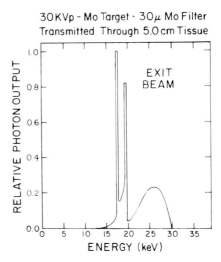

Fig. 4-4 This x-ray spectrum was obtained under conditions identical to the spectrum in Figure 4-3, except that the x-ray beam has traveled through 5 cm of tissue. The vertical scale in this figure has been magnified by a factor of 167 compared with Figure 4-3 in order to compensate for the large amount of x-ray attenuation caused by the tissue. (Adapted from Birch et al,[8] with permission.)

of 167 to compensate for the large amount of attenuation of the x-ray beam in the tissue. Note that since the lower energy photons are more heavily attenuated than the higher energy photons, the higher energy photons now make up a much greater fraction of the entire x-ray spectrum even with the 30 μm molybdenum filter. A reduction of the thickness of the molybdenum filtration would further increase this fraction of photons above 20 keV and thus reduce the image contrast.

What effect does kVp and kV ripple have on image quality and patient dose? Raising the kVp raises the average energy of the x-ray photons emitted by the x-ray tube. Higher energy photons are less affected by their passage through tissue and thus are more weakly attenuated compared with lower energy photons. This means that less patient dose results if higher energy photons are used, but the very fact that these higher energy photons are less affected by the tissue also means that the image they produce will contain less image contrast. The choice of kVp in diagnostic imaging always involves a compromise between image contrast and patient dose. The use of higher kVp lowers patient dose but reduces the image contrast. Lower kVp improves image contrast at the cost of increased patient

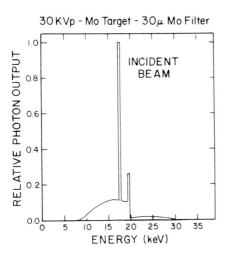

Fig. 4-3 The x-ray spectrum of the x-ray beam exiting a mammographic tube having a beryllium window. The tube anode surface is molybdenum and the filter is 30 μm of molybdenum. The kVp is set at 30 kVp. A constant potential generator is used. The spectrum gives the relative number of photons exiting the tube at different photon energies. (Adapted from Birch et al.,[8] with permission.)

dose. In screen-film mammography this compromise between image contrast and patient dose usually results in a choice of 26 to 30 kVp.

The amount of kV ripple also affects the average energy of the x-ray photons. For a given kVp, the larger the ripple, the lower the average photon energy. Thus single-phase units will produce x-ray beams whose photons have lower average energy than those from a three-phase unit operating at the same kVp.

What are the clinical differences between single-phase, three-phase, and constant potential generators in screen-film mammography? First, there is a difference in the effective x-ray output. Systems with three-phase or constant potential generators provide higher effective x-ray output than single-phase units. This allows the use of shorter exposure times with less chance of image blurring due to patient motion. A second distinction is that systems with three-phase or constant potential generators produce lower patient doses than single-phase units when the exposure techniques are set to give images of similar quality and density. Since single-phase units have the largest kV ripple, during much of the exposure time the actual potential across the x-ray tube is significantly below the kVp value. This, of course, reduces the x-ray output but also produces an x-ray beam that contains a larger portion of photons with energies below 15 keV. Since these photons are almost completely absorbed in the breast tissue, they do not contribute to forming the image but only increase the patient dose.

What about the differences between three-phase and constant potential units? It is true that when operated at the same kVp setting, a constant potential unit will produce a somewhat greater x-ray output and lower patient dose than a three-phase unit. However, the constant potential unit will also produce slightly lower image contrast. When the kVp of the constant potential unit is lowered to yield equal image contrast, the differences in x-ray output and patient dose between the constant potential and three-phase units become less significant. To produce images of equal contrast, the kVp on a constant potential unit needs to be set from 1 to 3 kV lower than that on a three-phase unit.

Single-phase units do have the advantage of not requiring three-phase power for their operation. However, there are now available other generator types (such as medium- or high-frequency invertor units) that can operate using single-phase power and that offer kV ripple similar to three-phase or even constant potential units.

The X-Ray Tube and Filter

As explained previously, screen-film mammography is most commonly performed using an x-ray tube with a molybdenum anode together with a molybdenum filter. The molybdenum (Mo) filter is used to reduce the proportion of photons in the x-ray beam with energies less than 15 keV and greater than 20 keV. To adequately accomplish this task the thickness of the Mo filter must be at least 25 μm (0.025 mm). Mo filters up to 50 μm are sometimes used. The problem with the thicker filters is that they reduce the usable x-ray output and can result in excessively long exposure times. For this reason the usual Mo filter thickness is 25 to 30 μm.

Most tubes with an Mo anode have a tube window made of beryllium (Be) foil. The attenuation of this Be foil to the 15 to 20 keV photons most useful for imaging is negligible; thus the full useful output of the x-ray tube is allowed to exit the tube. Some Mo anode tubes are made in a more conventional manner with a thin glass window. In the best of these tubes the effective filtration of the tube port is 0.5 to 0.7 mm aluminum equivalent. In this case the attenuation of the output beam is significant; the number of "imaging" photons from 15 to 20 kev is cut in half. However, some of these glass window tubes have effective filtration of up to 1.5 mm aluminum equivalent or more, due to the glass and the oil surrounding the tube insert. These tubes may only transmit 10 to 30 percent of the "imaging" photons through the tube window. The result is that effective tube output is drastically reduced and a significant part of the x-ray spectrum is now made up of photons above 20 kev, which produce noticeably lower image contrast. Since these x-ray tubes are often coupled to low power x-ray generators, their lowered output is more acutely felt. To compensate for the reduced output, the user will end up either raising the kVp, which further reduces image contrast, or using very long exposure times, which increases the chances of blurring due to patient motion and raises patient exposure due to film reciprocity failure (this phenomenon will be discussed in the section on screen-film cassettes). Some manufacturers have compounded the problems with these glass window tubes by removing most of the added Mo filtration in an attempt to increase tube output. The remaining Mo filtration of 15 or even 7.5 μm is too thin to be effective. The result is a further degradation of image contrast.

Another possible filtration problem is the use of too little filtration with a Be window tube. Either the added filtration is totally missing, or the thickness of the added Mo filter is less than 25 μm. The raw, unfiltered x-ray beam leaving the tube anode always contains a very large amount of very low energy photons, below 10 keV, which normally are totally removed from the x-ray beam by the tube window (if made of glass) and/or by the added beam filter. Since a Be window provides very little attenuation even for extremely low energy x-rays, if no added filtration is used, these low energy photons are allowed to exit the tube and expose the patient. The increase in patient dose, particularly to the skin of the breast, due to these low energy photons can be extreme. In all cases it is very important that the correct thickness of Mo filtration be used: from 25 to 50 μm.

One important test of proper beam filtration is the *half-value layer* (HVL) of the x-ray beam. The HVL is defined as the amount of aluminum that when added to the x-ray beam will reduce the x-ray intensity by one-half. For optimum operation, the HVL of a screen-film mammography system at the kVp normally used should be less than 0.40 mm aluminum. The U.S. government requires that the HVL in mm aluminum for mammographic units operating below 50 kVp be no less than the kVp value at which the HVL is measured divided by 100; for example, if measured at 28 kVp, the minimum allowed HVL is 0.28 mm aluminum. Values less than the required minimum may indicate lack of proper filtration, while values above 0.40 mm can indicate excessive inherent filtration in the x-ray tube or excessively high kVp. Increased filtration of the x-ray beam can also be caused by the collimator mirror if it remains in the x-ray beam during the exposure and is not suitably constructed to minimize its x-ray attenuation. Ten years ago it was common to find screen-film mammography performed with systems having much higher HVLs, up to 1.0 mm and greater. The improvement in image contrast and image quality at the lower, recommended, HVLs is dramatic.

One aspect of filter characteristics that is rarely mentioned is filter uniformity and *filter mottle*. In conventional radiography, minor defects or scratches on the aluminum filter are of no consequence, since they do not appear in the images. In screen-film mammography, any defects in the surface of this filter are more than 100 times more significant due to the much higher attenuating power of the filtration material, particularly at the low energies used in mammography. In fact, the surface defects of the Mo filters commonly used are easily seen in images made of uniform phantoms. Figure 4-5 shows images of a mammographic phantom exposed with and without a Mo filter. The mottle added by the presence of the filter is readily apparent and definitely interferes with the perception of the masses in this phantom. In this case the mottle is a result of the filter production method. More serious image artifacts can result if the delicate filter is actually damaged by handling (this can happen during installation). This mottle is one example of the structure noise previously discussed. It can vary significantly with different filters. If filter mottle appears excessive or if damage artifacts are apparent, the filter should be replaced.

It is possible to successfully use tube anode/filtration combinations other than Mo/Mo. One useful combination is a tungsten anode with variable k-edge filters. K-edge filters have the special property of strongly attenuating any x-ray photons with energies just above the k-edge energy of the filter material. Mo is an example of a k-edge filter whose k-edge is at 20.0 keV. The proponents of this system point out that it allows a greater control of the x-ray spectrum for better optimization to different patient thicknesses. (Imaging theory predicts that the optimum energy for breast imaging increases as the breast size increases.) The spectrum can be effectively controlled by filter selection, since the tungsten tube does not give off a large peak of characteristic radiation below 20 keV as Mo does. Some of the filters that are used (along with their k-edge energies) are: Mo (20.0 keV), rhodium (Rh) (23.2 keV), and palladium (Pd) (24.3 keV). The Mo filter would be used for thin breasts and would provide the lowest energy x-ray beam. The Pd filter would be used for thick/dense breasts and would provide an x-ray beam with higher energy photons. While the theory of this imaging system appears sound, with currently available screen-film systems it produces images of lower contrast, which may not be acceptable to the radiologist.

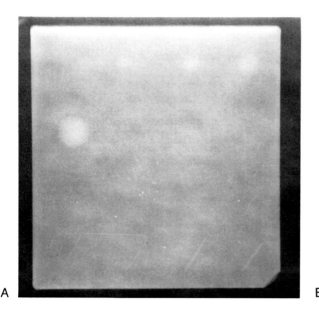
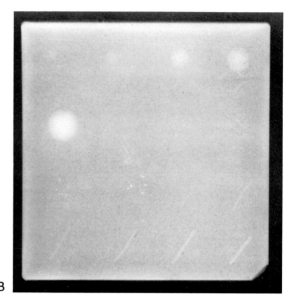

A   B

Fig. 4-5. An example of "filter mottle": artifacts resulting from irregularities in the surface of the filter. An RMI 152C mammography phantom was used in producing these images. These are radiographs of the wax block containing the test objects: **(A)** image made using the normal 30 μm molybdenum filter and **(B)** image made with the filter removed. Of course, in clinical use the molybdenum filter is essential for two reasons: (1) to improve image contrast by removing most of the higher energy x-ray photons above 20 keV and (2) to protect the patient from excess radiation exposure by removing most of the very low energy x-ray photons that are emitted from a beryllium window x-ray tube. However, these images illustrate the artifacts that can arise when the molybdenum filter is not of the highest quality. They also demonstrate some of the test objects present in the RMI 152 mammography phantom. This phantom contains test objects simulating microcalcifications, fibrils, and masses of various sizes.

Another system that has been used with some success is a mammographic tungsten anode tube with a glass window having an inherent filtration equivalent to about 0.5 mm of aluminum but with no other added filtration. This system can produce satisfactory images if operated at lower kVp settings, from 22 to 26 kVp.

A very important x-ray tube characteristic is the *focal spot size.* It is a major contributor to the overall image sharpness. The specification of focal spot size is normally given by the manufacturer as "nominal focal spot size." This is a specification standardized by the National Electrical Manufacturers Association (NEMA). This specification contains tolerance factors that allow the actual focal spot size as measured with a pinhole or slit camera (this is also called the "effective" focal spot size) to be substantially larger than the specified "nominal" size. As an example, a focal spot specified as

0.3 mm nominal is allowed to have an "effective" focal spot size as large as 0.45 mm × 0.65 mm. In addition, the pinhole camera measurement, using the NEMA standards, is made at the highest kV rating of the tube, typically 49 kV, and at one-half of the maximum tube current (mA) allowed at an exposure time of 0.1 seconds. At clinical settings of about 28 kVp and maximum mA, the focal spot may be significantly larger, an effect known as focal spot blooming. (As a rule, the actual focal spot size increases somewhat as the mA is raised or the kVp is lowered.) Thus it is possible for two tubes, both with the same nominal focal spot size and both satisfying NEMA standards, to produce noticeably different image sharpness in clinical use. Even if the focal spots of the two tubes have identical "effective" dimensions at clinically used technique settings, these tubes may still produce different image sharpness due to different distributions of x-ray emission intensity from within the focal spot.

The easiest way to measure the focal spot size in the clinical setting is by means of a resolution pattern, or "siemens star" pattern, which is positioned in the x-ray beam so that it is imaged with substantial magnification (2× or more). By determining the resolution limit in this test image, one can derive an actual focal spot size by assuming that the focal spot emits x-rays uniformly from within a rectangular area. The dimensions of this rectangular area are referred to as the "equivalent" focal spot size. This "equivalent" focal spot size is much easier to measure than the "effective" focal spot size obtained using a pinhole camera. These two types of focal spot measurement will usually disagree somewhat because the real focal spot does not emit x-rays uniformly from a rectangular source. Although the "equivalent" focal spot size is not identical to the actual focal spot size, it more directly indicates the effect of the focal spot on image sharpness due to both the overall size and the distribution of x-ray intensity from within the focal spot.

Using the "siemens star" resolution pattern method, the calculated "equivalent" focal spot size of focal spots that satisfy NEMA standards for "effective" focal spot size can measure from one to nearly two times the specified nominal size. The best way of ensuring that a particular x-ray tube provides the desired level of image sharpness is to specify that it must meet a certain specification of "equivalent" focal spot size using the star resolution pattern method of focal spot measurement at clinical technique settings of kVp and mA.

Figure 4-6 shows two test images of a siemens star

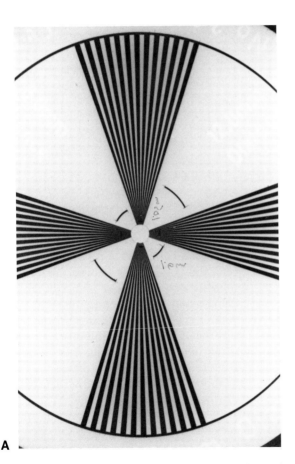

A

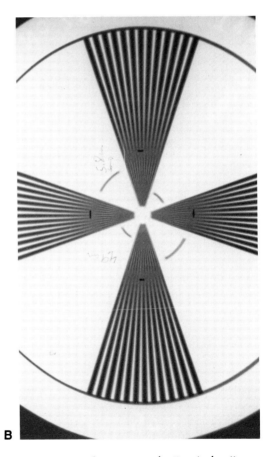

B

Fig. 4-6. These images are magnification radiographs of a siemens star pattern used to measure the "equivalent" focal spot size. **(A)** Image made using a focal spot with a nominal size of 0.1 mm. **(B)** Image made using a focal spot with a nominal size of 0.4 mm. The points of limiting resolution used to make the focal spot size determination are marked on the films with short black lines.

Table 4-3 Equivalent Focal Spot Sizes Required to Provide Specified Values of Image Resolution

Image Resolution:	5 lp/mm		10 lp/mm		15 lp/mm		20 lp/mm	
	Equivalent Focal Spot Size (mm) that Will Yield the Resolution Given Above							
2× magnification	0.2		0.1		0.07		0.05	
1.5× magnification	0.4		0.2		0.13		0.1	
	NG	G	NG	G	NG	G	NG	G
50 cm (20″) FFD	1.8	1.5	0.9	0.75	0.6	0.5	0.45	0.35
60 cm (24″) FFD	2.2	1.8	1.1	0.9	0.75	0.6	0.55	0.45
65 cm (26″) FFD	2.4	2.0	1.2	1.0	0.8	0.65	0.6	0.5
75 cm (30″) FFD	2.8	2.3	1.4	1.2	0.95	0.75	0.7	0.6

This table gives the equivalent focal spot sizes that would yield the specified values of resolution in the image for different imaging geometries in the absence of other limiting factors such as screen-film resolution. Focal spot resolutions greater than 10 to 15 lp/mm are unlikely to provide much improvement in the image quality of clinical images due to the limitations of image noise, screen-film sharpness, and patient motion. Focal spot resolutions of less than 10 lp/mm will probably result in some degradation of clinical images.

The measured equivalent focal spot size of a focal spot may range up to two times the specified nominal size. The resolution provided by a focal spot depends both on its size and on the image magnification. For typical "nonmagnification" mammographic imaging, there is still some minimal magnification, which depends on the focal spot to film distance (FFD) and on the distance between the object to be imaged and the image receptor. In this table the distance between the object of interest and the image receptor is taken as 5 cm for the nongrid (NG) technique (or "contact" technique—no grid, or a stationary grid placed within the film cassette) and 6 cm for the moving grid (G) technique. (The presence of a moving grid mechanism typically adds a distance of 1 cm between the breast and the film cassette. Stationary grids placed within the cassette do not add this extra distance.)

pattern used to measure the "equivalent" focal spot sizes of a dual focal spot x-ray tube. The greater resolution obtained in the test image using the smaller focal spot is readily apparent. From the measured resolution limit, the "equivalent" focal spot sizes can be determined.

Both the "equivalent" focal spot size measured with a resolution pattern and the "effective" focal spot size measured with a pinhole or slit camera are simplified descriptions of the focal spot and have limitations. Occasionally, they may provide somewhat misleading information concerning the image sharpness characteristics of a specific tube. The most complete description of the effect of the focal spot on image sharpness is the MTF of the focal spot. Accurately determining the MTF is a difficult process, so in the clinical setting the simpler test methods must normally suffice.

What size focal spots are required to provide images with good image sharpness? The answer depends on the imaging geometry of the mammography system (Table 4-3). In the normal, nonmagnified imaging mode this is determined by the focal spot to film distance (FFD) and by the distance between the breast and the image receptor. This last item is affected by the presence of a moving grid mechanism between the breast and the screen-film cassette. If the FFD is decreased or the breast-to-film distance is increased by grid use, then a smaller focal spot is required to maintain the same image sharpness. For an FFD of 50 cm without the use of moving grid or an FFD of 60 cm with a moving grid, an "equivalent" focal spot size of 0.6 to 0.9 mm is about optimal. This is usually accomplished with a nominal focal spot size of 0.3 to 0.5 mm. The use of a larger focal spot will probably cause a significant degradation of image quality. The use of too small a focal spot can also compromise image quality by limiting the maximum mA that can be used. This will require either the use of a longer exposure time, with the added chance of blur due to patient motion, or the use of higher kVp, which will reduce the image contrast.

In a magnification imaging mode, the required focal spot size depends on the degree of magnification. For 1.5× magnification, the optimal "equivalent" focal spot size is about 0.2 mm, while for 2× magnification the optimal "equivalent" focal spot is about 0.1 mm. This means that if a mammography unit is to perform both standard and magnification imaging, a dual focus x-ray tube is essential. Some mammography systems sold in the past have tried to perform both standard and magnification imaging using a single focal spot, such as 0.3 mm nominal. The magnification images from such units have a quite noticeable lack of sharpness. In fact, the resolution in these systems can actually be better in the standard imaging mode than in the magnification mode!

Off-focus radiation is another aspect of x-ray tube performance that, like focal spot size, significantly affects image quality. It is much less discussed and harder to measure. Not all of the radiation that leaves the x-ray tube is emitted from the focal spot. Some of the radiation comes from other locations within the tube. This "off-focus" or "extra-focal" radiation may comprise from 5 to 25 percent of the total radiation output. Like scatter radiation, off-focus radiation adds an overall haze to the image, reducing the image contrast. The fraction of off-focus radiation is not generally reported as part of the technical specifications of the x-ray system, but it is an important factor in determining overall image quality. Some manufacturers of mammographic tubes do claim that their tube designs significantly reduce off-focus radiation. Such tubes would be expected to give improved image quality.

Off-focus radiation can be reduced somewhat by techniques exterior to the x-ray tube. A basic principle for reducing off-focus radiation is to perform any collimation of the x-ray beam as close as possible to the focal spot. This is the rationale for placing fixed lead apertures within the tube port.

Mammography x-ray tubes are available with either a stationary anode or a rotating anode. Tubes with a rotating anode have the distinct advantage of being able to operate at higher tube loadings. This means higher mA settings are possible with the result that exposure times can be reduced. Since the rotating anode provides a larger source of off-focus radiation, rotating anode tubes have the potential for producing larger amounts of off-focus radiation than stationary anode tubes.

However, the actual amount of off-focus radiation produced by a specific tube depends on its particular design.

The Collimator

The purpose of the x-ray collimator is to restrict the x-ray field to the area of interest. Reducing the area of the radiation field has two beneficial effects: a reduction in the radiation exposure to the patient, and a reduction in the amount of scattered radiation produced. This reduction in scatter produces an improvement in image contrast. Mammographic systems employ either continuously adjustable collimation or collimation using a set of fixed apertures of various sizes. Most collimators also use a light field to indicate the area of x-ray exposure. With these units the position of the light field should be adjusted so that it precisely coincides with the radiation field. In all cases it is important that the position of the x-ray field with respect to the film cassette be properly adjusted, particularly at the chest wall. Exposing the chest wall beyond the edge of the film simply produces unnecessary radiation exposure to the patient and increased scatter to the film, which degrades the image. If the radiation field does not extend to the edge of the film at the chest wall, important pathology may be missed.

Compression

Proper, vigorous compression is essential to the screen-film mammographic examination for a number of reasons: improved image sharpness, scatter reduction, dose reduction, maintaining a uniform film density over the image, and improving the separation and visibility of tissue structures.

By compressing the breast, all structures in the breast are moved closer to the film cassette. In this way, blurring due to the focal spot size is reduced. Breast compression immobilizes the breast and reduces blur due to patient motion. By decreasing the thickness of the imaged tissue, compression reduces the amount of scattered radiation produced, thereby improving image contrast. The decrease in breast thickness also reduces the radiation exposure required to produce an image. This lowers the radiation dose to the patient. It also decreases the exposure time, which further reduces the chances of motion blur. The compression device should be made of material that produces little attenuation of the x-ray beam. Excessive attenuation will reduce image contrast and lengthen exposure times.

To provide proper compression of the breast, the compression device should be stiff and parallel to the film cassette. The compression device should angle sharply at the chest wall; its posterior part should *not* slope upwards. If such a compression device with posterior sloping were used, part of the breast tissue would be pushed back out of the image. Also, the resultant increased thickness of the posterior part of the breast would cause that part of the breast to image with too low a density. A proper compression device should grab the part of the breast nearest the chest wall and pull it into the imaging area. It should also maintain equal tissue thickness so that a relatively uniform film density is achieved over the image.

To provide the most complete imaging of the breast tissue closest to the chest wall, it is also important that the focal spot of the tube be positioned over the extreme posterior part of the film cassette, close to the chest wall. The focal spot should *not* be positioned over the center of the film cassette.

The Antiscatter Grid

As the x-ray beam emitted by the x-ray tube passes through the patient, many of the x-ray photons are totally absorbed by the tissue and removed from the x-ray beam. The differing amount of absorption produced by the structures in the breast produces a varying x-ray intensity exiting the breast at different positions, and thus different densities on the x-ray film. This variation in density, which constitutes the x-ray image, is somewhat compromised by a phenomenon called x-ray scattering. Some of the x-ray photons that enter the breast experience a second type of interaction with the breast tissue in which the photons are not totally absorbed; this is called scattering. These photons lose only a fraction of their energy and are then deflected into another direction. When these "scattered" x-ray photons reach the film cassette, they add an overall haze to the x-ray image and thus reduce image contrast.

Two methods exist to reduce the amount of scattered radiation reaching the film cassette. One method is to use an air gap between the breast and the cassette. In this way, much of the scattered radiation produced in the breast misses the film cassette. This geometry occurs

with magnification imaging. A second method is to utilize an antiscatter grid. A grid is composed of a series of parallel, thin lead strips separated by a spacing material. The grid is oriented so that radiation emitted by the focal spot and passing undeflected through the patient (called primary radiation) is mostly able to pass through the grid, while scattered radiation approaching the grid from a different direction is absorbed by the lead strips. An ideal grid would absorb all of the scattered radiation and none of the primary. Such an ideal device, however, is impossible. In practice, some of the primary beam is absorbed by the lead strips and the interspace material, and some of the scattered radiation will get through the grid. Real grids can still provide a significant increase in image contrast by reduction of the scattered radiation reaching the film cassette. Because a grid absorbs much of the scattered and some of the primary radiation, its use requires an increase in mAs technique and patient dose. This increase (the Bucky factor) is typically a factor of two to three times in mammography.

Either stationary or moving grids can be used successfully in mammography. Moving grids require an additional mechanism to provide the motion and this is an added expense. It is important that this mechanism not add significant distance between the breast and film cassette, otherwise image sharpness may suffer (see the previous discussion on focal spots). In well-designed units the grid mechanism adds only about 1 cm to this distance. Stationary grids have thin, closely spaced lead strips (up to 200 per inch), so that the grid lines are not very apparent in the images. These grids can be rather easily damaged by handling. One solution is to permanently place a grid in each mammography film cassette, although this also increases costs.

The grids used in conventional radiography (60 to 140 kVp) typically have covers and interspaces made of aluminum. At these higher x-ray photon energies, the attenuation of the aluminum is not very significant. At the x-ray energies used in screen-film mammography, however, the use of aluminum is generally unacceptable. Grids used in mammography should optimally have fiber interspaces and a low attenuation carbon fiber cover. It is important to note that the specification that a grid has a carbon fiber cover *does not* necessarily indicate that the grid uses fiber interspaces. There are presently grids sold for use in mammography that advertise the features of carbon fiber covers but use aluminum rather than fiber interspaces. These grids require increased patient dose and produce images with reduced contrast compared with similar fiber interspaced grids, due to significant attenuation of the low energy photons: they absorb more than 50 percent of the primary x-ray photons with energies between 15 and 20 keV, which are most useful in producing good image contrast. Thin, fine-line, stationary grids generally use aluminum interspaces for needed mechanical stability. The thinness of these grids reduces the aluminum's attenuation somewhat so that the grids may be useful for mammographic imaging. However, the interspace attenuation in these grids is still greater than that of thicker fiber interspaced grids.

Grids are most effective in improving image quality when the amount of scattered radiation is high, i.e., imaging thick or dense breasts. In the imaging of predominately fatty breasts that can be compressed rather thinly, the use of a grid is much less helpful and may not be worth the increase in radiation exposure; in such a case, an aluminum interspace grid, in particular, might not improve image quality at all and may even hurt it. The breakpoint in breast thickness and density at which grid use is recommended is a matter of active current debate. A significant complication is the variation in the quality of available grids. A good fiber interspaced grid would be useful with much smaller breast thicknesses than would a similar aluminum interspaced grid.

Grids should never be used in magnification mammography, since the scattered radiation reaching the film cassette is already greatly reduced by the air gap. Adding a grid in this case would increase patient dose without a significant change in image quality.

For optimal results the specified focal distance of the grid should match the FFD of the imaging system. If the mammography unit has a variable FFD, there is normally a recommended FFD to be used with the grid. For example, if the grid is focused at 65 cm, an FFD of 65 cm should be used, but an FFD of 50 cm should not. Focused grids need to be placed with a specified side toward the x-ray tube. It is important that any grid be properly aligned with respect to the tube; a small tilt may significantly degrade image quality and require increased radiation exposure. Mishandling or denting of the grid can cause grid damage, resulting in artifacts in the radiograph. The thin, fine-line grids intended for

stationary use are particularly susceptible to damage from mishandling. Occasionally, grid lines may be seen with moving grids, due to breakdowns in the Bucky mechanism. Possible problems include total lack of grid motion, improper synchronization of the grid motion with the exposure time, and binding of the grid so that part of its normal motion is stopped or slowed.

The Screen-Film Cassette

Although I have referred to it as the film cassette in this chapter for brevity, the cassette actually contains two essential elements: the radiographic film and an intensifying screen. Initially, many years ago, mammography was performed using film alone. While film is capable of providing very high quality images, it is not very efficient in capturing x-ray energy. Thus much higher radiation exposures were required to produce these images. In an attempt to reduce the radiation exposure, intensifying screens were introduced into mammographic imaging. These screens are very efficient in capturing the x-ray energy and then converting it into visible light that exposes the film. However, the screens used in conventional radiography were found to produce unacceptable image blurring. To produce diagnostic images, special high-resolution screens have been developed for mammography.

The design of a screen-film system is always a compromise between three characteristics: *system speed, image sharpness,* and *image noise.* The speed is a measure of the sensitivity of the system to radiation and thus will affect patient dose. If the speed of system A is twice that of system B, then system A will require only one-half the radiation exposure of system B to produce an image with similar image density.

As x-rays are absorbed in different parts of the intensifying screen, light is emitted. This light must travel through part of the intensifying screen to reach the film. As the light travels through the screen it spreads out. This means that a precise, point x-ray exposure on the intensifying screen produces a small blur on the x-ray film. The size of this blur depends on the average distance the light must travel to exit the screen and thus depends on the thickness of the screen. To reduce the amount of image blurring, mammography screens are made very thin. The penalty for this is a reduction in the speed of the screen: since it is thinner, it absorbs a smaller fraction of the x-ray energy.

Image sharpness is also affected by the degree of contact between the intensifying screen and the film. Any small gap between the screen and the film will allow the light emitted by the screen to spread out before hitting the film. This produces additional image blurring. Well-designed cassettes ensure intimate contact between the film and the screen. Even with such cassettes, screen-film contact can be compromised by the presence of dust on the screen surface. Frequent, even daily, cleaning of the screens is recommended both to ensure proper screen-film contact and to eliminate image artifacts from the dust particles.

In addition to screen properties, the speed of a screen-film system is also affected by the sensitivity of the film. Increasing the sensitivity of the film will increase the system speed but at the same time will increase the image noise.

The contrast of the x-ray image is partly determined by the inherent film contrast. Increasing the film contrast will increase image contrast but will also increase image noise. The above is true whether the increase in sensitivity or contrast is achieved by using a different film or by changing the film processing conditions. Increasing film contrast also reduces the exposure latitude and thus makes the task of obtaining useful film densities over the entire image more difficult. Some manufacturers provide a selection of films for mammography so that the clinician can choose the film best suited for his/her needs. For example, Kodak supplies the following single emulsion films for mammography, listed in order of increasing sensitivity and increasing contrast: Min-R, NMB, and OM-1. Of these three films, OM-1 is most commonly chosen for optimal sensitivity and contrast.

One more item of importance to screen-film speed is a phenomenon called *reciprocity failure.* This refers to the loss of speed that occurs when long exposure times are used. In a sense, during a long exposure the film partially "forgets" about the radiation it received at the start of the exposure. Because of this "lost" radiation, the film requires a greater total amount of radiation to obtain a particular density compared with that required using a higher x-ray intensity and a shorter exposure time. Consider two mammography systems that differ only in the mA used: system A uses 100 mA, while system B uses 50 mA. Suppose a typical exposure technique with system A is 28 kVp and 200 mA. With this technique, system A will require a 2 second exposure time. System B would require a 4 second exposure time if reciprocity failure did not exist, but in reality it will require a longer exposure time. System B will therefore produce a greater patient exposure and a greater chance of motion blur. With exposure times of several seconds common in mammography, the required increase in exposure time due to reciprocity failure can be greater than a factor of two.

In general radiography, screen-film cassettes normally use double emulsion film sandwiched between a pair of intensifying screens. Ideally, each screen exposes only the film emulsion in contact with it. The use of two screens increases the speed of the system by absorbing more of the x-ray photons without increasing the thickness of the individual screens. This would seem an ideal situation, except that in reality some of the light emitted by each screen is able to penetrate through the film and expose the emulsion on the opposite side. As the light passes through the film it spreads out and produces a blurred density on the opposite emulsion. For applications like mammography that require very high image sharpness, it has generally not been possible to achieve acceptable image quality using dual screen and double emulsion film because of this phenomenon of *crossover exposure.* The typical mammography cassette consists of a single screen used with single emulsion film within a cassette of low attenuation material. The film is placed on top of the screen with the emulsion side down, facing the screen. In this way the part of the screen first hit by the x-rays, and emitting the brightest light, is closest to the film; blurring is therefore reduced.

Within the last few years mammography systems utilizing dual screens and double emulsion film have been introduced. The films used in these systems are specially designed to have a low degree of crossover exposure. The use of these special films improves image sharpness over older film types, but the images are still inferior to single screen systems, since the crossover exposure is only reduced, not eliminated. Just recently a new film has been introduced by Kodak that claims to almost totally eliminate crossover exposure and thus provide improved image sharpness at reduced dose. By the use of dual screens, Kodak claims a gain in system speed of about a factor of 2 compared with its Min-R/OM-1 system.

In addition to affecting image sharpness, dual screen systems affect image contrast and noise in the following way. Both single and dual screen systems absorb the lower energy photons efficiently. The biggest difference in x-ray absorption between these two systems is with the higher energy photons that carry less image contrast. By absorbing a greater fraction of these higher energy photons, the image contrast is reduced somewhat with dual screen systems. This contrast loss can be recovered by increasing the inherent film contrast, but then the image noise is increased. To maintain the same ratio of image contrast to image noise it would be necessary to decrease the kVp setting somewhat when using dual screens. Because of these considerations it is not clear whether the newer dual screen systems will prove optimal for mammographic imaging. To some extent, the decision to use a dual screen system is affected by the type of mammography unit being used. If the unit provides a rather low x-ray output, the clinician may find that thicker, denser breasts require an increase in kVp and/or exposure time beyond recommended limits in order to obtain a useful film density. The increase in kVp further reduces image contrast in a radiograph that starts out with poor contrast. The long exposure time risks blurring due to patient motion and causes loss of speed due to reciprocity failure. In this case the use of a faster dual screen system is particularly beneficial in allowing lower kVp settings and shorter exposure times.

Film Processing

Proper film processing is *essential* for maintaining optimal image quality in mammography. The single emulsion films used in mammography are usually more sensitive to variations in processor temperature and developer activity than the double emulsion films used in general radiography. Scratches and other developer marks can be more troublesome with the demanding mammographic examination. Very often, image quality and patient dose problems can be traced back to problems with the film processor.

Common processor problems include incorrect developer temperature and improper developer dilution or replenishment. Often, complaints of poor image contrast or high patient doses result from the use of too low a developer temperature. While the recommended developer temperature depends on the particular combi-

nation of film, developer, and processor, 95°F is a typical value. It is not uncommon to see processors run at developer temperatures of 90°F to 92°F, when 95°F is the recommended temperature. Similar problems can be produced by improper developer dilution or replenishment. If there is a question as to whether the processor is being supplied with properly diluted solutions, the manufacturer of the processor chemistry may be willing to test the solutions for you to determine if a problem exists. The degree of dilution of processor solutions can be determined by measurement of the specific gravity of the solutions with a hydrometer. Improper replenishment rates may be a particular problem with processors that are not dedicated to mammography but that process both single and double emulsion films. It can be difficult to maintain proper replenishment in this case, since the replenishment requirements of the different film types can vary significantly.

Increasing the time that the film spends in the developer solution, and thereby extending the processing time from the usual 90 seconds up to 180 seconds, has been suggested by some as a means of improving mammographic imaging. This extended processing can increase film speed and film contrast with some films. As a result, such films may have a more appealing, higher contrast appearance, and patient dose will be somewhat reduced. There is also a down side to this technique. The increased contrast will result in reduced exposure latitude. As discussed previously, increasing either film speed or contrast by changing the film type or processing methods will also increase image noise by increasing the quantum mottle. Thus extended processing will generally increase quantum mottle in the image and can decrease the ratio of image contrast to image noise. Extended processing has both advantages and disadvantages; its suitability for a particular application depends on the unavoidable compromise between image contrast, image noise, exposure latitude, and patient dose.

To maintain proper operation of the processor, daily quality assurance testing is recommended. Films exposed in a sensitometer should be processed and examined every day. These films are read out using a densitometer to obtain readings of base + fog, speed index, and contrast index. If serious problems are encountered with variations in film contrast or density during the working day, it may be useful to expose three separate films in the sensitometer at the beginning of the day and then develop these test films at three different times during the day. In this way processor variations during the day can be monitored.

The processor temperature should also be monitored daily. The thermometer that is built into some processors may not be accurate enough for proper monitoring. For best results, a metal stem or electronic thermometer should be used to monitor the temperature. A liquid-filled glass thermometer should *never* be used, since breakage could permanently contaminate the processor. The processor should be cleaned on a regular schedule to prevent residue buildup that can scratch or mark the film.

To avoid fogging the x-ray film, the darkroom should be checked for any light leaks and for safelight adequacy. Most of the film used in mammography is orthochromatic: it is sensitive to both green and blue light. Such film requires the use of a red safelight. The amber safelights used with blue-sensitive film will fog orthochromatic film.

I strongly recommend that those responsible for the daily processor quality assurance and maintenance obtain literature containing more complete information on the proper processor testing and maintenance methods. Some books and articles on these subjects are included in the references at the end of this chapter. The manufacturers of x-ray film and film processors (and some distributors of densitometers and sensitometers) are also good sources of information on these topics.

The Phototimer

Although phototiming can be a useful feature of a mammographic system, the performance of many of the phototimers found in mammography units is rather disappointing. The problems arise because, unlike general radiographic systems, the phototimer sensor in mammography systems is normally positioned in back of the film cassette rather than in front of it. The mammographic imaging process is so sensitive that it would be difficult to avoid imaging the phototimer sensors if they were placed in front of the cassette. Phototimer sensors in this position would also filter the x-ray beam, thereby reducing image contrast and requiring an in-

crease in patient dose. Finally, a phototimer sensor in front of the cassette would increase the distance between the breast and the cassette and thus degrade image sharpness. The problem with placing the phototimer sensor behind the cassette is that the sensors then see only the leftover radiation that passes through the cassette; they do not directly sense the x-ray intensity incident on the cassette. As the thickness of the breast being imaged increases, the attenuation of the x-ray beam increases. Lower energy photons are attenuated more than the higher energy photons. Thus the average energy of the photons incident on the film cassette increases as the breast thickness increases. These higher energy photons penetrate more effectively through the film cassette and cause the phototimer to terminate the exposure prematurely. The result is that as the breast thickness increases, the film density decreases. This mistracking with thickness variation can be dramatic: if the phototimer is set up to give proper exposure with an average breast, the image of a large, dense breast may be underexposed by a factor of two, while the image of a small, predominately fatty breast may be overexposed by a factor of two.

If you have such a phototimer with poor thickness tracking, it is important that you make liberal use of the phototimer's density control adjustment to maintain proper film density. It is common to find films of large dense breasts, taken with a phototimer, that are either too light or too low contrast. In these cases the density control adjustment was not set high enough for proper film density or the kVp was significantly raised in an attempt to correct the film density. Sometimes these poorly exposed films are used to demonstrate the superiority of Xerography in imaging large breasts. The poor quality of these images does not indicate an inherent problem with the performance of the screen-film imaging system, but rather a simply correctable problem with exposure techniques.

Over the last 2 years many manufacturers of mammographic units have used improved phototimer designs that correct these problems with thickness tracking. These units give much improved performance in maintaining correct film densities.

Most phototimers allow adjustment of the position of the sensor so that its distance from the chest wall can be varied. Careful adjustment of the sensor position is important for proper phototimer operation. If the phototimer sensor is not placed under the thickest part of the breast, underexposure of that part of the breast may result. Another problem can occur with breasts containing islands of glandular tissue: if the phototimer sensor is under an area of predominately fatty tissue, it will try to set the correct density for that area. This will cause the areas of glandular tissue to be underexposed. In some mammographic units, if a large area of the film outside the breast is exposed, scatter from the high intensity radiation hitting that part of the cassette may reach the phototimer sensor; this will cause the phototimer to terminate the exposure prematurely and result in a light film.

All phototimers employ a "backup timer" that prevents the mAs or exposure time from exceeding some set maximum value. This protects against excessive patient exposure or x-ray tube damage from too long exposure times. The backup timer acts as a fail-safe to terminate the exposure if the phototimer should fail to do so. The back-up timer may also be occasionally activated when imaging large, dense breasts that require long exposures to obtain a proper film density. If this is more than a rare occurrence, it indicates that a higher kVp setting is required for these difficult-to-image breasts, or that the backup time or mAs is set to a value that is too low. Other possible causes are low x-ray output due to a malfunction of the generator or tube, incorrect kVp or mA calibration, or excessive tube filtration.

A display of the actual mAs or exposure time is very helpful when the mammographic system is used in phototimed mode. This will allow the radiographer to become aware of the level of radiation exposure given to each patient and also to better select suitable kVp values for differing breast types. Without knowledge of the actual exposure times or mAs, the radiographer will not know when the exposure time or mAs approaches the backup limit and may defensively select higher kVps than actually required in order to prevent reaching this limit.

The Viewbox

The excellent film results produced by a well-functioning mammographic system can be wasted without proper conditions for viewing the films. Stray light is the principle culprit in degrading viewing conditions. Even when ambient lighting is reduced, the viewboxes themselves remain a major source of stray light. The viewing room should be arranged so that stray light from surrounding viewboxes is minimized. Of crucial impact in viewing mammographic images is the light from the light panels directly in front of the radiologist, including the panel(s) illuminating the film(s) under inspection. The ability to detect subtle structures in the film images is greatly affected by this stray light. One solution is to turn off all light panels except the one or two in use for a specific examination, and to additionally cover all areas of the remaining panel(s), outside of the film(s) being read, with black cardboard or black, overexposed film. This last suggestion is not trivial: it can make a dramatic effect in the perceived image quality, particularly with films of higher density.

In addition to reducing stray light, the viewboxes themselves should be maintained by cleaning any marks from the viewing surfaces and repairing any panels that begin to show flickering or dimming.

MAGNIFICATION IMAGING

The use of magnification can provide images with additional information, but great care must be exercised in the selection and maintenance of the imaging equipment and in performing the examination. Because of the technical difficulties in producing a magnification image in mammography, it is not uncommon to find no actual increase or even a degradation of image quality compared with the nonmagnified study. As discussed previously, focal spot size is critical. Magnification mammography requires extremely small focal spots to achieve the added resolution expected of this technique. Since these small focal spots can only be used at relatively low mA settings, long exposure times, up to 10 seconds or longer, can result. The higher potential resolution limit and longer exposure times make patient motion a particularly difficult problem to overcome. Motion unsharpness in magnification imaging can also result from any instability in the breast support table or in the tube-cassette holder assembly. To achieve high-quality magnification images, every effort must be made to assure an absolute minimum of patient and equipment motion during the exposure.

Magnification mammography results in increased radiation dose to the tissue within the x-ray field. A magnification of 2× increases the dose by about a factor of 2 to 4 compared to a grid technique. The use of an antiscatter grid in magnification mammography is *not* recommended. Scatter clean-up is effectively achieved by means of the air gap. The addition of a grid would not change the scatter reaching the cassette by a significant amount but would further increase patient dose unnecessarily.

The advantages of magnification mammography in producing improved image quality are (1) increased image resolution, (2) improved low contrast detectability, and (3) a reduction of x-ray scatter reaching the film. The magnified image directly produces an increase in the effective image resolution and sharpness when measured relative to sizes in the tissue, *as long as the focal spot size is sufficiently small.* The improvement in low contrast detectability is due to the larger number of photons used to form the enlarged image. With a magnification of 2×, the area of any structure in the image is increased by a factor of 4; thus four times as many photons are used to form the image. Ignoring the effects of scatter, the combination of increased image resolution and improved low contrast detectability using a magnification of 2× theoretically should allow the detection of microcalcifications that are about 70 percent of the size (in linear dimension) of those that could be detected without the use of magnification.

Scatter reduction in magnification mammography is achieved by means of the air gap which is introduced between the breast and the film cassette. If the air gap is large enough, scatter reduction comparable to that produced by antiscatter grids is possible. Better scatter reduction is obtained with mammography units that use larger focal spot to film distances and larger magnification factors, since in these cases the size of the air gap is increased.

Scatter reduction by means of an air gap has the advantage of not causing any additional attenuation of the primary x-ray beam. Grids do cause some attenuation of the primary beam due to x-ray absorption in the lead strips, the interspace material, and the grid cover. This primary beam attenuation in the grid produces some reduction in image contrast and also an increase in patient dose.

Most mammographic units that permit magnification imaging utilize a magnification factor between 1.4 and 2.0. Setting aside questions of patient dose for the moment, one can ask what magnification factor will give the best image quality with a given mammographic unit. Increasing the magnification factor improves scatter rejection and low contrast detectability; however, image sharpness and resolution are only improved up to a certain magnification factor. Increasing the magnification beyond that point will reduce sharpness and resolution because of the effects of focal spot size. In determining which magnification factor will yield the optimum overall image quality, one must consider all of the above image quality components. With a particular mammographic unit it is quite possible that image resolution may be somewhat better at a magnification of 1.5× than of 2.0× but that microcalcifications are better imaged using the 2.0× magnification technique. In this case, improved low contrast detectability and improved scatter reduction at the 2.0× magnification technique more than compensate for the reduced image sharpness. To properly determine optimal magnification factors, it is very helpful to evaluate images of a phantom that simulates breast tissue and the structures of interest, such as microcalcifications.

All of the above image quality advantages of magnification imaging are tempered by the increased radiation dose this technique normally delivers. Partly because of this increased dose, magnification imaging is not normally used for the initial screening examination, but is reserved for evaluating suspicious areas in the hope of obtaining an image containing more definitive diagnostic information. With the use of higher speed screen-film systems that utilize dual screens and double emulsion film with extremely low crossover characteristics, the patient dose with magnification imaging can be similar to that obtained with more conventional nonmagnification techniques using single screens and an antiscatter grid. This new screen-film technology, opens up new possibilities for the use of magnification in standard mammographic imaging.

CAUTIONS IN EQUIPMENT COMPARISONS

In comparing the technical specification of different x-ray units it is important to use care in interpreting the numbers. We have already seen that the specification of the nominal focal spot is not by itself an adequate indication of the potential image sharpness capability of the x-ray system. The image sharpness depends on such items as the actual "equivalent" focal spot size and the system geometry. The following is another example showing some of the possible pitfalls in comparing x-ray systems.

Suppose we are evaluating two hypothetical mammographic systems with the following specifications:

System A: Rotating anode, Mo anode, 30 μm Mo filter, glass tube window, 0.6 mm nominal focal spot size, 0.9 mm equivalent focal spot size, single-phase, 160 mA, 75 cm FFD.

System B: Stationary anode, Mo anode, 30 μm Mo filter, Be tube window, 0.4 mm nominal focal spot size, 0.75 mm equivalent focal spot size, three-phase, 40 mA, 50 cm FFD.

On superficial analysis, looking only at the mA rating, one might conclude that system A would have the higher x-ray output and would be able to produce images using much shorter exposure times than system B. One might also conclude that system B would be able to produce sharper images because of its smaller nominal focal spot size. Both of these conclusions are in fact wrong.

Although system A does use much higher mA, its useful radiation output at the film cassette is reduced compared with system B by three design characteristics: the glass tube window absorbs a significant amount of radiation, the single-phase generator produces less radiation than a three-phase generator at the same mA, and the amount of radiation that reaches the film is reduced by the larger FFD of system A. Each of these characteristics separately reduces the radiation output to the film by about one-half. The total effect is approximately:

$$160 \text{ mA} \times \tfrac{1}{2} \times \tfrac{1}{2} \times \tfrac{1}{2} = 20 \text{ mA effective}$$

Thus system A actually delivers to the film cassette only about one-half the radiation intensity as system B.

Though system B has the smaller nominal focal spot size, a look at Table 4-2 indicates that system A can actually produce a sharper image. A focal spot with an equivalent size of 0.75 mm used at an FFD of 50 cm produces sharpness similar to a focal spot with an equivalent size of 1.2 mm used at an FFD of 75 cm.

Table 4-4 Quality Assurance Testing by the Radiologists and Radiographers

Test	Recommended Testing Frequency
Film processor monitoring: base + fog, speed index, contrast index, developer temperature, etc. (requires a sensitometer, densitometer, and thermometer)	Daily
Inspection and cleaning of intensifying screens	Daily
Inspection of condition of viewboxes	Daily
Image quality evaluation with imaging phantom	Monthly, after repair or maintenance of the x-ray equipment and whenever suspicions of reduced image quality arise
Evaluation of patient dose using TLDs	Monthly
Testing of each cassette for film/screen contact and image artifacts (requires perforated metal, film/screen contact test tool)	Annually

Abbreviations: TLDs, thermoluminescent dosimeter chips.

QUALITY ASSURANCE METHODS

After a mammographic system has been selected and properly installed, there remains the task of maintaining optimal system performance. To achieve this, a program of quality assurance (QA) is essential. A QA program will identify performance problems, monitor that repairs are quickly accomplished, and verify that any repairs or calibration have been properly performed. In order to identify potential problems, a mechanism should be established that will allow for easy reporting of any problems encountered with the clinical images. In addition, a program of equipment testing should be set up to monitor equipment performance. This testing can be done in a cooperative effort between the radiologists/radiographers and the physicist. For example, the radiologists and radiographers can perform the more frequently required testing, while the physicist comes in once or twice a year to perform more comprehensive testing. Tables 4-4 and 4-5 are examples of a practical testing program for a mammographic installation.

Table 4-5 Quality Assurance Testing by a Physicist

Test	Recommended Testing Frequency
Image quality evaluation with imaging phantom	Annually or semiannually
Measurement of surface exposure with ion chamber or TLDs and calculation of mean glandular dose (using a patient equivalent or imaging phantom)	Annually or semiannually
Measurement of half-value layer (HVL) (requires an ion chamber/exposure meter and high purity aluminum filters)	Annually or semiannually
Measurement of focal spot size (requires a star resolution pattern—a focal spot test tool containing a bar resolution pattern can be used to test focal spot sizes of 0.3 mm or greater)	Annually or semiannually
Collimation: light field accuracy and alignment of x-ray field to cassette	Annually or semiannually
kVp Accuracy and reproducibility (requires a mammography kVp meter or kVp cassette)	Annually or semiannually
mAs linearity (and timer accuracy if time is set separately) (requires an ion chamber/exposure meter and a timer test tool)	Annually or semiannually
Exposure output and reproducibility (requires an ion chamber/exposure meter)	Annually or semiannually
Phototimer performance: tracking with kVp and phantom thickness, density level, density adjustment controls, reproducibility (requires a patient equivalent or imaging phantom and a densitometer)	Annually or semiannually
Evaluation of clinicians' test results and analysis of imaging problems and retakes	Ongoing—as required

SUGGESTED READINGS

1. Alcorn FS, Gold RH, Paulus DD Jr: Mammographic phantoms and image quality control. p. 609. In Feig SA, McLelland R (eds): Breast Carcinoma. Masson, New York, 1983

2. Arnold BA, Eisenberg H, Bjarngard BE: Magnification mammography: a low dose technique. Radiology 131:743, 1979

3. Arnold BA, Webster EW, Kalisher L: Evaluation of mammographic screen-film systems. Radiology 129:179, 1978

4. Barnes GT, Brezovich IA: The intensity of scattered radiation in mammography. Radiology 126:243, 1978

5. Barnes GT, Chakraborty DP: Radiographic mottle and patient exposure in mammography. Radiology 145:815, 1982

6. Beaman S, Lillicrap SC, Price JL: Tungsten anode tubes with K-edge filters for mammography. Br J Radiol 56:721, 1983

7. Bencomo JA, Haus AG, Paulus DD, et al: Method to study the effect of controlled changes of breast image total system modulation transfer function (MTF) on diagnostic accuracy. SPIE Vol. 347, Application of Optical Instrumentation in Medicine X:84, 1982

8. Birch R, Marshall M, Ardran GM: Catalogue of Spectral Data for Diagnostic X-Rays. Scientific Report Series No. 30. The Hospital Physicists Association, London, 1979

9. Burgess A: A mammography quality assurance test program. Radiology 133:491, 1979

10. Burkhart RL: A Basic Quality Assurance Program for Small Diagnostic Radiology Facilities. HHS Publication FDA 83-8218. U.S. Department of Health and Human Services, National Center for Devices and Radiological Health, Rockville, MD, 1983

11. Boag JW, Stacey AJ, Davis R: Radiation exposure to the patient in xeroradiography. Br J Radiol 49:253, 1976

12. Chan H-P, Frank PH, Doi K, et al: Ultra-high-strip-density radiographic grids: a new antiscatter technique for mammography. Radiology 154:807, 1985

13. Chang CHJ, Sibala JL, Martin NL, Riley RC: Film mammography: new low radiation technology. Radiology 121:215, 1976

14. De Paredes ES, Frazier AB, Hartwell GD: Development and implementation of a quality assurance program for mammography. Radiology 163:83, 1987.

15. Dershaw DD, Malik S: Stationary and moving mammography grids: comparative radiation dose. AJR 147:491, 1986

16. Dershaw DD, Masterson ME, Malik S, Cruz NM: Mammography using an ultrahigh-strip-density, stationary, focused grid. Radiology 156:541, 1985

17. Doi K, Chan H-P: Evaluation of absorbed dose in mammography: Monte Carlo simulation studies. Radiology 135:199, 1980

18. Egan RL, McSweeney MB, Sprawls P: Grids in mammography. Radiology 146:359, 1983

19. Evans AL, James WB, McLellan J, Davison M: Film and xeroradiographic images in mammography. A comparison of tungsten and molybdenum anode materials Br J Radiol 48:968, 1975

20. Fatouros PP, Goodman H, Rao GU, et al: Absorbed dose and image quality in xeromammography. SPIE Vol. 419, Application of Optical Instrumentation in Medicine XI:37, 1983

21. Feig SA: Low-dose mammography: assessment of theoretical risk. p. 69. In Feig SA, McLelland R (eds): Breast Carcinoma. Masson, New York, 1983

22. Feig SA: Mammographic screening: benefit and risk. p. 351. In Feig SA, McLelland R (eds): Breast Carcinoma. Masson, New York, 1983

23. Feig SA: Screening mammography: benefits and risks. p. 75. In Moskowitz M (ed): Diagnostic Categorical Course in Breast Imaging. Radiological Society of North America, Oak Brook, IL, 1986

24. Fewell TR, Shuping RE: A comparison of mammographic x-ray spectra. Radiology 128:211, 1978

25. Fewell TR, Shuping RE: Handbook of Mammographic X-Ray Spectra. HEW Publication (FDA) 79-8071. U.S. Department of Health, Education, and Welfare, Bureau of Radiological Health, Rockville, MD, 1978

26. Fitzgerald M: Mammography. p. 446. In McAinsy (ed): Physics in Medicine and Biology Encyclopedia. Vol. 1. Pergamon Press, Oxford, 1986

27. Gannon FE, Fields T, Griffith CR, et al: Breast radiology: phantom, equipment performance, and radiation dosage comparisons for twenty-eight major mammography centers in the midwest. Radiology 149:579, 1983

28. Gohagan JK, Darby WP, Spitznagel EL, et al: Radiogenic breast cancer effects of mammographic screening. J Natl Cancer Inst 77:71, 1986

29. Gray JE: Photographic Quality Assurance in Diagnostic Radiology, Nuclear Medicine, and Radiation Therapy – Volume I – The Basic Principles of Daily Photographic Quality Assurance. HEW Publication (FDA) 76-8043. U.S. Department of Health, Education, and Welfare, Bureau of Radiological Health, Rockville, MD, 1976

30. Gray JE: Photographic Quality Assurance in Diagnostic Radiology, Nuclear Medicine, and Radiation Therapy – Volume II – Photographic Processing, Quality Assurance, and the Evaluation of Photographic Materials. HEW Publication (FDA) 77-8018. U.S. Department of Health, Education, and Welfare, Bureau of Radiological Health, Rockville, MD, 1977

31. Gray JE, Winkler NT, Stears J, Frank ED: Quality Control in Diagnostic Imaging. University Park Press, Baltimore, 1983

32. Hammerstein GR, Miller DW, White DR, et al: Absorbed radiation dose in mammography. Radiology 130:485, 1979

33. Haus AG, Cowart RW, Dodd GD, Bencomo J: A method of evaluating and minimizing geometric unsharpness for mammographic x-ray units. Radiology 128:775, 1978

34. Haus AG, Doi K, Metz CE, Bernstein J: Image quality in mammography. Radiology 125:77, 1977

35. Haus AG, Erickson L: Image quality factors and radiation dose in mammography. J Imaging Technol 10:29, 1984

36. Haus AG, Metz CE, Chiles JT, Rossmann K: The effect of x-ray spectra from molybdenum and tungsten target tubes on image quality in mammography. Radiology 118:705, 1976

37. Haus AG, Metz CE, Doi K, Bernstein J: Determination of x-ray spectra incident on and transmitted through breast tissue. Radiology 124:511, 1977

38. Haus AG, Meyer J, Guebert DK: Evaluation of the resolution limit for radiological procedures. SPIE Vol. 273, Application of Optical Instrumentation in Medicine IX:177, 1981

39. Hessler C, Depeursinge C, Grecescu M, et al: Objective assessment of mammography systems. Part I: Method. Radiology 156:215, 1985

40. Hessler C, Depeursinge C, Grecescu M, et al: Objective assessment of mammography systems. Part II: Implementation. Radiology 156:221, 1985

41. Jaeger SS, Cacak RK, Barnes JE, Hendee WR: Optimization of xeroradiographic exposures. Radiology 128:217, 1978

42. Jans RG, Butler PF, McCrohan JL Jr, Thompson WE: The status of film/screen mammography. Results of the BENT study. Radiology 132:197, 1979

43. Jenkins D: Radiographic Photography and Imaging Processes. University Park Press, Baltimore, 1980

44. Jennings RJ, Eastgate RJ, Siedband MP, Ergun DL: Optimal x-ray spectra for screen-film mammography. Med Phys 8:629, 1981

45. Johnson GA, O'Foghludha F: Stimulation of mammographic x-ray spectra. Med Phys 7:189, 1980

46. Jones CH: Methods of breast imaging. Phys Med Biol 27:463, 1982

47. Karila KTK: Performance of x-ray generators and unnecessary dose in mammography. Radiology 14:395, 1982

48. Kimme-Smith C, Bassett LW, Gold RH, et al: Mammographic dual-screen dual-emulsion-film combination: visibility of simulated microcalcifications and effect on image contrast. Radiology 165:313, 1987

49. Kimme-Smith C, Bassett LW, Gold RH: Evaluation of radiation dose, focal spot, and automatic exposure of newer film-screen mammography units. AJR 149:913, 1987

50. Kirkpatrick AE, Law J: The usefulness of a moving grid in mammography. Br J Radiol 58:257, 1985

51. Kirkpatrick AE, Law J: A comparative study of films and screens for mammography. Br J Radiol 60:73, 1987

52. Kulkarni RN, Supe SJ: Monte Carlo calculations of mammographic x-ray spectra. Phys Med Biol 29:185, 1984

53. Kulkarni RN, Supe SJ: Radiation dose to the breast during mammography: a comprehensive, realistic Monte Carlo calculation. Phys Med Biol 29:1257, 1984

54. LaFrance R, Gelskey DE, Barnes GT: A circuit modification that improves mammographic phototimer performance. Radiology 166:773, 1988

55. Lassen M, Bloch P: Theoretical considerations of effects of x-ray film-screen characteristics on threshold detectability of small low contrast objects. Med Phys 5:146, 1978

56. Logan WW, Muntz EP (eds): Reduced Dose Mammography. Masson, New York, 1979

57. Malik S, Masterson ME, Hunt M: Effects of kVp variation and x-ray tube filtration on the mammographic examination. SPIE Vol. 419, Application of Optical Instrumentation in Medicine XI:42, 1983

58. McSweeney MB, Sprawls P, Egan RL: Mammographic grids. p. 169. In Feig SA, McLelland R (eds): Breast Carcinoma. Masson, New York, 1983

59. Muntz EP, Logan WW: Focal spot size and scatter suppression in magnification mammography. AJR 133:453, 1979

60. Muntz EP, Wilkinson E, George FW: Mammography at reduced doses: present performance and future possibilities. AJR 134:741, 1980

61. National Council on Radiation Protection and Measurements. Mammography. NCRP Report No. 66. National Council on Radiation Protection, Washington, DC, 1980

62. National Council on Radiation Protection and Measurements: Mammography—A User's Guide. NCRP Report No. 85. National Council on Radiation Protection. Bethesda, MD, 1986

63. Niklason LT, Barnes GT, Rubin E: Mammography phototimer technique chart. Radiology 157:539, 1985

64. Oestmann JW, Kopans DB, Linetsky L, et al: Comparison of two screen-film combinations in contact and magnification mammography: detectability of microcalcifications. Radiology 168:657, 1988

65. Ostrum BJ, Becker W, Isard HJ: Low-dose mammography. Radiology 109:323, 1973

66. Pochon Y, Depeursinge C, Hessler C, et al: Simulta-

neous objective measurements of dose and image quality in mammography. SPIE Vol. 347, Application of Optical Instrumentation in Medicine X:238, 1982

67. Price JL, Butler PD: The reduction of radiation and exposure time in mammography. Br J Radiol 43:251, 1970

68. Ramsden JA, Moores BM, Asbury DL: The dose to the patient and the quality of the image in xeromammography. Br J Radiol 52:804, 1979

69. Rosenstein M, Andersen LW, Warner GG: Handbook of Glandular Tissue Doses in Mammography. HHS Publication FDA 85-8239. U.S. Department of Health and Human Services, Center for Devices and Radiological Health, Rockville, MD, 1985

70. Rothenberg LN: Physical aspects of mammography. Ch. 9. In Taveras JM, Ferrucci JT (eds): Radiology. Diagnosis-Imaging-Intervention. Vol. 1. JB Lippincott, Philadelphia, 1988

71. Rothenberg LN, Kirch RLA, Snyder RE: Patient exposures from film and xeroradiographic mammographic techniques. Radiology 117:701, 1975

72. Sickles EA, Weber WN: High-contrast mammography with a moving grid: assessment of clinical utility. AJR 146:1137, 1986

73. Sickles EA, Doi K, Genant HK: Magnification film mammography: image quality and clinical studies. Radiology 125:69, 1977

74. Shrivastava PN: Model to analyze radiographic factors in mammography. Med Phys 7:222, 1980

75. Shrivastava PN: Radiation dose in mammography: an energy balance approach. Radiology 140:483, 1981

76. Siedband MP, Jennings RJ, Eastgate RJ, Eastgate RJ, Ergun DL: X-ray beam filtration for mammography. SPIE Vol. 127, Optical Instrumentation in Medicine VI:204, 1977

77. Skubic SE, Fatouros PP: Absorbed breast dose: dependence on radiographic modality and technique, and breast thickness. Radiology 161:263, 1986

78. Speiser RC, Zanrosso EM, Jeromin LS, Carlson RA: Dose comparisons for mammographic systems. Med Phys 13:667, 1986

79. Stanton L, Day JL, Brattelli SD, Lightfoot DA: Comparison of ion chamber and TLD dosimetry in mammography. Med Phys 8:792, 1981

80. Stanton L, Day JL, Villafana T, et al: Screen-film mammographic technique for breast cancer screening. Radiology 163:471, 1987

81. Stanton L, Villafana T, Day JL, Lightfoot DA: A breast phantom method for evaluating mammography technique. Invest Radiol 13:291, 1978

82. Stanton L, Villafana T, Day JL, Lightfoot DA: Dosage evaluation in mammography. Radiology 150:577, 1984

83. Stanton L, Villafana T, Day JL, et al: A study of mammographic exposure and detail visibility using three systems: Xerox 125, Min-R, and Xonics XERG. Radiology 132:455, 1979

84. Tabar L, Dean PB: Screen/film mammography: Quality control. p. 161. In Feig SA, McLelland R (eds): Breast Carcinoma. Masson, New York, 1983

85. Van de Riet WG, Wolfe JN: Dose reduction in xeroradiography of the breast. Am J Roentgenol 128:821, 1977

86. Yaffe MJ, Mawdsley GE, Nishikawa RM: Quality assurance in a national breast screening study. SPIE Vol. 419, Application of Optical Instrumentation in Medicine XI:23, 1983

87. Zamenhof RGA: Mammography. p. 1840. In Webster JG (ed): Encyclopedia of Medical Devices and Instrumentation. Vol. 3. John Wiley & Sons, New York, 1988

5
Before the Mammogram

Margaret I. Fagerholm

Appropriate clinical information and a physical examination of the breast are an integral part of the mammographic study. These data are often needed to clarify abnormal radiographic findings, since benign and malignant changes may mimic one another. A patient information sheet is used to record the necessary information needed by the mammographer. This sheet is filled out at the time of the baseline mammogram and should request all information needed for adequate assessment of the mammogram as well as determination of the patient's relative risk for breast cancer. An example of the patient information sheet used in our institution is shown in Figure 5-1. In a follow-up study, additional pertinent information can be added to the existing data sheet.

A major risk factor for breast cancer is aging. Various medical organizations including the American College of Radiology, the American College of Obstetricians and Gynecologists, the American Medical Association, and the American Academy of Family Physicians have compiled specific recommendations, which differ slightly, for screening of asymptomatic patients. They have all accepted various parts of the recommendations put forth by the American Cancer Society (ACS). The ACS recommends a baseline examination between the ages of 35 and 39, annual or biannual screening between the ages of 40 and 49, and annual mammograms after the age of 50. Regular physical examination is also recommended regularly beginning in the 20s.

It has been well established that the benefits of screening mammography in patients over the age of 50 far outweighs the theoretical risk of radiation exposure. The frequency of screening in the 40 to 49-year-old age group is currently under discussion. Moskowitz[5] has suggested that yearly screening be performed in this age group. He also concludes that biannual screening may be more appropriate than yearly screening after the age of 50. Routine screening of asymptomatic patients below the age of 35 years is generally not accepted. Patients in this age group have a much lower incidence of breast cancer, and the risk/benefit ratio is not appropriate for routine screening. Abnormalities of the breast in this age group are also more difficult to image because generally the parenchyma is less fatty replaced. Glandular elements of younger patients are also more radiosensitive. The National Cancer Institute estimates the risk of developing breast cancer from radiation exposure secondary to mammography in women over the age of 35 is 3.5 excess cancers/million women/year/rad. The risk to women under the age of 35 is theorized to be twice this estimate. This information is based on extrapolation from linear models derived from patients receiving high doses of radiation. These figures are currently disputed and are thought to greatly overestimate the radiation risk. A more appropriate estimate of the radiation risk is believed to be obtained by using the linear-quadratic or quadratic model, which would decrease the estimates for low-dose risk by a factor of one-half or greater.

```
┌─────────────────────────────────────────────────────────────────────┐
│ PATIENT INFORMATION SHEET FOR MAMMOGRAPHY                             │
│                                                                       │
│ Instructions:  Fill in information or check appropriate answer(s).    │
├─────────────────────────────────────────────────────────────────────┤
│ NAME:_____     DATE:_____      │
│                                                                       │
│ HISTORY #:_____  AGE:____  SEX: __Female __Male            │
└─────────────────────────────────────────────────────────────────────┘
```

I. REASON FOR CURRENT EXAM:	IV. FAMILY HISTORY

___Screening, no known problems
___Lump felt
___Discharge from nipple
___Pain or sensation
___Skin change
___Change in appearance of nipple
___Abnormality on previous mammogram
___Other:_____
	Is there breast cancer in your
	   family?.................__Y __N
	If yes, list age and relationship:
	  (Note if maternal or paternal side)
	   _____
	   _____
	   _____
	   _____

II. MENSTRUAL/PREGNANCY HISTORY:

Are you pregnant now?...........__Y __N
Last menstrual period_____
Number of births_____
Age at first pregnancy_____
Did you breast feed?............__Y __N
Have you had a hysterectomy?....__Y __N
 If yes, why?_____
Were your ovaries removed?......__Y __N

V. BIOPSY HISTORY:

#	Date	R/L	Method*	Diagnosis
1				
2				
3				
4				
5				

*Method: Surgical(S) or Needle(N)

III. PERSONAL HISTORY

Have you ever had breast cancer?__Y __N
 If yes, when? (date) _____
 Mark the location with a circle:

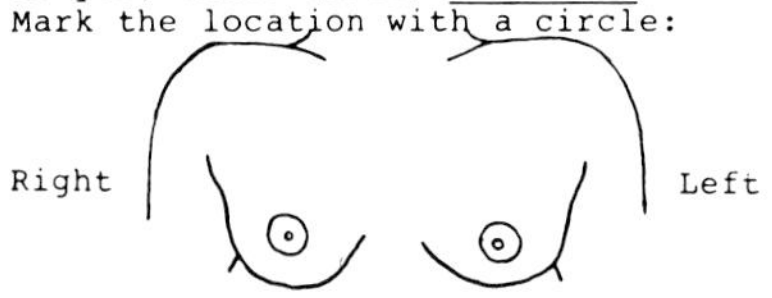

Right   Left

Size when found:_____
Who discovered it?
 __X-ray __Physician __Patient
Were lymph nodes involved?....__Y __N
Treatment:
 ___None
 ___Mastectomy
 ___Local removal of lump
 ___Radiotherapy (dates)_____to_____
 ___Surgery
 ___Chemotherapy (dates)_____to_____

Have you had any other cancer?..__Y __N
 If yes, what kind? _____
 When? _____

Are you on any of the following medicine?
 ___Birth control pills
 ___Estrogen
 ___Progesterone
 ___Thyroid medication

FOR PHYSICIAN'S USE ONLY

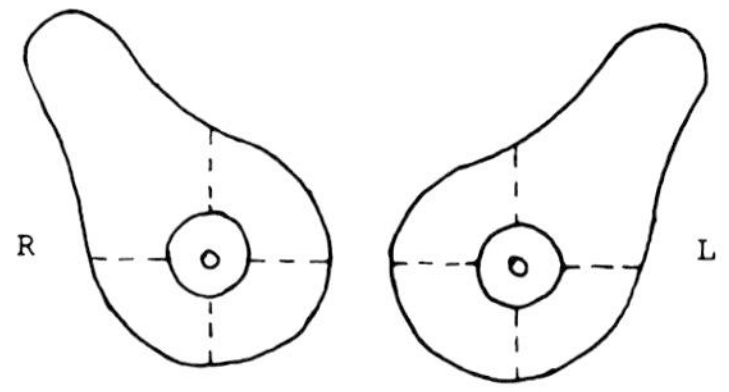

R   L

Have you ever taken female hormones?
.........................__Y __N
If so, when? _____

Have you ever been treated for
 fibrocystic disease?......__Y __N

Have you ever had breast reduction
 or augmentation surgery?.__Y __N
If so, when? _____

Have you had previous mammograms or
 ultrasound of the breasts?__Y __N
 If so, when and where?

   _____

Fig. 5-1 Patient information sheet for mammography.

Mammography in patients between the ages of 30 and 35 can be helpful in symptomatic patients, in those with a personal history of breast cancer, and in those with a strong family history of premenopausal breast cancer. Under the age of 30, most breast problems can be evaluated without mammography. The majority of patients in this age group are referred for a palpable lump, which can be easily evaluated with aspiration, biopsy, or ultrasound. Mammography in this age group may not be helpful in evaluating soft tissue masses, since normal breast parenchymal elements can obscure masses of similar density. The great majority of masses in this age group are of a benign origin. Most often the palpated abnormality is secondary to normal lumpy breast tissue or fibroadenomas. Mammography may be needed if the surgeon suspects malignancy and wishes to evaluate for calcifications or other signs of malignancy prior to biopsy. Other appropriate indications include bloody nipple discharge, axillary adenopathy, or personal history of breast cancer.

Women are at much greater risk for breast cancer than are men; however, male breast cancer accounts for 1 out of every 100 breast cancers. Indications for mammography in males are similar to that in females, including changes in the skin or nipple, palpable lump, and nipple discharge. Male patients often also present with unilateral or bilateral breast enlargement secondary to gynecomastia. Gynecomastia may be idiopathic or may be caused by several commonly prescribed drugs, including hormones to treat prostatic cancer. Chronic liver disease and developmental abnormalities have also been associated with gynecomastia. More information on male breast cancer is included in Chapter 17.

Other major risk factors for breast cancer besides age and sex are personal or family history of breast cancer and specific pathologic findings on biopsy, including atypical hyperplasia. If a patient has a personal history of breast cancer, it is helpful to know when the diagnosis was made as well as the location of the cancer, extent of involvement, and treatment performed. Surgery and radiation cause changes in the remaining breast tissue of patients who have had conservative therapy. The timing of the mammogram in relation to this treatment is important, since both postsurgical and radiation changes will alter the breast structure for several months.

All biopsies should be recorded and their location marked for review by the mammographer. This procedure will help to prevent unnecessary follow-up or biopsy for unrecognized, surgically induced architectural distortion, masses, or fat necrosis.

The patient with a family history of breast cancer will be at greatest risk if the cancer was detected in a first-degree relative, specifically a sister or mother.

Minor risk factors for breast cancer include early age of menarche and late age of menopause. A women who is less than 18 years of age at her first childbirth has a smaller risk, compared with the woman who gives birth for the first time after the age of 30. Other minor risk factors are histories of gynecologic tumors, radiation exposure for treatment of tuberculosis, and multiple films for scoliosis evaluation.

A history of the patient's hormonal therapy is needed. Parenchymal changes are seen in the breast with the onset of hormonal therapy, demonstrated as diffuse increased density with or without cyst formation.

Finally, in addition to a clinical history and physical examination, previous ultrasounds and mammograms of the breasts should be obtained. Subtle changes may only be identifiable when comparison is made with previous studies. Unnecessary biopsy may also be avoided if previous mammograms have shown that an area of suspicion has been stable over a long period of time.

SUGGESTED READINGS

1. Feig S: Mammographic screening: benefit and risk. p. 351. In Feig S, McLellan R (eds): Breast Carcinoma: Current Diagnosis and Treatment. Masson Publishing, New York, 1983
2. Feig S: Low dose mammography in the question of radiation risk. p. 101. In: Syllabus for the Categorical Course on Mammography. American College of Radiology, 1984
3. McLellan R: Screening for breast cancer. p. 117. In: Syllabus for the Categorical Course on Mammography, American College of Radiology, 1984
4. McLellan R, Feig S: Guidelines for mammography. p. 365. In Feig S, McLellan R (eds): Breast Carcinoma: Current Diagnosis and Treatment. Masson Publishing, New York, 1983
5. Moskowitz M: Breast cancer: age-specific growth rates and screening strategies. Radiology 40:37, 1986
6. National Cancer Institute: The Breast Cancer Digest (2). Office of Cancer Communications, National Cancer Institute, Bethesda, MD, 1984
7. Whitehouse GH, Leinster SJ: Variation of breast parenchymal patterns with age. Br J Radiol 58:315, 1985

6
Positioning for the Mammogram

Lucinda K. Prue

Mammography is currently the single most effective imaging modality for detecting breast cancer. There are two methods of mammography in use today: one method utilizes a screen-film combination, and the other employs the Xerox process to produce the final image.

Since interpretation is dependent on the quality of the mammogram, the technologist plays a major role in diagnostic accuracy. To obtain an optimum examination, the patient must be relaxed and cooperative. A brief explanation of the mammographic procedure is required to place the patient at ease.

Because rigorous compression is used, patients with tender breasts may find mammography momentarily uncomfortable. However, compression is necessary, as it reduces the radiation dose and enhances image quality. The technical improvements resulting from compression include (1) reduction of motion artifact by immobilizing the breast; (2) reduction of geometric blur by bringing the breast parenchyma as close to the film as possible; (3) reduction in the change of radiographic density from the nipple to the chest wall by producing a more uniform breast thickness; and (4) reduction of the ratio of scattered to primary radiation by decreasing breast thickness, resulting in better subject contrast.

Enhanced contrast can also be achieved by the use of a reciprocating grid. At our institution, all mammograms are performed with the use of a grid.

The basic screening mammographic views are the craniocaudal and mediolateral oblique views. Once the standard views have been obtained, the radiologist may find it necessary to visualize the breast parenchyma in a different projection for evaluation of a suspected mass, parenchymal distortion, or microcalcifications. Complementary views include the Cleopatra, 90 degree lateral, lateral medial, and coned compression with or without microfocus magnification.

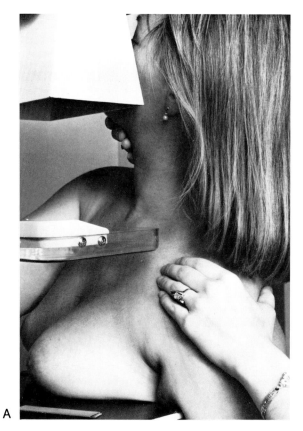

A

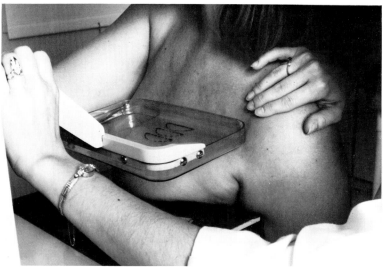

B

Fig. 6-1. (A) The craniocaudal view is performed with the cassette holder beneath the breast and the x-ray beam directed in a cranial-to-caudal direction. The patient turns her head away from the breast being imaged, which enables the chest wall to come into direct contact with the cassette holder. She may wish to grasp the machine to steady herself. **(B)** The shoulder on the side of the breast being positioned is relaxed down as the compression paddle is lowered, and the patient leans slightly forward. This is a modification of the standard craniocaudal view in which the shoulder is not dropped. More of the lateral portion of the breast can be imaged using this modified projection. *(Figure continues.)*

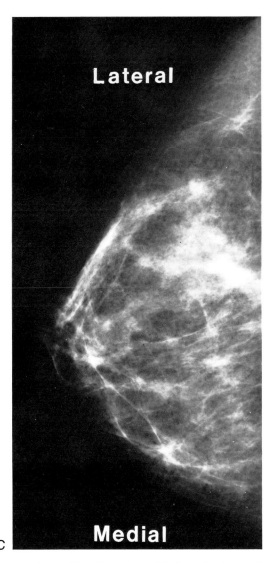

C

Fig. 6-1 *(Continued)*. **(C)** A correctly positioned craniocaudal view. As the result of rigorous compression, the breast parenchyma is dispersed, which increases the detectability of masses and parenchymal distortion. The craniocaudal view best images the medial, central, and subareolar portions of the breast. With the use of the modified craniocaudal projection, a major portion of the lateral breast can also be visualized. However, not all of the axillary tail will be seen on this projection. In some cases, the pectoralis muscle can be visualized.

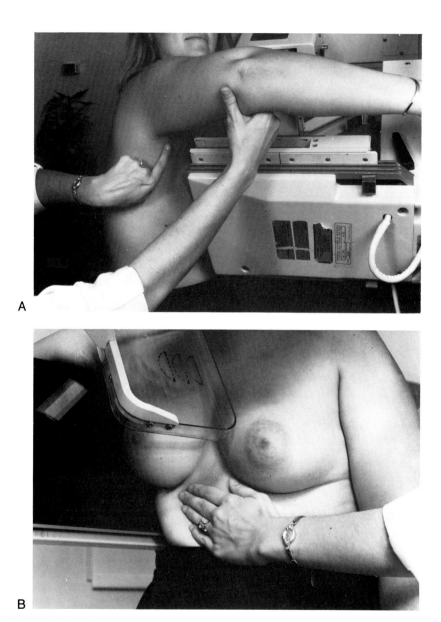

Fig. 6-2. (A) The mediolateral oblique view is performed with the C arm of the mammographic unit between 40 and 60 degrees. This placement is determined by the angle of the pectoralis muscle. The breast must be placed on the cassette holder parallel to the long axis of the pectoralis muscle, which enables the compression paddle to displace the breast away from the ribs. **(B)** The beam is directed from superomedial to inferolateral, allowing visualization of the entire breast including the axillary tail. The patient's arm rests on the cassette holder; the arm is lowered and bent so that the entire breast is in direct contact with the holder. Abdominal tissue must be tucked behind the holder to prevent skin folds from obscuring the breast parenchyma. *(Figure continues.)*

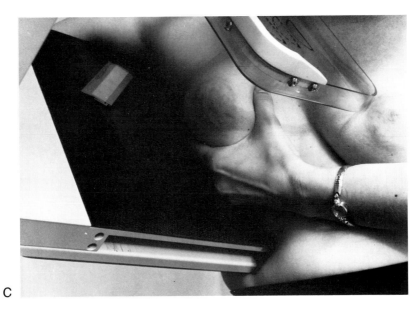

C

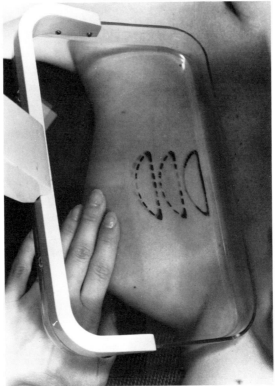

D

Fig. 6-2 *(Continued).* **(C)** The breast is pulled forward from the rib cage and held in place by the technologist's hand. **(D)** The compression paddle is placed so that it extends from beneath the clavicle to the most inferior portion of the breast. As the paddle takes over the support of the breast, the technologist moves her hand toward the nipple allowing the paddle to complete the compression. *(Figure continues.)*

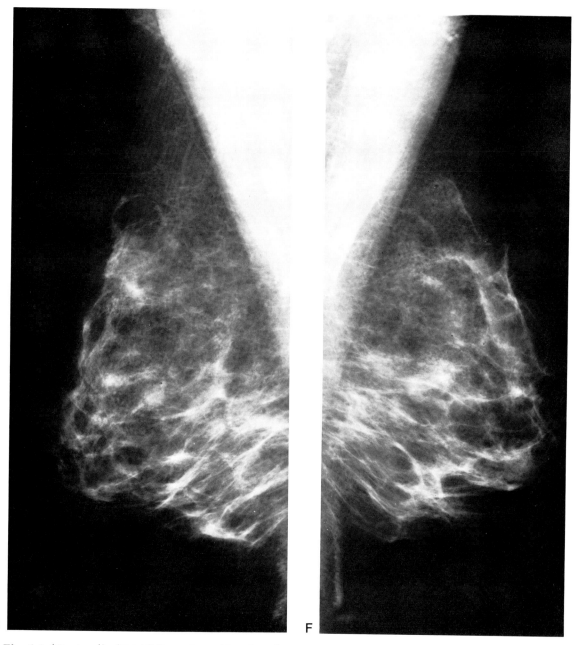

E   F

Fig. 6-2 *(Continued).* **(E & F)** Properly positioned 60 degree mediolateral oblique views. The pectoralis muscle should be visualized to approximately the level of the nipple. On screen-film technique, the ribs are not visualized.

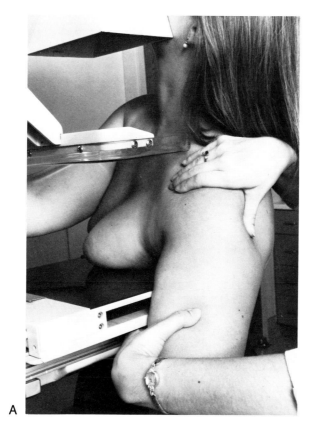

A

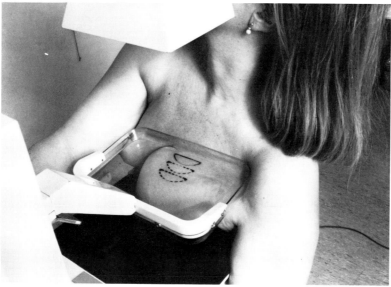

B

Fig. 6-3. **(A)** For the Cleopatra view, the breast is placed on the cassette holder in much the same manner as the craniocaudal view. The ipsilateral shoulder, however, is in an exaggerated down and forward position, bringing the tail of the breast onto the film. **(B)** The medial section of the breast will not be completely imaged in this position. The patient's chin is raised so that she may relax her shoulder as much as possible into a reclining position. Note the extensive compression of the axillary tail. *(Figure continues.)*

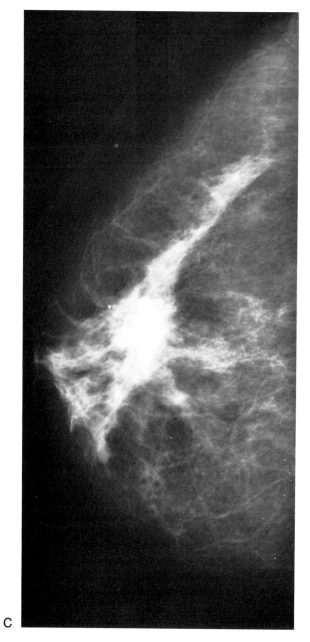

C

Fig. 6-3 *(Continued).* **(C)** Craniocaudal view. *(Figure continues.)*

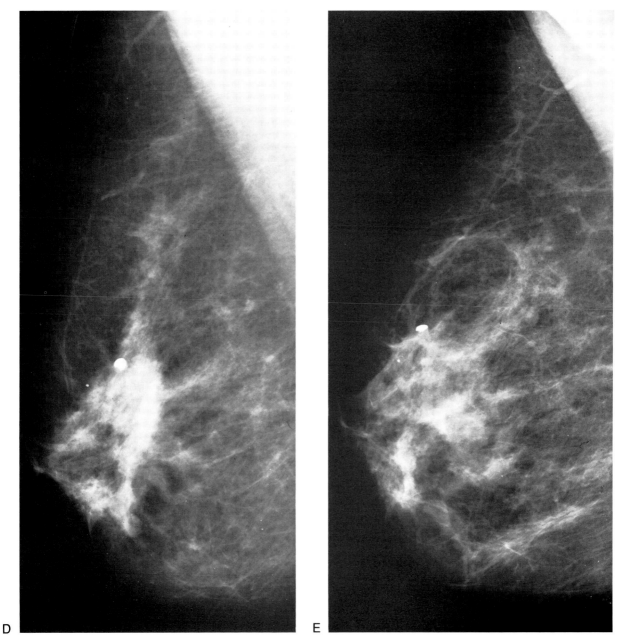

D E

Fig. 6-3 *(Continued)*. **(D)** A correctly positioned Cleopatra view. The entire axillary tail, including a portion of the pectoralis muscle, has been imaged. Lesions lying close to the pectoralis muscle on the mediolateral oblique view and not seen on the craniocaudal view can be visualized in this manner. **(E)** A properly positioned 60 degree mediolateral oblique view. Note that the Cleopatra view resembles it.

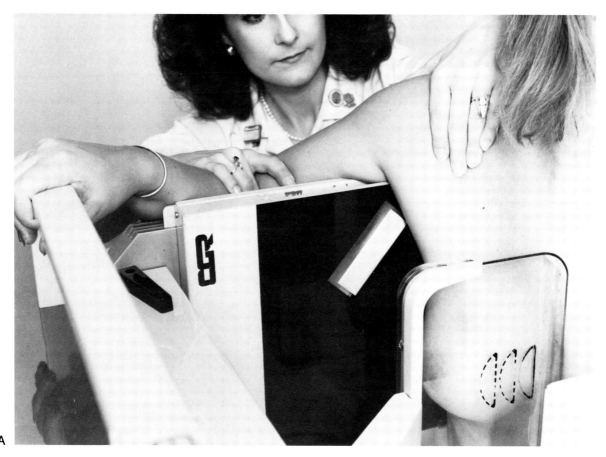

A

Fig. 6-4. (A) Positioning for the 90 degree mediolateral view is similar to the mediolateral oblique view with the x-ray beam directed from medial to lateral. However, the 90 degree angle does not correspond to the long axis of the pectoralis muscle, so it cannot be compressed. To obtain adequate compression of the breast, the pectoralis muscle will not be entirely positioned on the cassette holder. *(Figure continues.)*

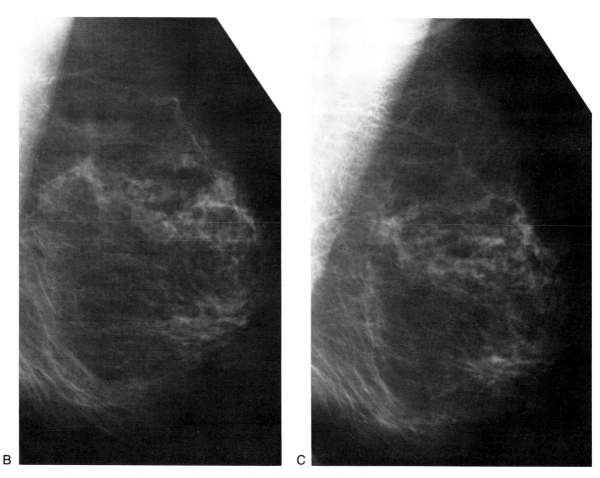

B

C

Fig. 6-4 *(Continued)*. **(B)** A correctly positioned 90 degree mediolateral view. Note the difference in the amount of pectoralis muscle visualized on this view in comparison with the 60 degree mediolateral oblique view **(C)**. **(C)** A correctly positioned 60 degree mediolateral oblique view.

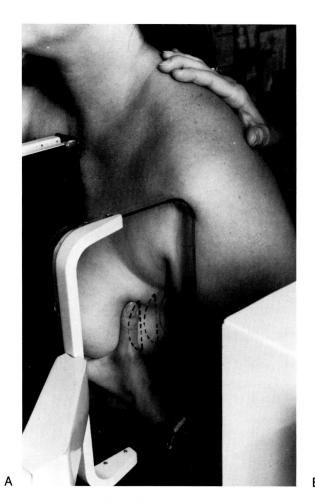

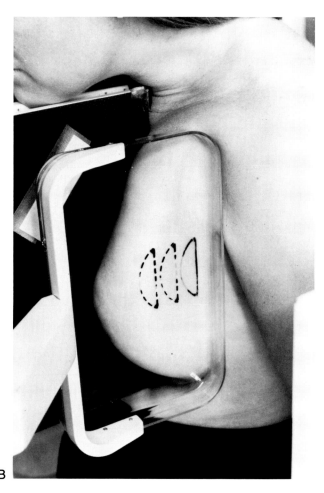

A   B

Fig. 6-5. (A) The lateral medial view can be used in evaluating medial lesions. The patient stands facing the machine with the C arm at 90 degrees. The medial surface of the breast is placed on the cassette holder with the compression paddle against the lateral aspect of the breast. **(B)** To optimally visualize the superior portion of the breast, the patient rests her chin on the cassette holder. This brings the superior portion of the breast in close approximation to the holder. *(Figure continues.)*

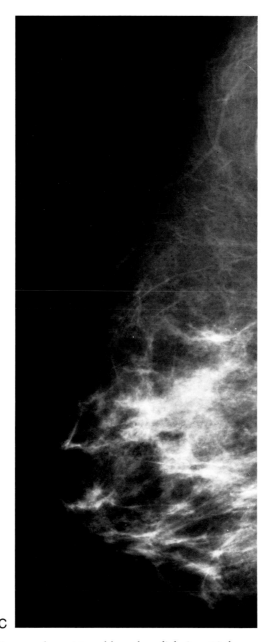

C

Fig. 6-5 *(Continued).* **(C)** A correctly positioned lateral medial view. Little or no pectoralis muscle is seen.

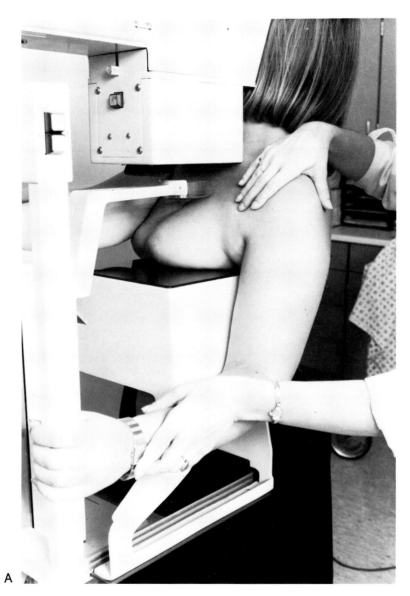

A

Fig. 6-6. **(A)** For the coned view with or without microfocus magnification, the technologist must first localize the suspicious area on the original craniocaudal or oblique radiograph, depending on which best demonstrates the lesion. The breast must be positioned in the same manner as the original view was obtained. For the magnification view, the breast is placed on the mammographic tower. *(Figure continues.)*

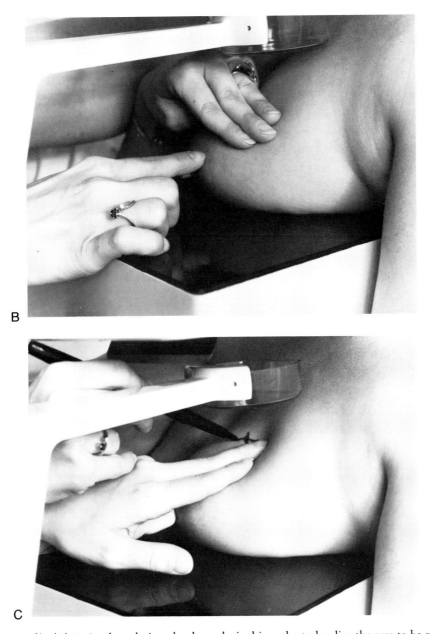

B

C

Fig. 6-6 *(Continued)*. **(B)** A simple technique has been devised in order to localize the area to be radiographed: Using your fingers as a guide, duplicate the distance from the nipple as you did on the mammogram. **(C)** Also, measure from the nipple to the medial or lateral side just as you did on the radiograph. By placing a mark on the skin, you can localize the area to be focally compressed. *(Figure continues.)*

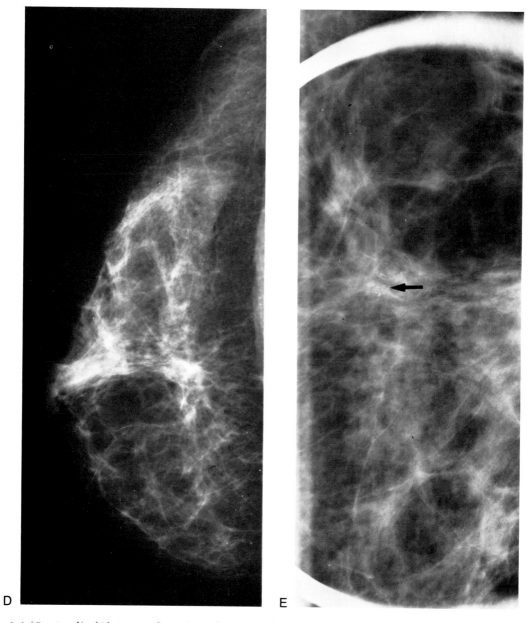

D

E

Fig. 6-6 *(Continued).* **(D)** A properly positioned craniocaudal view shows an area of increased density posterior to the nipple. **(E)** Microfocus magnification image positioned from the craniocaudal view. It demonstrates the increased density with small microcalcifications *(arrow).* The microfocus magnification view increases resolution and reduces image noise.

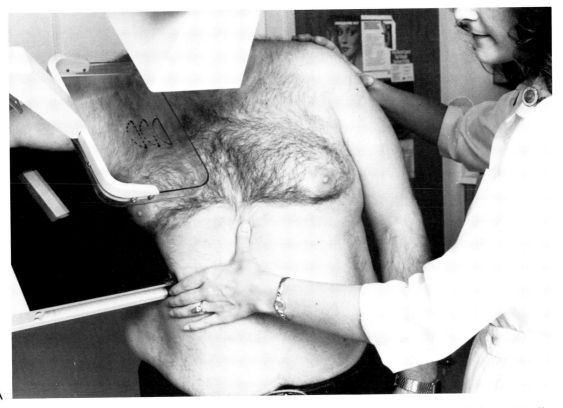

A

Fig. 6-7. (A) Positioning of the male breast is performed in much the same manner as the female breast. Usually only mediolateral oblique views are obtained. The technologist chooses an angle between 40 and 60 degrees corresponding to the long axis of the pectoral muscle. *(Figure continues.)*

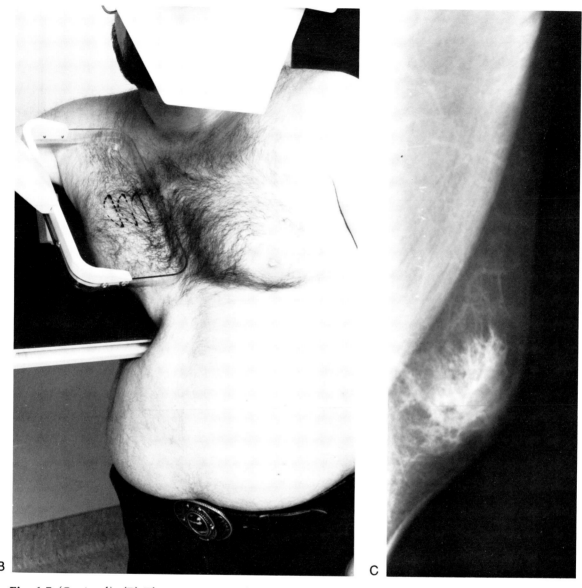

Fig. 6-7 *(Continued)*. **(B)** The compression paddle extends from just beneath the clavicle to the most inferior portion of the breast. **(C)** A properly performed 45 degree mediolateral oblique view of a male breast.

SUGGESTED READINGS

1. Andersson I: Mammography in clinical practice. Med Radiogr Photogr 62:1, 1986
2. Bassett LW, Gold RH: Breast radiography using the oblique projection. Radiology 149:585, 1983
3. Council's Scientific Committee 72 on Radiation Protec- tion in Mammography: Mammography—A User's Guide. National Council on Radiation and Protection and Measurements, Bethesda, MD, 1986
4. Egan RL, McSweeney MB, Sprawls P: Grids in mam- mography. Radiology 146:359, 1983
5. Feig SA: Mammography equipment: principles, features, selection. Radiol Clin North Am 25:897, 1987
6. Goodrich WA, Jr.: The Cleopatra view in xeromam-

mography: a semi-reclining position for the tail of the breast. Radiology 128:811, 1978

7. Haus AG: Recent advances in screen film mammography. Radiol Clin North Am 25:913, 1987

8. Logan WW: Screen/film mammography. pp. 141. In Feig SA, McLelland (eds): Breast Carcinoma. Masson, Publishing, New York, 1983

9. Logan WW: Use of special mammographic views to maximize radiographic information. Radiol Clin North Am 25:953, 1987

10. Seago K: Breast imaging centers and patient emotions: niceness counts. Appl Radiol Nov/Dec:59, 1986

11. Sickles EA, Webber WN: High-contrast mammography with a moving grid: assessment of clinical utility. AJR 146:1137, 1986

7

Evaluating the Mammogram

Mary Ellen Peters

Attention to minute detail and a systematic approach are the keys to mammographic interpretation. Normal breast parenchyma is usually symmetrical. This is assessed by placing the craniocaudal and mediolateral oblique views adjacent to one another for comparison (Fig. 7-1). Compare the mammograms, gathering an overall impression of the parenchyma and scanning for masses or asymmetry which may indicate carcinoma.

After the general inspection, mask the comparison views to more completely examine for masses and asymmetry (Figs. 7-2 and 7-3). Be sure to inspect the skin and areolar-nipple complex for clues of an underlying malignancy. (These findings are described in subsequent chapters.) In properly exposed screen-film mammograms, a bright light is often required to visualize the skin. Then search for calcifications by scrutinizing all of the films with a magnifying glass. Finally, evaluate the size, configuration, and density of the axillary nodes.

Comparison with previous studies is mandatory. If those studies have been performed at an outside hospital, the radiologist is obligated to obtain them. If the patient has had previous serial mammograms, never stop with comparison of the most recent examination.

Breast carcinoma can grow slowly, and comparison of serial studies can demonstrate minimal progressive changes.

All calcifications and masses need to be characterized. Although some masses and calcifications are obviously benign or malignant, a large number are indeterminate in appearance. For the latter group, careful characterization may prevent unnecessary biopsy or may indicate that it is necessary. (Characterization of masses and calcifications will be discussed in the ensuing chapters.)

If the initial study is not adequate for diagnostic purposes, obtain further views. For instance, a coned compression view will often help define the margins of a mass by displacing the surrounding fibroglandular tissues, which allows for better characterization. This view can also be used to determine if a "mass" is real or represents superimposed fibroglandular structures. Another method of solving the problem of "mass" versus superimposition of normal structures is to obtain a view projected at a different angle of obliquity. Magnification views frequently prove beneficial in the evaluation of calcifications and masses. A lateromedial rather than a mediolateral view can be helpful in defining medial lesions. Tangential views may be helpful in localizing masses and calcifications within the skin. If a lesion is

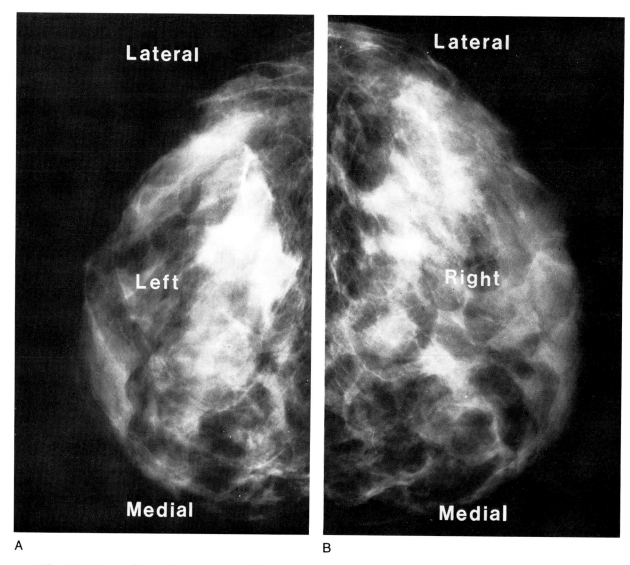

A   B

Fig. 7-1. A normal screening mammogram in a parous 31-year-old woman who breast fed. The left **(A)** and right **(B)** craniocaudal and left **(C)** and right **(D)** mediolateral oblique views have been placed adjacent to one another for comparison. Note that the craniocaudal views have been placed with the medial side down. As the mammogram is viewed, the left breast is on your left. This is the format that is used throughout the book. When viewing follow-up studies, ipsilateral views are compared with the previous study to the left. (The arrows on the mediolateral oblique views point to the pectoralis muscle.) *(Figure continues.)*

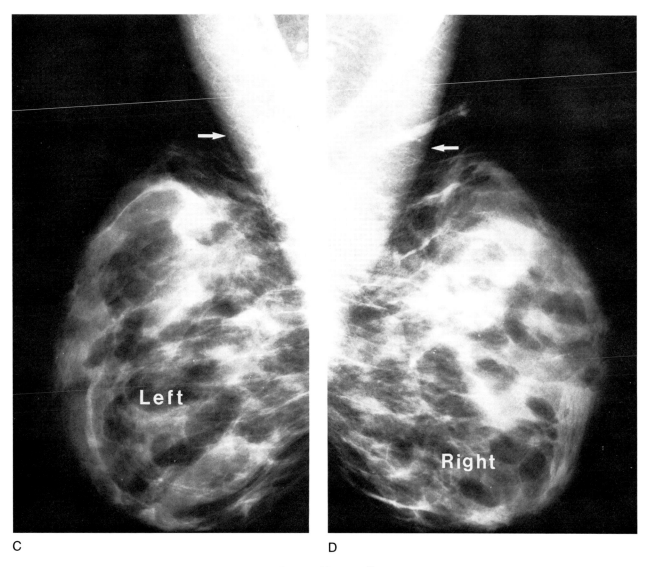

C D

Fig. 7-1 *(Continued)*.

seen on only one standard projection, further views will be necessary to localize it. The additional time and radiation "spent" obtaining these additional views is worthwhile.

When describing the location of a lesion, it is customary to localize it according to the quadrant of the breast. Common terminology is superolateral, superomedial, inferolateral, and inferomedial; equally descriptive is upper-outer, upper-inner, lower-outer, and lower-inner. A third method describes the lesion according to

the hands of a clock, with 3 o'clock being medial on the right and lateral on the left.

The denseness of the fibroglandular tissue on the mammogram is extremely variable. During lactation, the fibroglandular tissue is very dense, which is generally also true for the young patient. With advancing age and following pregnancy and lactation, the breast parenchyma usually becomes more fatty replaced. Involution first occurs inferomedially, progressing inferolaterally and superomedially; the fibroglandular tissue in the

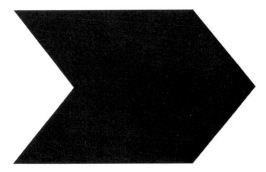

Fig. 7-2. A simple device for use in masking the mammogram (Fig. 7-3) can be made by cutting an "arrow" out of cardboard and gluing exposed film to it. (Adapted from Tabar and Dean,[18] with permission.)

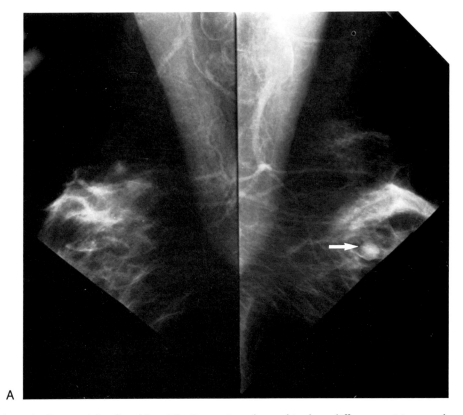

A

Fig. 7-3. (A–C) The principle of masking. The "arrow" can be used in three different positions, as shown. Place the mask at the top of the comparison views and move it down slowly, while carefully looking for asymmetry. Note the asymmetrical mass on the right *(arrow)*. Dashed line in Fig. C indicates arrow placement. (Adapted from Tabar and Dean,[18] with permission.) *(Figure continues.)*

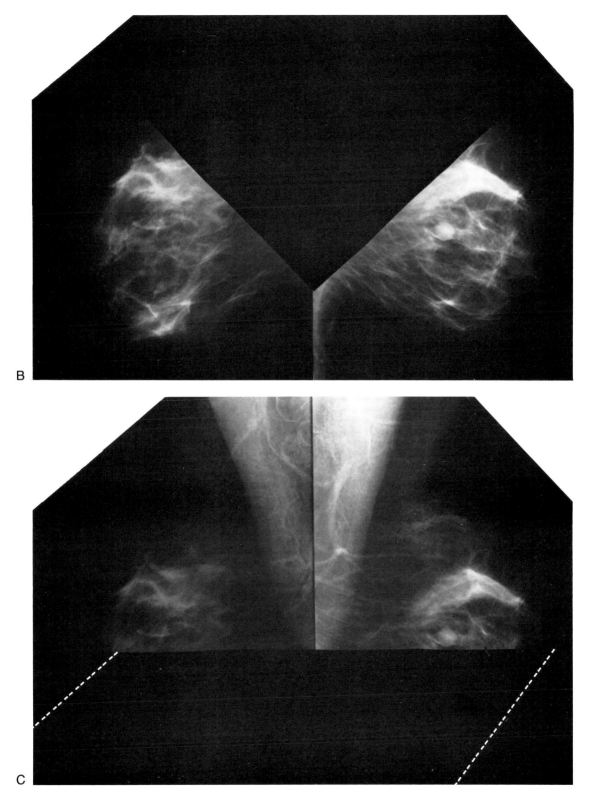

Fig. 7-3 *(Continued)*.

superolateral quadrant is the last to involute. There is, however, a wide variation of denseness of the fibroglandular tissue irrespective of age, past history of pregnancy and lactation, and body habitus (Figs. 7-4 to 7-14).

Wolfe[20-22] has classified breast parenchymal patterns into four categories, depending upon the degree of fatty replacement. He believes that the more epithelial and connective tissue within the breast, the greater the risk of developing cancer, particularly after the age of 35 years. Although his work has been corroborated by some, other studies dispute it. Because of the disagreement, the utility of this classification is not universally accepted. The following is an outline of Wolfe's breast parenchymal classification.

N1: The breast is primarily fatty replaced, and it may have a trabeculated appearance

P1: One-fourth or less of the breast is involved with prominent ducts

P2: More than one-fourth of the breast is involved with prominent ducts

DY: Severe "mammary dysplasia" is present

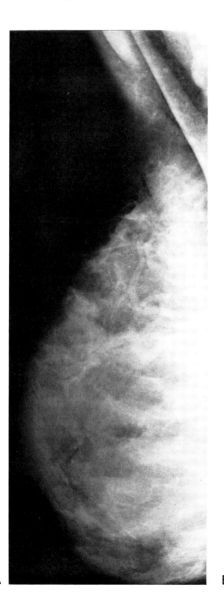
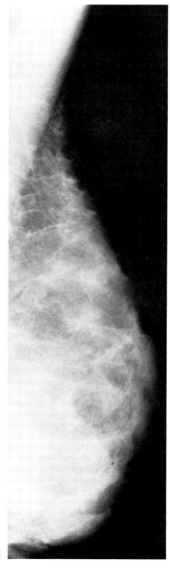

A   B

Fig. 7-4. (A & B) Normal left and right mediolateral oblique views in a parous 36-year-old woman who breast fed. The fibroglandular tissues are dense. The left breast is larger than the right. Discrepancy in size is most often a variant of normal, but occasionally an underlying pathologic process is the cause. Note the prominent axillary extension (tail of Spence) of the breast parenchyma.

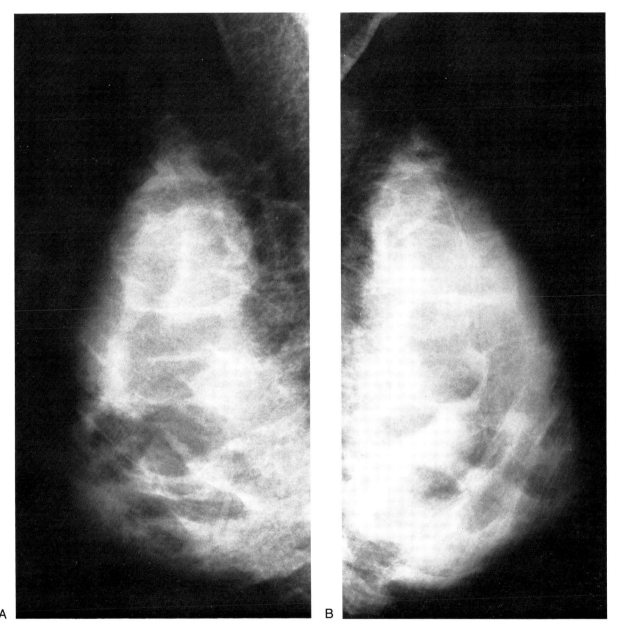

A B

Fig. 7-5. (A & B) Normal left and right mediolateral oblique views in a nulliparous 21-year-old woman. The study demonstrates a marbled appearance of the parenchyma secondary to fatty replacement.

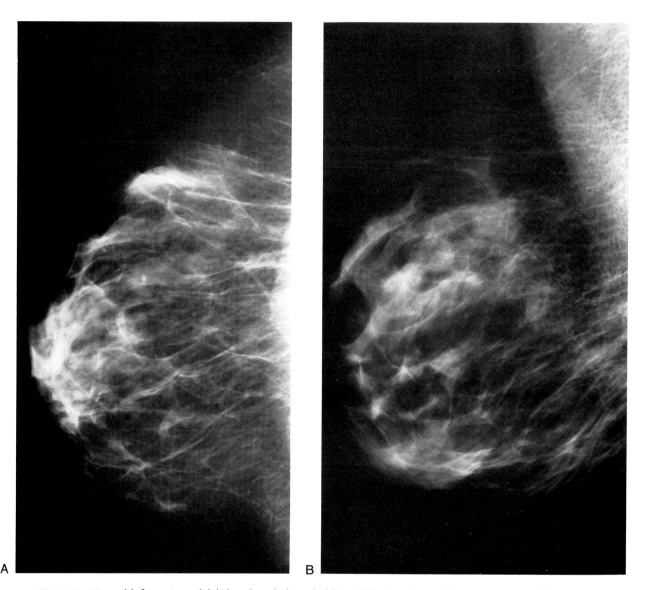

A   B

Fig. 7-6. Normal left craniocaudal **(A)** and mediolateral oblique **(B)** views in a nulliparous 35-year-old woman. The majority of the residual fibroglandular tissue is in the superolateral quadrant, as is usually seen in the partially fatty replaced breast.

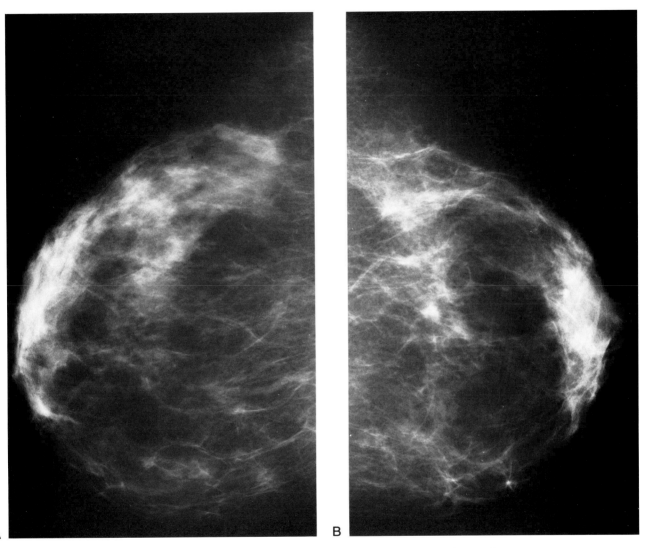

Fig. 7-7. Normal left and right craniocaudal **(A & B)** and mediolateral oblique **(C & D)** views in a parous 41-year-old woman who breast fed. The study demonstrates asymmetry of the residual fibroglandular tissues in the superolateral quadrants. Asymmetry of the fibroglandular tissues in most cases is a variant of normal. However, carcinomas can produce fibrotic reactions, causing the fibroglandular tissues to appear asymmetric. If the mammographic findings are inconclusive and no palpable masses are present to warrant prompt biopsy, a 3- to 4-month follow-up study can be obtained. (Note that asymmetry of the fibroglandular tissues is *not* the same as an asymmetrical mass density.) *(Figure continues.)*

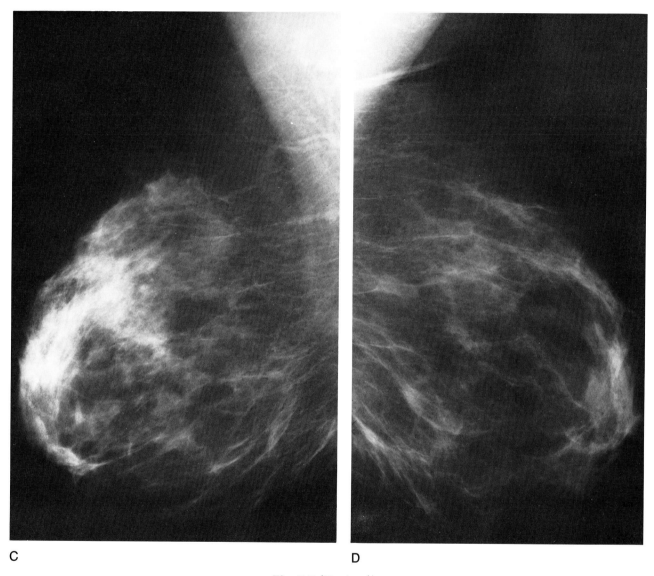

C

D

Fig. 7-7 *(Continued)*.

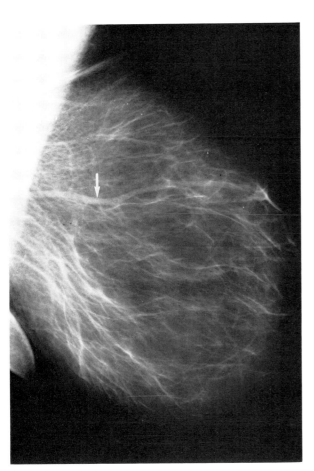

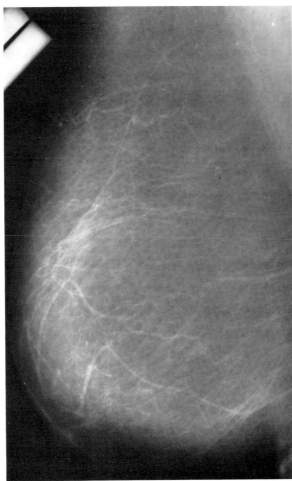

Fig. 7-8. Normal mediolateral oblique view in a parous 40-year-old woman who did not breast feed. The parenchyma is almost totally fat replaced, with only fibrous trabeculae remaining. The arrow points to a normal vein.

Fig. 7-9. Normal mediolateral oblique view in a parous 57-year-old woman who did not breast feed. The parenchyma is fat replaced. Several normal veins are seen.

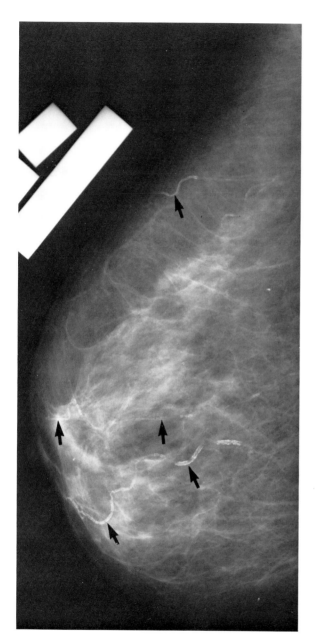

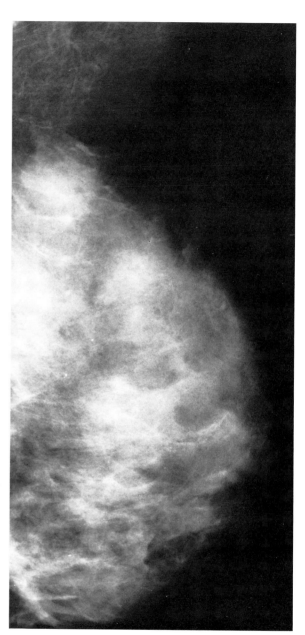

Fig. 7-10. Normal craniocaudal view in a parous 80-year-old woman who breast fed. The study demonstrates residual fibroglandular tissues in the superolateral quadrant. Arterial calcification *(arrows)* is present.

Fig. 7-11. Normal mediolateral oblique view in a parous 45-year-old woman who had been breast feeding for 7 years. The parenchyma is dense, as is seen during lactation.

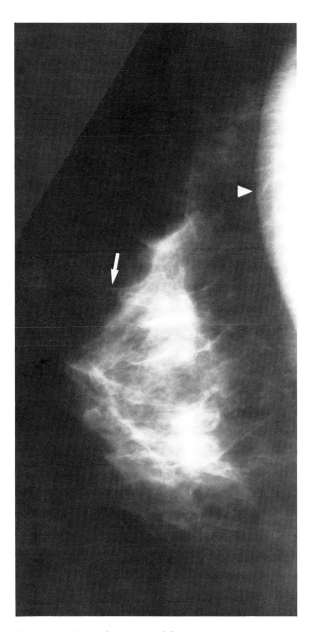

Fig. 7-12. Normal craniocaudal view in a parous 45-year-old woman who did not breast feed. The study demonstrates normal Cooper's ligaments *(arrow)*. The pectoralis muscle *(arrowhead)* can be visualized.

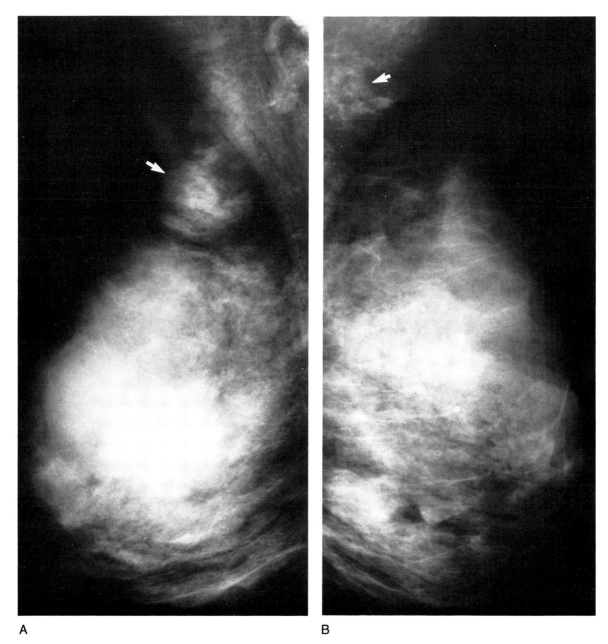

A   B

Fig. 7-13. (A & B) Normal left and right mediolateral oblique views in a parous 47-year-old woman who breast fed. Normal accessory fibroglandular tissue is present in the axillae. Note that the accessory tissue is separate from the main parenchymal mass. This normal variant can be seen bilaterally, in which case it may be symmetric or asymmetric (as in this case), or it may be present unilaterally.

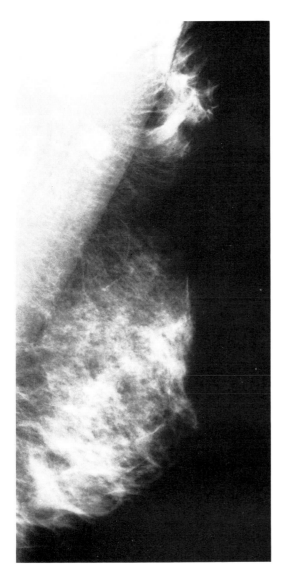

Fig. 7-14. Normal mediolateral oblique view in a parous 47-year-old woman who breast fed. Normal accessory fibroglandular tissue is present in the axilla.

SUGGESTED READINGS

1. Adler DD, Rebner M, Pennes DR: Accessory breast tissue in the axilla: mammographic appearance. Radiology 163:709, 1987
2. Andersson I, Janzon L, Petterson H: Radiographic patterns of the mammary parenchyma. Radiology 136:59, 1981
3. Chaudary MA, Gravelle IH, Bulstrode JC et al: Breast parenchymal patterns in women with bilateral primary breast cancer. Br J Radiol 56:703, 1983
4. Dewhurst J: Breast disorders in children and adolescents. Pediatr Clin North Am 28:287, 1981
5. Eagan RL: Breast Imaging: Diagnosis and Morphology of Breast Diseases. WB Saunders, Philadelphia, 1988
6. Ernster VL, Sacks ST, Peterson CA, Schweitzer RJ: Mammographic parenchymal patterns and risk factors for breast cancer. Radiology 134:617, 1980
7. Feig SA: The importance of supplementary mammographic views to diagnostic accuracy. AJR 151:40, 1988
8. Gravelle IH, Bulstrode JC, Bulbrook RD: The relation between radiological patterns of the breast and body weight and height. Br J Radiol 55:23, 1982
9. Grove JS, Goodman MJ, Gilbert FI, Mi MP: Factors associated with mammographic pattern. Br J Radiol 58:21, 1985
10. Hainline S, Myers L, McLelland R et al: Mammographic patterns and risk of breast cancer. AJR 130:1157, 1978
11. Leinster SJ, Whitehouse GH: The mammographic breast pattern and oral contraception. Br J Radiol 59:237, 1986
12. Martin JE: Atlas of Mammography: Histologic and Mammographic Correlations. Williams & Wilkins, Baltimore, 1982
13. Moskowitz M, Gartside P, McLaughlin C, Programmer S: Mammographic patterns as markers for high-risk benign breast disease and incident cancers. Radiology 134:293, 1980
14. Sickles EA: Microfocal magnification mammography using xeroradiographic and screen-film recording systems. Radiology 131:599, 1979
15. Sickles EA: Further experience with microfocal spot magnification mammography in the assessment of clustered breast microcalcifications. Radiology 137:9, 1980
16. Sickles EA: Practical solutions to common mammographic problems: tailoring the examination. AJR 151:31, 1988
17. Tabar L, Dean PB: Mammographic parenchymal patterns: risk indicator for breast cancer. JAMA 247:185, 1982
18. Tabar L, Dean PB: Teaching Atlas of Mammography. Thieme-Stratton, New York, 1983
19. Whitehouse GH, Leinster SJ: The variation of breast parenchymal patterns with age. Br J Radiol 58:315, 1985
20. Wolfe JN: Xeroradiography of the Breast. 2nd Ed. Charles C Thomas, Springfield, IL, 1983
21. Wolfe JN, Albert S, Belle S, Salane M: Breast parenchymal patterns: analysis of 332 incident breast carcinomas. AJR 138:113, 1982
22. Wolfe JN, Albert S, Belle S, Salane M: Breast parenchymal patterns and their relationship to risk for having or developing carcinoma. Radiol Clin North Am 21:127, 1983

8
Skin

Mary Ellen Peters

Evaluation of the mammogram should always include careful inspection of the skin, since abnormalities can direct attention to an underlying malignancy. Conversely, unrecognized skin masses and calcifications can lead to the mistaken diagnosis of breast carcinoma.

Willson et al.[17] report that with a 0.6 focal spot the range of normal skin thickness is between 0.8 and 3 mm, with skin medially and inferiorly thicker than laterally and superiorly. This range is slightly greater than in the Pope et al.[11] series. They conclude that skin thickness greater than 2.5 mm using a microfocus focal spot should be suspect as being abnormal. The skin often appears denser and thicker in the smaller breast, compared with the larger breast. Often small, round, or ovoid lucencies in close approximation are seen over the entire breast or localized to a small area. They represent normal skin pores (sebaceous glands) (Fig. 8-1).

A large number of pathologic conditions can produce skin thickening. Bilateral generalized skin thickening can result from anasarca, obstruction of mediastinal lymphatics, central venous obstruction, and extensive pleural disease. The thickening associated with anasarca sometimes involves one breast more than the other because of patient positioning (Fig. 8-2). Unilateral generalized thickening can be caused by inflammatory breast carcinoma, lymphoma, leukemia, metastatic extramammary carcinoma, acute mastitis, radiation therapy, cellulitis, unilateral venous obstruction, pleural disease, and obstruction of a lymphatic chain that drains the breast (Fig. 8-3). The contralateral

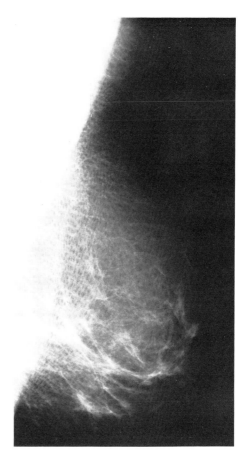

Fig. 8-1. Normal mediolateral oblique view in an asymptomatic 40-year-old woman. Numerous small radiolucencies, representing skin pores, can be seen over the entire breast. They are more pronounced posteriorly, as is seen in most cases.

93

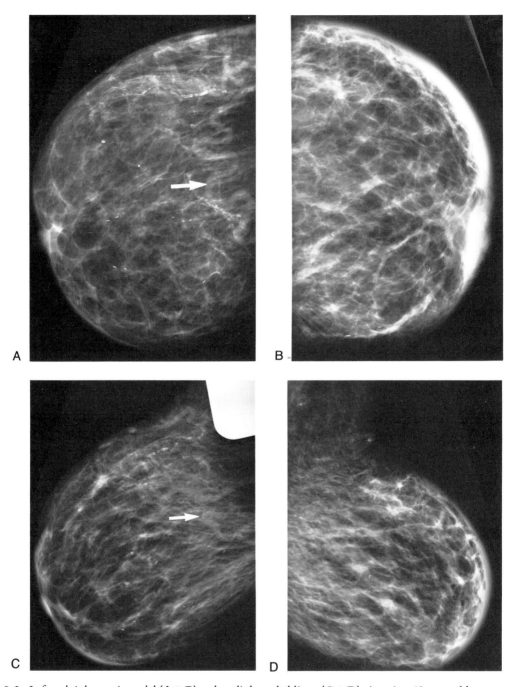

Fig. 8-2. Left and right craniocaudal **(A & B)** and mediolateral oblique **(C & D)** views in a 68-year-old woman with a history of congestive heart failure (CHF) and recent onset of right breast enlargement. Extensive skin thickening is present on the right and inferomedially on the left. Clinically, the enlargement of the right breast resolved with improvement of the CHF. The discrepancy of the skin edema was probably the result of dependent edema. On the left, the arrow points to a normal, tortuous vein.

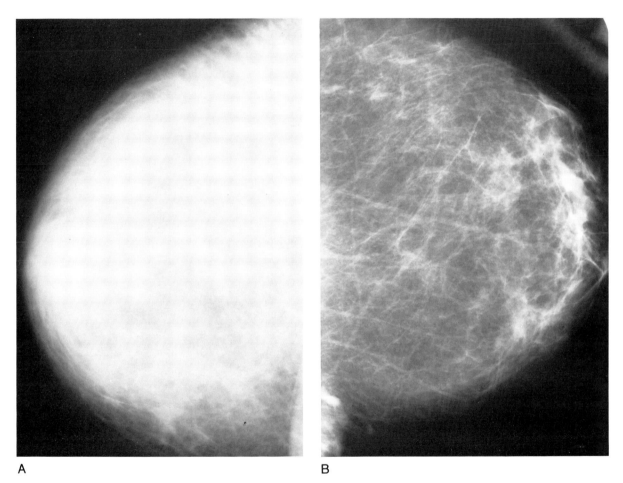

A   B

Fig. 8-3. (A & B) Left and right craniocaudal views in a 30-year-old woman with a painful erythematous left breast of acute onset. The study demonstrates an overall increased density of the left breast associated with skin thickening. Clinically, the patient had cellulitis. The right breast is normal.

spread of breast carcinoma also causes unilateral thickening, but the effects are usually more pronounced medially.

Etiologies for localized skin thickening include carcinoma, abscess, plasma cell mastitis, trauma, fat necrosis, dermatitis, and metastatic extramammary carcinoma. Postbiopsy skin thickening is usually localized, but in the immediate postoperative period the thickening can involve a major portion of the breast. Commonly, the postsurgical thickening never completely resolves. Mondor's disease, a thrombophlebitis of superficial veins, can be associated with generalized or localized skin thickening. Paget's disease can cause thickening of the nipple, but usually this is not evident on the mammogram.

Retraction of the skin can occur as the result of carcinoma, fat necrosis, postinflammatory change, and postsurgical change. Often the retraction is accompanied by skin thickening.

Nipple retraction is most often a variant of normal. It can be seen in the older woman as the result of fibrosis, in which case it is almost always bilateral and of a mild degree (Fig. 8-4). Unilateral or bilateral retraction can be of developmental origin. Inflammatory processes and surgical intervention can also be the cause of nipple retraction. If retraction is of recent onset and the patient gives no relevant past history, careful search must be made for a carcinoma as the underlying etiology.

Superficial skin and intradermal lesions can simulate breast masses, and it is important to recognize them as such to prevent an unnecessary attempt at needle localization. In addition, the nipple should be profiled in at least one view, preferably both, so that it is not mistaken for a breast mass or does not obscure a retroareolar carcinoma.

Skin lesions, such as moles and warts, viewed en face are often defined by a rim of radiolucency (Figs. 8-5 and 8-6). If there is question that a "mass" on the mammogram represents a known skin lesion, a repeat mammogram with a small lead marker placed on the lesion will clarify the problem. Warts seen en face commonly have a distinctive, variegated appearance — small linear lucencies intertwined with small radiopacities (Fig. 8-7). Accessory nipples are uncommon, but can also simulate

breast masses when viewed en face. Because of their sloping margins, they are often not as well defined as other skin lesions. Viewed tangentially, they present no problem in differential diagnosis.

Sebaceous cysts (epidermoid inclusion cysts) are most often located in the periareolar region or in a lower quadrant. Some grow quite large and can appear very dense. Viewed en face they are often well defined but are not as distinctly outlined as lesions on the skin (Fig. 8-8). When viewed tangentially, they produce a localized area of skin thickening. If infected, their margins can become indistinct (Fig. 8-9).

Metastatic lesions can occur intradermally; the diagnosis is usually clinically evident, however. Dermatofibrosarcoma protuberance, an uncommon, slow-growing tumor of the dermis, can also involve the breast. This tumor can be locally aggressive, but rarely metastatizes. On histopathologic examination, it has the appearance of a low-grade fibrosarcoma. The mammographic appearances of metastatic lesions and dermatofibrosarcoma protuberances are similar to the sebaceous cyst (Figs. 8-10 and 8-11).

Skin calcifications are common. The calcifications associated with sebaceous glands are round, oval, or dumbbell-shaped in configuration when viewed en face and measure approximately 1 to 1.5 mm. A central lucency can often be identified within them. In tangent, they appear discoid. They can be solitary, grouped, or scattered over the breast (Figs. 8-12 to 8-14). Those that appear tightly grouped can mimic the appearance seen in adenosis, which is described in Chapter 10. Occasionally the calcifications are punctate or linear with no central lucency, simulating those seen in malignancy. If their true nature is not recognized, unnecessary attempts at needle localization and biopsy may be performed. Tangential views may prove useful in localizing the calcifications within the skin. Calcifications can develop in the skin postsurgically and can be seen as early as 6 months after the procedure. They can be large and plaquelike or punctate in appearance.

Skin lesions, particularly warts, may be associated with calcifications. Tattoos, skin creams, and deodorants contain metallic salts that can mimic breast calcifications (Fig. 8-15). Large, benign-appearing calcifica-

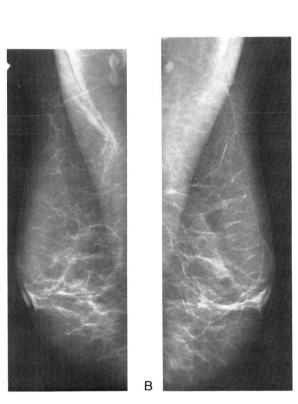

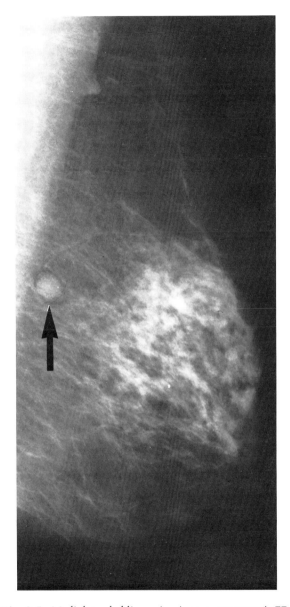

Fig. 8-4. (A & B) Left and right mediolateral oblique views in an asymptomatic 70-year-old woman. Both nipples are mildly retracted. The patient stated that the retraction had been present for a number of years. Diagnosis: normal mammogram.

Fig. 8-5. Mediolateral oblique view in an asymptomatic 77-year-old woman. There should be no question in this case that the mass *(arrow)* is on the skin, since a broad rim of radiolucency surrounds it. Intradermal and intraparenchymal masses are never associated with such a wide rim of lucency. A mole was present.

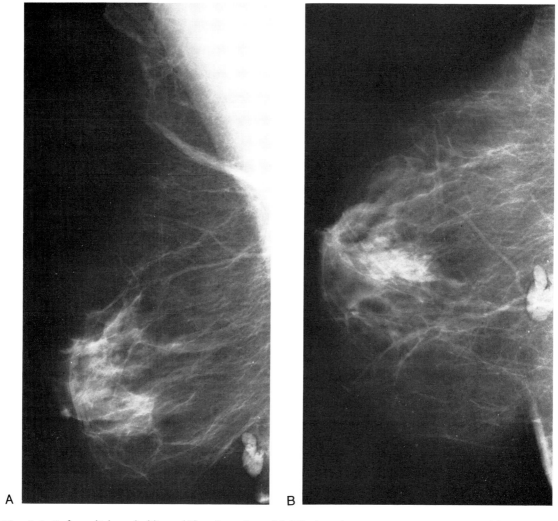

A   B

Fig. 8-6. Left mediolateral oblique **(A)** and craniocaudal **(B)** views in an asymptomatic 70-year-old woman. A lobulated mass, surrounded by a distinctive band of lucency, can be seen inferomedially. Diagnosis: skin lesion (mole).

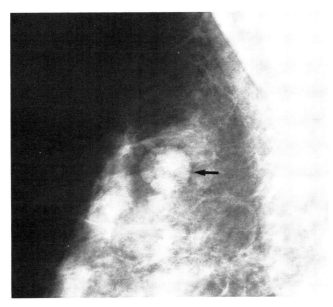

Fig. 8-7. Enlargement from a mediolateral oblique view in an asymptomatic 56-year-old woman, demonstrating the typical varigated appearance of a wart *(arrow)*.

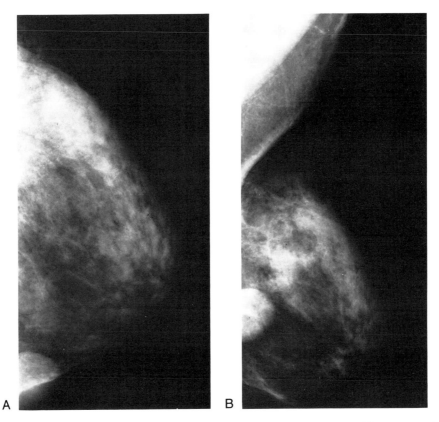

Fig. 8-8. Right craniocaudal **(A)** and mediolateral oblique **(B)** views in a 45-year-old woman with a palpable intradermal mass. A round, well-defined mass is seen inferomedially. If the clinical findings were not known, this could be mistaken for a parenchymal mass. Diagnosis: sebaceous cyst.

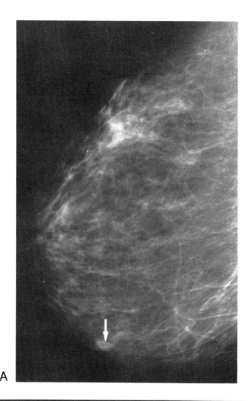

A

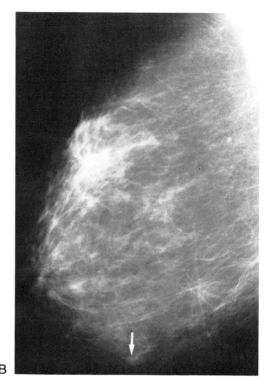

B

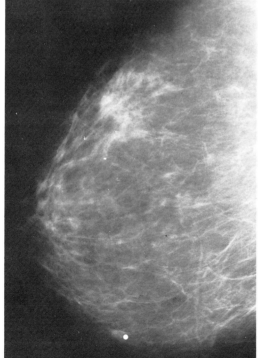

C

Fig. 8-9. Left craniocaudal **(A)** and mediolateral oblique **(B)** views in an asymptomatic 47-year-old woman. No clues are present on this study that the ill-defined density *(arrow)* is located in the skin. The technician noticed that an inflammatory intradermal lesion was present in the area. **(C)** A repeat left cranio-caudal view with a lead marker proved that the ill-defined density represented the intradermal lesion. Diagnosis: inflamed sebaceous cyst.

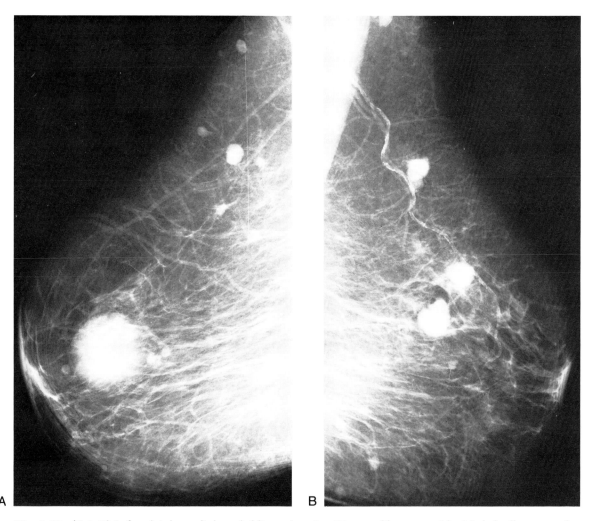

A

B

Fig. 8-10. (A & B) Left and right mediolateral oblique views in a 77-year-old woman with a Merkel cell tumor and multiple, bilateral, palpable, intradermal lesions. Multiple, well-defined, dense masses are present bilaterally. Unless they are viewed tangentially, it is impossible to distinguish them from intraparenchymal lesions. Histology: metastatic Merkel cell tumor.

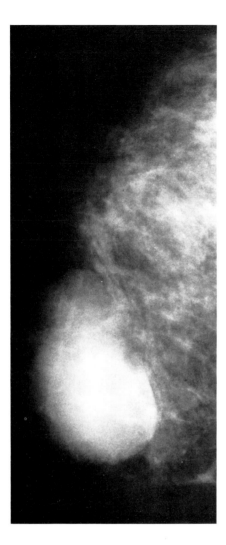

Fig. 8-11. Mediolateral view in a 57-year-old woman with a palpable intradermal mass. A large, well-defined density can be seen anteriorly. Histology: dermatofibrosarcoma protuberans.

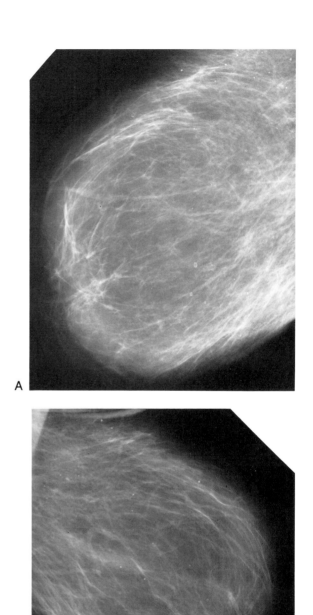

Fig. 8-12. (A & B) Left and right mediolateral oblique views in an asymptomatic 64-year-old woman. Numerous small, round-to-ovoid calcifications are scattered over both breasts. A central lucency can be identified within some of the calcifications. These are the typical calcifications that occur in sebaceous glands.

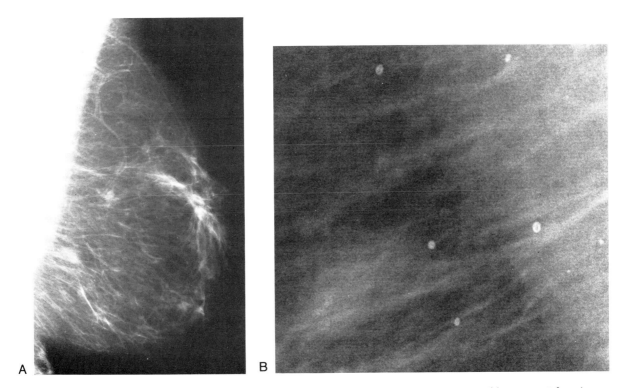

Fig. 8-13. (A) Mediolateral oblique view and an enlargement in an asymptomatic 53-year-old woman. Often the calcified sebaceous glands are more numerous posteriorly, as is evident in this case. **(B)** The enlargement shows the central lucencies well.

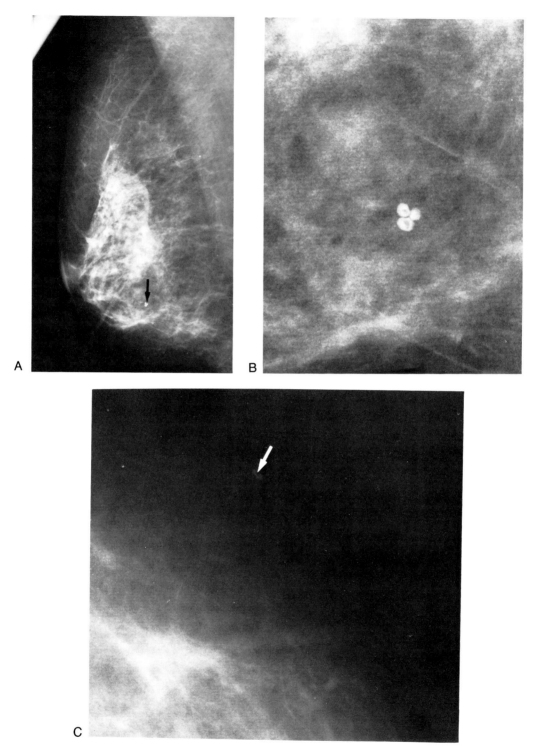

Fig. 8-14. (A) Mediolateral oblique view in a 55-year-old woman. A group of calcifications *(arrow)* is seen inferiorly. **(B)** An enlargement of the calcifications demonstrates a calcified rim with a central radiolucency. **(C)** The craniocaudal view demonstrates that they are located within the skin *(arrow)*.

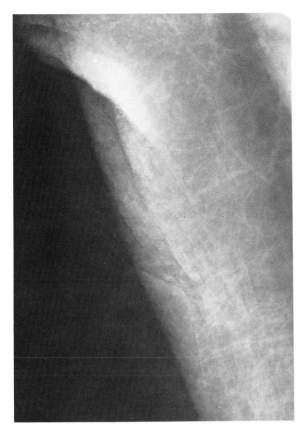

Fig. 8-15. Enlargement of the axilla from a mediolateral oblique view. Deodorant has produced numerous small radiopacities on the skin.

tions can be observed within the nipple secondary to the debris within the ducts calcifying. Calcifications can also be seen within the nipple secondary to Paget's disease, but these have a characteristic malignant appearance that will be discussed in Chapter 13.

SUGGESTED READINGS

1. Brown RC, Zuehlke RL, Ehrhardt JC, Jochimsen PR: Tattoos simulating calcifications on xeroradiographs of the breast. Radiology 138:583, 1981

2. Egan RL: Breast Imaging: Diagnosis and Morphology of Breast Diseases. WB Saunders, Philadelphia, 1988

3. Gold RH, Montgomery CK, Minagi H, Annes GP: The significance of mammary skin thickening in disorders other than primary carcinoma: a roentgenologic-pathologic correlation. AJR 112:613, 1971

4. Homer MJ: Mammary skin thickening. Contemp Diagn Radiol 4:1, 1981

5. Kopans DB, Meyer JE, Homer MJ, Grabbe J: Dermal deposits mistaken for breast calcifications. Radiology 149:592, 1983

6. Kowand LM, Verhulst LA, Copeland CM, Birewsar B: Epidermal cyst of the breast. Can Med Assoc J 131:217, 1984

7. Kushner LN: Hodgkins disease simulating inflammatory breast carcinoma on mammography. Radiology 92:350, 1969

8. Lanyi M: Diagnosis and Differential Diagnosis of Breast Calcifications. Springer-Verlag, New York, 1986

9. Martin JE: Atlas of Mammography: Histologic and Mammographic Correlations. Williams & Wilkins, Baltimore, 1982

10. Paulus DD: Benign diseases of the breast. Radiol Clin North Am 21:27, 1983

11. Pope TL, Read ME, Medsker T et al: Breast skin thickness: normal range and causes of thickening shown on film-screen mammography. J Can Assoc Radiol 35:365, 1984

12. Sadowsky N, Kopans DB: Breast cancer. Radiol Clin North Am 21:51, 1983

13. Shukla HS, Gravelle IH, Hughes LE et al: Mammary skin oedema: a new prognostic indicator for breast cancer. Br Med J 288:1338, 1984

14. Shukla HS, Hughes LE, Gravelle IH, Satir A: The significance of mammary skin edema in noninflammatory breast cancer. Ann Surg 189:53, 1979

15. Sickles EA: Breast calcifications: mammographic evaluation. Radiology 160:289, 1986

16. Tabar L, Dean PB: Teaching Atlas of Mammography. Thieme-Stratton, New York, 1983

17. Willson SA, Adam EJ, Tucker AK: Patterns of breast skin thickness in normal mammograms. Clin Radiol 33:691, 1982

18. Wolfe JN: Xeroradiography of the Breast. 2nd Ed. Charles C Thomas, Springfield, 1983

9
Lymph Nodes

Mary Ellen Peters

Lymph nodes are commonly seen on mammograms. Axillary nodes are the most frequently visualized, but intramammary and lateral thoracic lymph nodes are also commonly seen. Characteristically, lymph nodes appear as round, ovoid, or bean-shaped well-defined densities. They often contain a central or umbilicated lucency secondary to fat in the hilum.

Normal axillary nodes usually measure 1 to 1.5 cm, but those with a large fatty hilus often measure up to 3 to 4 cm (Figs. 9-1 to 9-5). Fatty replacement of nodes occurs with obesity and increasing age. In the younger patient, multiple, nonmatted, solid nodes measuring up to 2 cm can be seen and are normal. Frequently axillary nodes are not symmetrical in size and number.

Axillary nodes that are replaced by metastatic disease lose their radiolucent hilum and are dense (Fig. 9-6). They do not necessarily appear enlarged. Usually metastatic nodes are well defined, and it is only in advanced disease that the margins become ill defined (Fig. 9-7). Occasionally, they are matted together. In metastatic breast carcinoma, microcalcifications may be observed within the nodes (Fig. 9-8). This is in contrast to the large, coarse calcifications seen in inflammatory diseases such as histoplasmosis. Some institutions employ ipsilateral axillary views for mastectomy patients to assist in detection of metastatic adenopathy (Figs. 9-9 and 9-10).

Other etiologies that should be considered in the presence of abnormal-appearing axillary nodes are leukemia, lymphoma, rheumatoid arthritis, sarcoidosis, dermatitis, and infectious disease processes (Figs. 9-11 to 9-13). Microcalcifications within axillary nodes have been described in patients with rheumatoid arthritis who are on parenteral gold therapy.

Intramammary lymph nodes are almost always located in the superolateral quadrant (Figs. 9-14 to 9-17). They are often bilateral and may be multiple. An intramammary lymph node that does not have a definable radiolucent hilum and measures 1 cm or greater should be considered abnormal. If there is no known cause for the enlargement (such as dermatitis and mastitis), the node should be biopsied to rule out the presence of an occult breast carcinoma (Figs. 9-18 and 9-19).

Lateral thoracic lymph nodes can be visualized lying far posteriorly on the mediolateral oblique view. They can also be visualized on a craniocaudal view that has been positioned with the shoulder dropped, but not on a straight craniocaudal view (Fig. 9-20). Unlike intramammary lymph nodes, lateral thoracic nodes are often unilateral and solitary. Commonly, the fatty hilum is not identifiable within them. A normal lateral thoracic lymph node can measure up to 1 cm (Fig. 9-21).

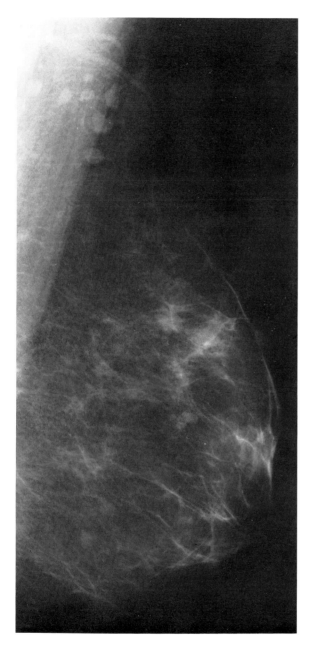

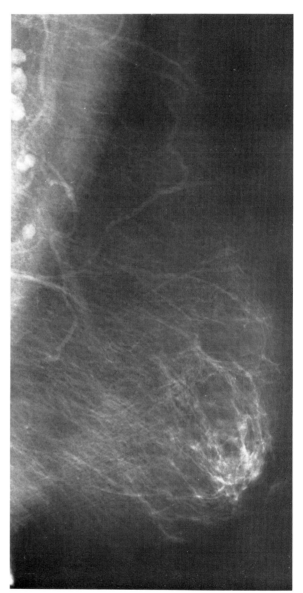

Fig. 9-1. Mediolateral oblique view in an asymptomatic 53-year-old woman. Multiple axillary nodes measuring up to 1.5 cm can be seen. Some of the nodes are of homogeneous density, and others contain fat in the hilum. The nodes are normal.

Fig. 9-2. Mediolateral oblique view in an asymptomatic 78-year-old woman. The study demonstrates normal axillary nodes.

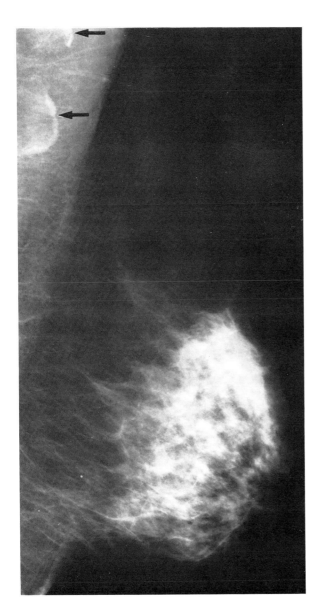

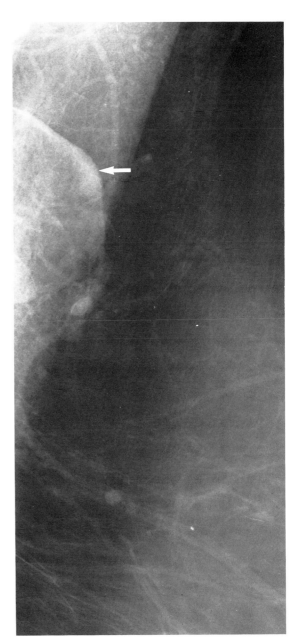

Fig. 9-3. Mediolateral oblique view in an asymptomatic 55-year-old woman. The curvilinear densities *(arrows)* in the axilla represent normal nodes that are largely fatty replaced.

Fig. 9-4. Enlargement of the axilla from a mediolateral oblique view in an asymptomatic 70-year-old woman. Multiple small, round nodes are present in addition to a large fatty replaced node *(arrow)*. The nodes are normal.

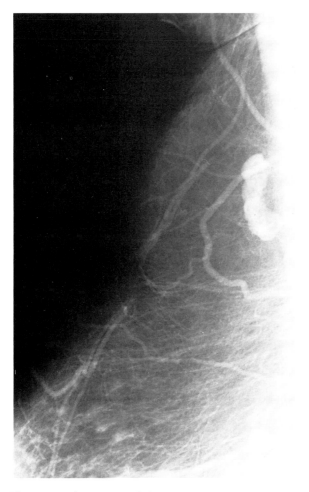

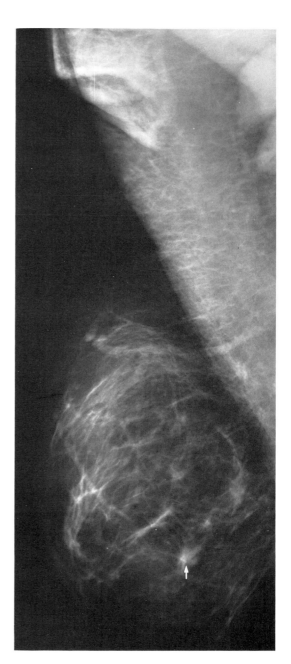

Fig. 9-5. Enlargement of the axilla from a mediolateral oblique view in an asymptomatic 65-year-old woman. The study demonstrates a large, fatty replaced node with a shell-like appearance.

Fig. 9-6. Mediolateral oblique view in a 63-year-old woman with a palpable breast mass. The axillary nodes are large and dense secondary to metastases from an infiltrating ductal carcinoma *(arrow)*.

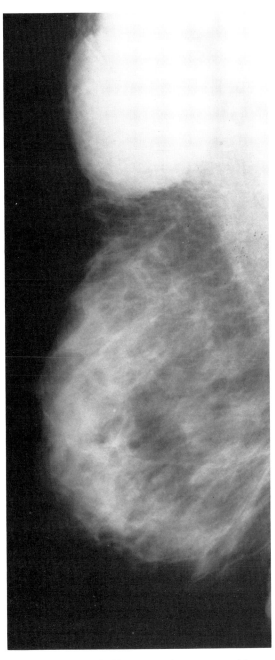

Fig. 9-7. Mediolateral oblique view in a 57-year-old woman with a history of a contralateral breast carcinoma. Huge, dense nodes involved with metastatic disease can be seen in the axilla. Portions of the lower node are ill defined.

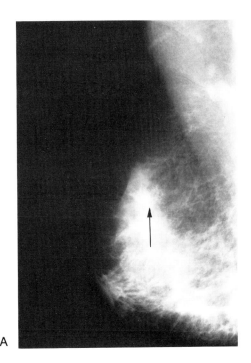

A

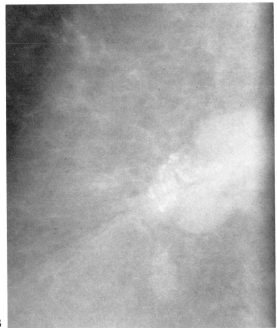

B

Fig. 9-8. (**A**) Mediolateral oblique view and (**B**) enlargement of the axilla in a 47-year-old woman with a palpable mass in the superolateral quadrant. The study demonstrates that three of the axillary nodes are dense and matted together. Small, irregular calcifications can be identified in one of the nodes. These findings indicate the presence of metastatic disease. The primary carcinoma is manifested by a spiculated mass that contains microcalcifications *(arrow)*.

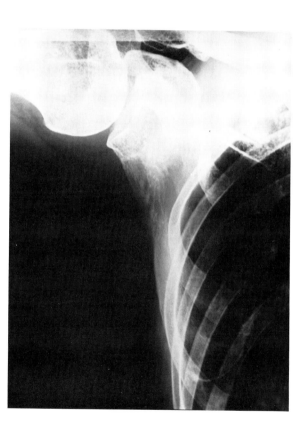

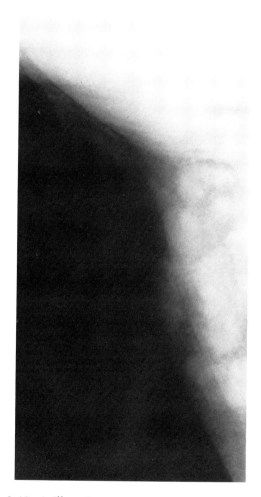

Fig. 9-9. Axillary view postmastectomy. This is a normal study with no evidence of adenopathy.

Fig. 9-10. Axillary view postmastectomy. Numerous, dense nodes are present, indicating metastatic disease.

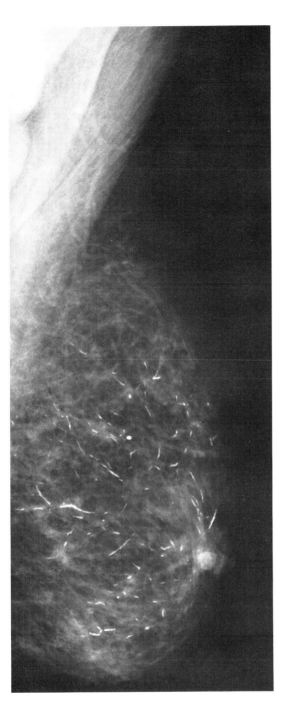

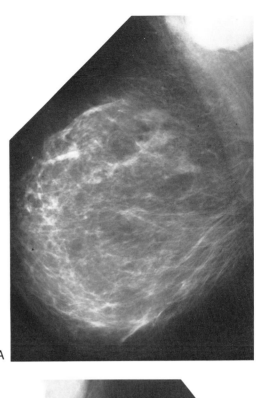

A

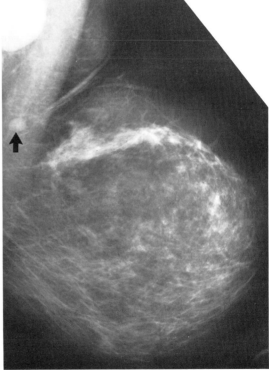

B

Fig. 9-11. Right mediolateral oblique view in a 73-year-old woman with leukemia and a negative breast examination. The axillary nodes are large and dense, secondary to the leukemia. Similar findings were present on the left. Diffuse secretory calcifications are present.

Fig. 9-12. (A & B) Left and right mediolateral oblique views in a 56-year-old woman with lymphoma and a normal breast examination. The axillary nodes are increased in size and density as the result of involvement with lymphoma. Radiographically, the lower axillary node *(arrow)* on the right does not appear to be involved because it is not dense.

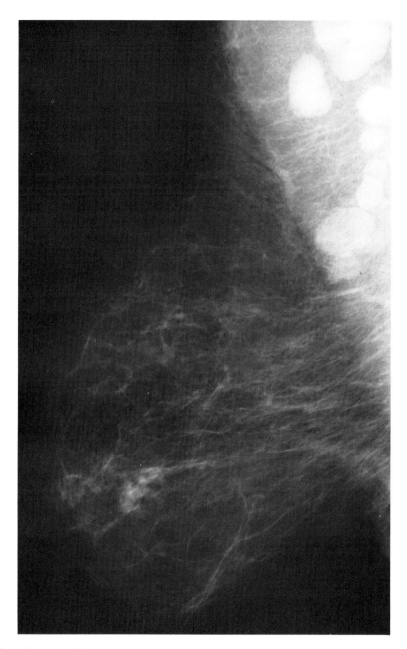

Fig. 9-13. Left mediolateral oblique view in a 70-year-old woman with a history of lymphoma and a normal breast examination. The nodes are extremely dense, indicating involvement with lymphoma. Note that not all of the nodes appear enlarged. Similar findings were present on the right.

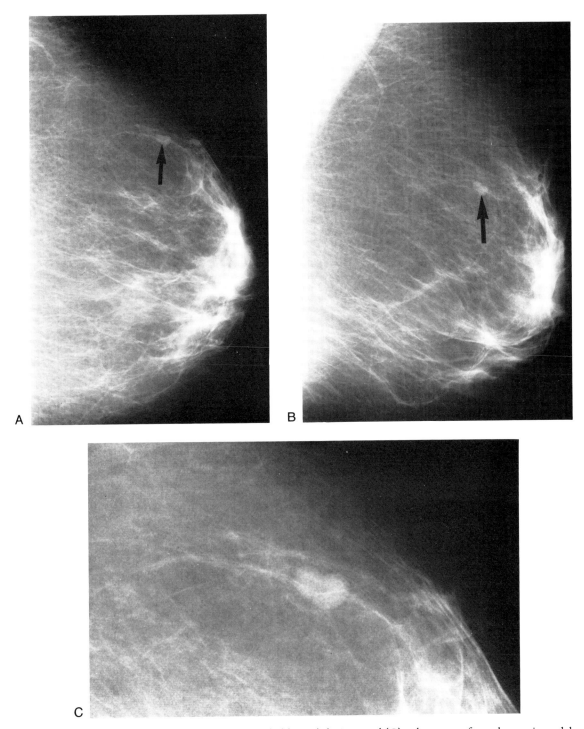

Fig. 9-14. Right craniocaudal **(A)** and mediolateral oblique **(B)** views and **(C)** enlargement from the craniocaudal view in a 45-year-old woman. A well-defined bean-shaped density, which is characteristic of an intramammary node, is present in the superolateral quadrant *(arrow)*.

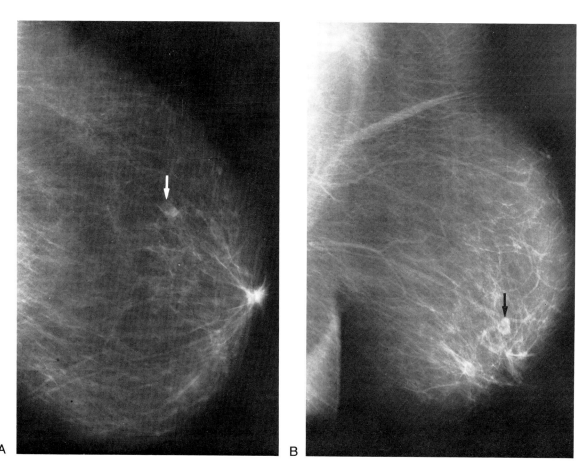

Fig. 9-15. Right craniocaudal **(A)** and mediolateral oblique **(B)** views in an 80-year-old woman. A small, well-defined "mass" *(arrow)* containing an eccentric area of lucency is seen in the superolateral quadrant. The findings are pathognomic of an intramammary node.

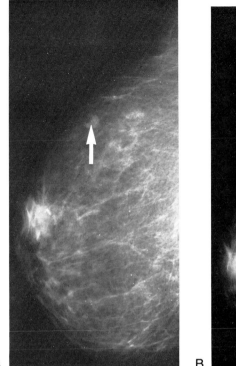

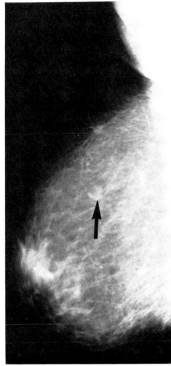

A   B

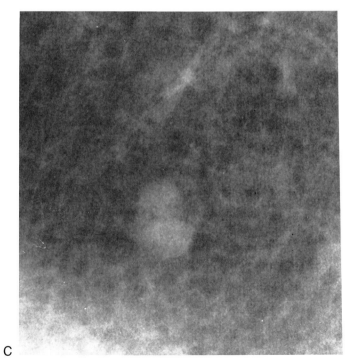

C

Fig. 9-16. Left craniocaudal **(A)** and mediolateral oblique **(B)** views and **(C)** enlargement from the mediolateral oblique view in a 78-year-old woman. A small, well-defined density *(arrow)* with an umbilicated lucency is located in the superolateral quadrant. These findings are typical of an intramammary node.

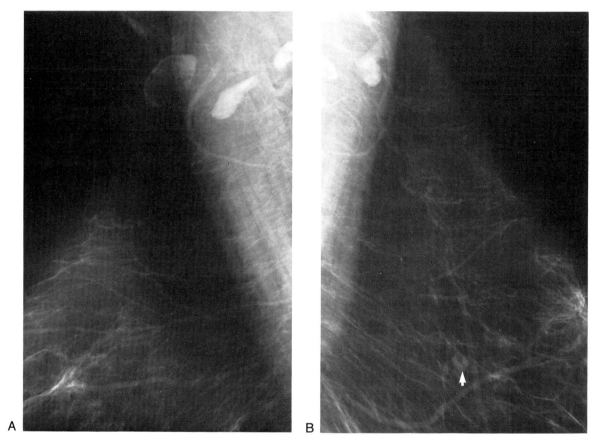

A   B

Fig. 9-17. (A & B) Enlargements from left and right mediolateral oblique views in a 42-year-old woman. The study demonstrates an intramammary node *(arrow)* with a fatty hilum on the right and bilateral axillary nodes of varying degrees of fatty replacement. All of the nodes are normal.

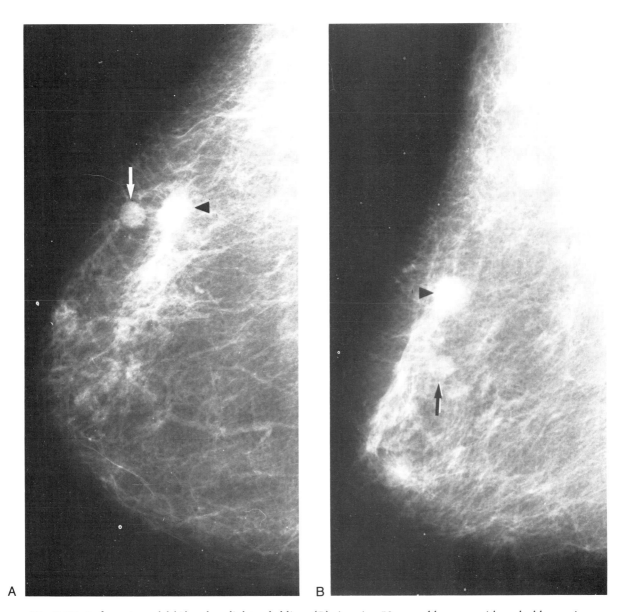

A

B

Fig. 9-18. Left craniocaudal **(A)** and mediolateral oblique **(B)** views in a 58-year-old woman with a palpable mass in the superolateral quadrant. A round, well-defined, homogeneous density *(white arrow)* measuring 12 mm in diameter is located in the superolateral quadrant, representing an intramammary node involved with metastases from an infiltrating ductal carcinoma *(black arrowhead)*. Also observe the dense lower axillary nodes, which are also involved with metastases.

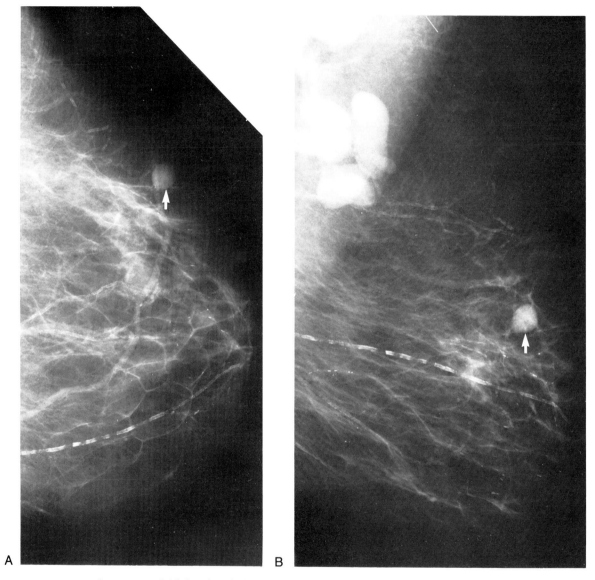

A

B

Fig. 9-19. Right craniocaudal **(A)** and mediolateral oblique **(B)** views in a 53-year-old woman with sarcoidosis and a negative breast examination. The intramammary *(arrow)* and axillary nodes are large and dense secondary to involvement with sarcoidosis. Axillary adenopathy was also present on the contralateral side.

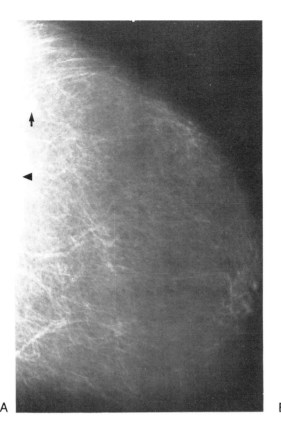

A

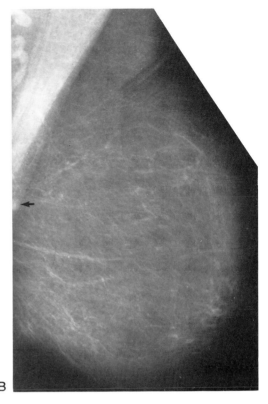

B

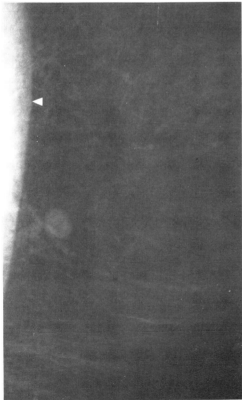

C

Fig. 9-20. Right craniocaudal **(A)** and mediolateral oblique **(B)** views and **(C)** enlargement from the craniocaudal view in an asymptomatic 65-year-old woman. A normal lateral thoracic node *(arrow)* can be seen lying far posteriorly. The coned view demonstrates fat within the hilum. The arrowhead on the craniocaudal view points to the pectoralis muscle.

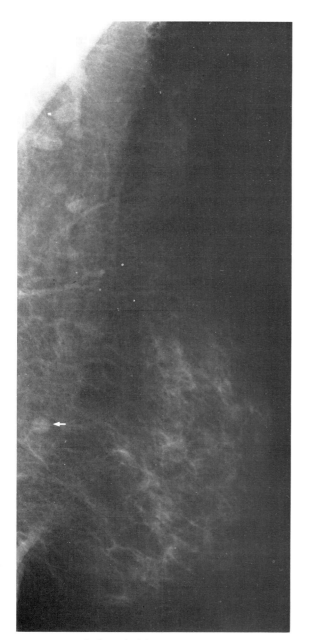

Fig. 9-21. Mediolateral oblique view in an asymptomatic 60-year-old woman. The study demonstrates a normal lateral thoracic node (*arrow*) as well as several normal axillary nodes.

SUGGESTED READINGS

1. Andersson I, Nilsson MB, Sjoblom K-G, Wollheim FA: Abnormal axillary lymph nodes in rheumatoid arthritis. Acta Radiol 21:645, 1980
2. Bjurstam N: The radiiographic appearance of normal and metastatic axillary lymph nodes. Recent Results Cancer Res 90:49, 1984
3. Bruwer A, Nelson GW, Spark RP: Punctate intranodal gold deposits simulating microcalcifications on mammograms. Radiology 163:87, 1987
4. Eagan RL, McSweeney MB: Intramammary lymph node. Cancer 51:1838, 1983
5. Heuser LS, Spratt JS, Kuhs JG et al: The association of pathologic and mammographic characteristics of primary human breast cancers with "slow" and "fast" growth rates and with axillary lymph node metastases. Cancer 53:96, 1984
6. Homer MJ: Imaging features and management of characteristically benign and probably benign breast lesions. Radiol Clin North Am 25:939, 1987
7. Kopans DB, Meyer JE, Murphy GF: Benign lymph nodes associated with dermatitis presenting as breast masses. Radiology 137:15, 1980
8. Leborgne R, Leborgne F, Leborgne JH: Soft tissue radiography of the axilla in cancer of the breast. Br J Radiol 36:494, 1963
9. Lindfors KK, Kopans DB, McCarthy KA et al: Breast cancer metastasis to intramammary lymph nodes. AJR 146:133, 1986
10. Martin JE: Atlas of Mammography: Histologic and Mammographic Correlations. Williams & Wilkins, Baltimore, 1982
11. McSweeney MB, Eagan RL: Prognosis of breast cancer related to intramammary nodes. Recent Results Cancer Res 90:166, 1984
12. Meyer JE, Kopans DB, Lawrence WD: Normal intramammary lymph nodes presenting as occult breast masses. Breast 40:30, 1982
13. Raytner Z, Williams J, Gazet J-C: The significance of lymph nodes detected by xeroradiography in cancer of the breast. Clin Oncol 7:39, 1981
14. Tabar L, Dean PB: Teaching Atlas of Mammography. Thieme-Stratton, New York, 1983
15. Wolfe JN: Xeroradiography of the Breast. 2nd Ed. Charles C Thomas, Springfield, IL, 1983

10
Fibrocystic Changes

Kathleen A. Scanlan

Fibrocystic change is a difficult label to analyze; it has been loosely used to identify a multitude of diverse entities, ranging from a spectrum of clinical symptoms to certain mammographic imaging characteristics. When asked to discuss fibrocystic change, which facets should be addressed? There are several relevant questions.

1. What does the term fibrocystic change indicate?
2. What is the symptomatology of fibrocystic change and how is it treated?
3. What comprises the histologic and clinical diagnosis of fibrocystic change?
4. How does the presence of fibrocystic change interfere with the clinical and radiographic diagnosis of breast cancer?
5. What does this diagnosis imply to the patient and her physician in reference to breast cancer risk?

To most people the term fibrocystic change indicates symptomatic breast alterations that include both the formation of cysts and the development of fibrotic tissue. These two components are only a small portion of the list of histologic breast alterations included under the title fibrocystic change. The term *disease* is probably not deserved in the majority of cases. This terminology is inadequate because the ubiquitous label *fibrocystic disease* has been used to include such an imposing variety of histologic and physiologic changes that it has ultimately become useless. If the term itself were not difficult enough, a long list of synonyms has been generated over the years. These include Schimmelbusch's dis-

ease, mazoplasia, cystic mastopathy, chronic mastitis, chronic cystic mastitis, cystic hyperplasia, bluedome cyst, and multiple permutations of these descriptors. All of these terms have been used to describe both the clinical symptoms of lumpy, swollen, painful breasts, often of a cyclic nature, as well as a mélange of benign histologic changes primarily of epithelial origin.

The term disease also overstates the case when one realizes that perhaps one-half of all women of reproductive age have palpably lumpy breasts, usually caused by an exaggerated response to normal physiology. In one series, 90 percent of women in the 30 to 50 age range demonstrated microscopic tissue findings that could be categorized as fibrocystic change. The physiologic alterations are not only troublesome to the patient because of the pain and tenderness that may interfere with a normal lifestyle, but also because of the palpable nodularity, which can cause clinical concern. The etiology of the changes seems related to a hormonal milieu as yet poorly understood or a heightened end-organ sensitivity present in some women. Whatever the etiology, the result is a variety of cellular alterations that may be accompanied by painful tissue edema and nodularity.

The treatment for these symptoms has been as murky as the definition of fibrocystic change itself and has covered the gamut of vitamin and hormonal therapy as well as dietary manipulation. Vitamin E therapy, abstinence from caffeine, and the antiestrogenic agent Danazol have all been used in an effort to treat fibrocystic symptoms. These therapies have resulted in variable degrees of success depending on the reported series.

The histologic alterations loosely clustered under the heading of fibrocystic change usually involve excessive cellular proliferation in terminal ducts, lobules, and connective tissues, as well as the development of fibrosis. Within this spectrum are changes both symptomatic and asymptomatic, ranging from changes that incur no increased cancer risk to lesions that are clearly premalignant. On mammographic examination, some of the alterations, such as dense fibrosis, may be clearly visible as increased density, masking normal breast parenchyma. On the other hand, lesions of pure epithelial proliferation are not mammographically visible.

Those who perform mammography are indebted to Azzopardi[2] and Wellings[24-26] for a clearer understanding of breast ultrastructure. A full discussion of breast anatomy can be found in Chapter 1; however, a review of microanatomy is helpful prior to a discussion of fibrocystic change.

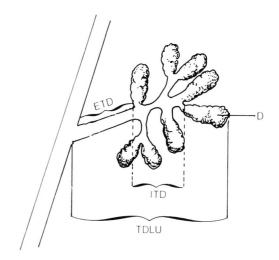

Fig. 10-2. Terminal ductal lobular unit (TDLU). *ETD*, extralobular terminal duct; *ITD*, intralobular terminal duct; *D*, ductule. The lobule consists of the intralobular terminal duct, ductules, and surrounding connective tissue. (Adapted from Wellings and Wolfe,[26] with permission.)

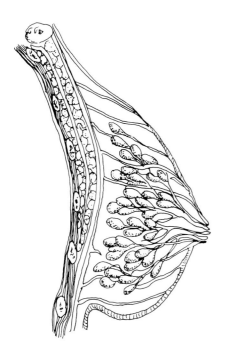

Fig. 10-1. Sagittal representation of the breast demonstrating multiple lobes, each with its own lactiferous duct. Expanded foci at the most proximal branch points of the ducts represent the terminal ductal lobular units.

The breast is composed of 15 to 18 lobar units, each draining via a lactiferous duct (Fig. 10-1). At the most terminal branch point of the ducts lies the terminal ductal lobular unit (TDLU) (Fig. 10-2). The TDLU concept is a useful bridge for discussion of both benign and malignant disease. This is the site of origin of most malignancies, as well as most of the histologic components of fibrocystic change. The TDLU is composed of an extralobular terminal duct and a lobule. The lobule consists of an intralobular terminal duct and multiple blunt ductules (termed *terminal acini* in some literature). The intralobular duct and blunt ductules are lined by cuboidal cells, while the extralobular duct is lined by columnar epithelium. Myoepithelial cells lie deep to the epithelium of both the intra- and extralobular ducts as well as the blunt ductules. The lobule itself is surrounded by a loose intralobular connective tissue; separating the lobules is a dense connective tissue, the interlobular connective tissue. The extralobular duct is also invested by elastic tissue.

Breast histology is not static but undergoes marked changes with each menstrual cycle under the influence of estrogen and progesterone. When estrogen levels rise at the end of the menstrual cycle, ductal and acinar epithelium proliferate, with resultant ductal and

TDLU dilatation and hypertrophy. Under the influence of progesterone in the latter half of the menstrual cycle, stromal growth and edema occur. With the onset of the menstrual cycle and falling estrogen and progesterone levels, intralobular connective tissue recedes, and edema diminishes. There may be some desquamation of epithelium as ductal and acinar size return to normal. In the late phases of the menstrual cycle, lymphocytes also accumulate in the periductal tissue. The remainder of the discussion of anatomic alterations will be based on this somewhat simplified concept of breast microanatomy. The following descriptions detail some of the histologic and clinical manifestations of several entities included under the umbrella of fibrocystic change.

CYSTIC DISEASE

True cysts arise from blunt ductules (terminal acini) and enlarge until they are palpable as dominant masses, usually at about 1 cm in diameter. The etiology of cyst development is not entirely clear. For unexplained reasons, in some patients microcysts (less than 3 mm and not evident on mammography) continue to enlarge, to become gross cystic disease. Macrocystic change is the most common benign palpable breast alteration, affecting about 7 percent of the adult women of the Western Hemisphere. The presence of microcysts alone is believed by most pathologists to be a normal finding. Although many small cysts regress and disappear, it is unusual for a cyst measuring greater than 2 cm to do so. Histologically, a simple cyst has a lining of flattened epithelium, which has its origin in the cuboidal lining of the lobule. Some authors believe that the simple cyst develops as a result of apocrine metaplasia of the lobular epithelium, causing increased fluid production. The lobule may then be blocked by either surrounding fibrosis or ductal epithelial hyperplasia. The "apocrine" cell of breast ductal epithelium is a large cylindrical cell with acidophilic cytoplasm and a basally located, inconspicuous nucleus. Its appearance is similar to that of cells comprising the apocrine sweat glands elsewhere in the body. The breast originates as a modified skin sweat gland. "Apocrine" metaplasia is a histologically evident change of the breast epithelium and is not mammographically visible as an isolated finding.

Cysts may be asymptomatic or may cause pain from enlargement or rupture. Although some authors report an increase of breast carcinoma with macrocystic disease, this finding is not supported by the consensus meeting of the American College of Pathologists. Categorization of cysts by their cation, steroid hormone, and pituitary hormone content is being pursued by some authors in order to better understand the dynamics and implications of cyst formation.

SUMMARY OF THE CONSENSUS MEETING: "IS FIBROCYSTIC DISEASE OF THE BREAST PRECANCEROUS?"

If the pathologic diagnosis FIBROCYSTIC DISEASE is used at all, or when the preferred terms *fibrocystic changes* or *fibrocystic condition* are used, the component elements should be specified.

RELATIVE RISK FOR INVASIVE BREAST CARCINOMA BASED ON PATHOLOGIC EXAMINATION OF BENIGN BREAST TISSUE

No Increased Risk

Women with any lesion specified below in a biopsy specimen are at no greater risk for invasive breast carcinoma than comparable women who have had no breast biopsy:

Adenosis, sclerosing or florid

Apocrine metaplasia

Cysts, macro and/or micro

Duct ectasia

Fibroadenoma

Fibrosis

Hyperplasia, mild (more than two but not more than four epithelial cells in depth)

Mastitis (inflammation)

Periductal mastitis

Squamous metaplasia

(Continued)

Slightly Increased Risk (1.5 to 2 times)

Women with any lesion specified below in a biopsy specimen are at slightly increased risk for invasive breast carcinoma relative to comparable women who have had no breast biopsy:

> Hyperplasia, moderate or florid, solid or papillary
>
> Papilloma with fibrovascular core

Moderately Increased Risk (5 times)

Women with a lesion specified below in a biopsy specimen are at moderately increased risk for invasive breast carcinoma relative to comparable women who have had no breast biopsy:

> Atypical hyperplasia (borderline lesion) (does not include frank carcinoma in situ)
>
> Ductal
>
> Lobular

(From Consensus Meeting, Oct. 3–5, 1985. Is "fibrocystic disease" of the breast precancerous? Arch Pathol Lab Med 110:171, 1986, with permission.)

The macrocyst previously discussed causes problems not only by obscuring parenchymal detail but also by presenting as a mammographic mass. The etiology of this solitary mass may be resolved by aspiration and/or ultrasound examination. When multiple benign-appearing masses are present, mammographic follow-up examination may be the only reasonable option. Ultrasound can be helpful, but it is not always conclusive. With increasing numbers of masses it is difficult to ensure that an area seen on ultrasound examination correlates specifically to a mass on the mammogram.

DUCTAL ECTASIA

Ductal ectasia is not a proliferative change per se but is discussed by many authors in conjunction with fibrocystic change. It occurs in peri- and postmenopausal women when the ducts beneath the nipple and areola become dilated and filled with cellular and fatty debris. The patient may present with nonbloody nipple discharge, and the breast may become painful if fluid leaks from the duct into surrounding tissues, inciting a sterile inflammatory response. Fluid collections in the tissue may occur, resulting in a palpable, painful mass near the areola. The inflammatory process may be complicated by reactive fibrosis. The enlarged ducts can sometimes be appreciated mammographically as linear densities extending posteriorly from the retroareolar area. Ultrasound examination can also be used to identify dilated ducts and associated parenchymal fluid collections.

FIBROADENOMA

The fibroadenoma is a common benign tumor of the breast with both glandular and fibrous components. As such it is included by many authors under the heading of fibrocystic change. Some believe the etiology is a focal glandular sensitivity to estrogen. The fibroadenoma presents clinically as a rubbery mobile mass, usually in a woman of reproductive age. Mammographically, it appears as an ovoid, well-circumscribed lesion often with a peripheral halo sign. Enlargement has been reported during pregnancy and during the menstrual cycle. Occasionally myxoid degeneration within the mass can cause retraction of the surrounding tissue and loss of the well-circumscribed characteristics, thus resulting in diagnostic confusion. Degeneration can also result in coarse, irregular dense calcification, which can aid in the diagnosis of fibroadenoma when the calcification is characteristic. Peripheral shell-type calcification also occurs. The presence of a benign fibroadenoma confers no increased risk of the development of invasive carcinoma. Unless the diagnosis of fibroadenoma can be made conclusively via the characteristic mammographic appearance or on fine-needle aspiration, surgical excision is usually warranted for histologic confirmation.

FIBROSIS

Dense fibrosis, or *fibrous mastopathy*, is incited by unknown factors and may present either diffusely in one or both breasts, or as a focal mass. Its presence decreases the sensitivity of the mammogram because of increased density, obscuring the normal glandular tissue (Figs. 10-3 and 10-4). When fibrosis presents as a focal mass, it can mimic the findings of carcinoma, and biopsy may be the only alternative (Fig. 10-5). Comparison with prior mammograms is invaluable in this situation. Fibrosis as an isolated entity occurs primarily during the menstrual years. Fibrotic change may also be reactive, caused by an irritating factor such as ductal inflammation. It can also accompany adenosis and epithelial hyperplasia. Dense, acellular hyalinized fibrosis may histologically result in obliteration of mammary lobules.

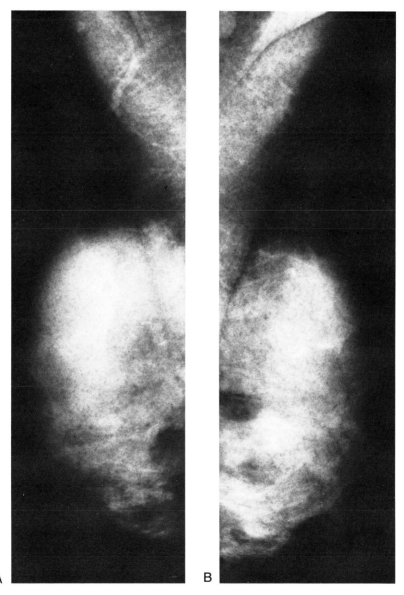

A   B

Fig. 10-3. (A & B) Left and right mediolateral oblique views in a 41-year-old woman with premenstrual breast tenderness. The breast tissue is extremely dense, a finding most marked in the upper-outer portions of both breasts. The pattern is that of dense fibrosis. Parenchymal detail is obscured by this process.

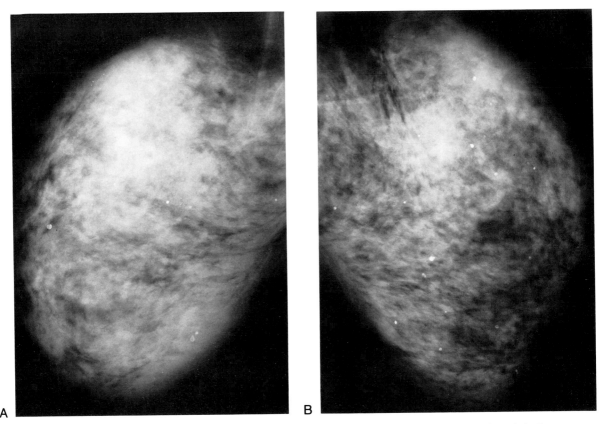

A   B

Fig. 10-4. (A & B) Left and right mediolateral oblique views in a 77-year-old woman with palpably nodular breasts. Radiographic density is increased diffusely, particularly considering the advanced age of the patient. The density is most marked in the upper-outer quadrant of the left breast. The findings are probably the result of a combination of adenosis and dense fibrosis. Scattered calcifications of secretory disease, fat necrosis, and adenosis are incidentally noted.

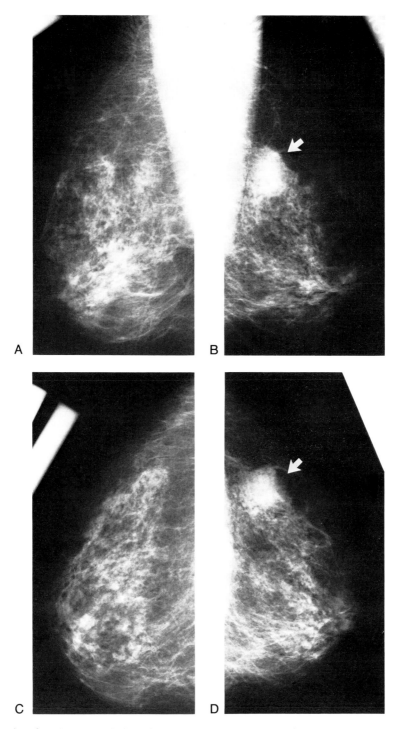

Fig. 10-5. **(A & B)** Left and right mediolateral oblique views in a 73-year-old asymptomatic woman. An irregular focus of increased density in the upper-outer quadrant on the right was considered suspicious for malignancy *(arrow)*. Open biopsy revealed only dense fibrosis. **(C & D)** Left and right craniocaudal views of the same patient. Upper-outer quadrant mass *(arrow)*.

ADENOSIS

Adenosis implies a proliferation of glandular structures resulting in new ductules and lobules. It also usually involves a proliferation of the epithelium and overgrowth of the myoepithelial cells (Fig. 10-6). If combined with a fibrous reaction of the stroma, it is termed sclerosing adenosis. Advanced fibrosis can cause distortion of the normal lobular pattern (Fig. 10-7). Although frequently resulting in diffuse change, sclerosing adenosis may produce a focal palpable mass that cannot be differentiated from malignant disease. Similarly, a focal area of increased density on the mammogram caused by sclerosing adenosis may be confused with a malignant mass. The intense fibrosis may simulate the desmoplastic changes of a scirrhous carcinoma. Often sclerosing adenosis is asymptomatic. The mammographic findings usually consist of increased radiographic density of either a diffuse or focal nature. On occasion, a "snowflake" pattern may be seen due to visualization of enlarged lobules (Fig. 10-8).

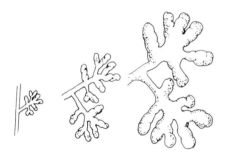

Fig. 10-6. Development of adenosis. The glandular structures proliferate, resulting in new ducts and lobules. Epithelial proliferation and overgrowth of myoepithelial cells usually occurs as well. (Adapted from Tabar and Dean,[22] with permission.)

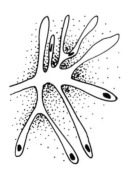

Fig. 10-7. Sclerosing adenosis. In addition to the changes of glandular proliferation, a fibrous reaction of the stroma has occurred, distorting and compressing the lobules. Small, smooth, calcific foci are seen in the blunt ducts. (Adapted from Tabar and Dean,[22] with permission.)

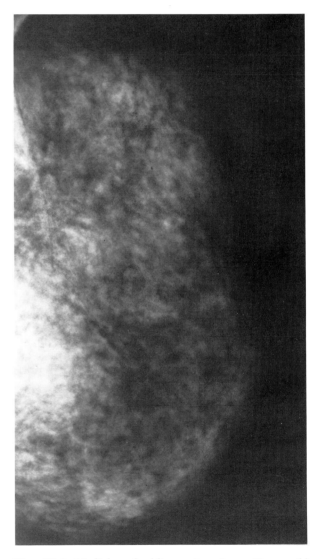

Fig. 10-8. Mediolateral oblique view in a 48-year-old asymptomatic woman. A patchy "snowflake" pattern of adenosis can be appreciated. This configuration of density is caused by the overlapping densities of multiple enlarged lobules.

Associated calcifications, if typical, may aid in the diagnosis. A wide range of calcifications seen on mammography can be produced by benign lobular disease. With adenosis, lobular calcification can occur, as fluid becomes inspissated in the terminal ductules, termed the "pearl" configuration by some authors (Fig. 10-9). Their smooth, rounded contour aids in differentiating this type of calcification from the more irregular clustered calcifications of malignancy. Lobular calcifications can be found in a diffuse distribution throughout the breast parenchyma (Fig. 10-10) or can be seen as one (Fig. 10-11) or several tight clusters (Figs. 10-12 and 10-13) when several TDLUs are involved.

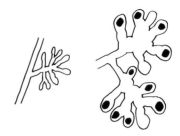

Fig. 10-9. Development of "pearl"-type calcifications in adenosis. Fluid stasis in enlarged blunt ducts ultimately leads to the formation of a small, dense, spherical calcification in the lumen of the blunt duct. (Adapted from Tabar and Dean,[22] with permission.)

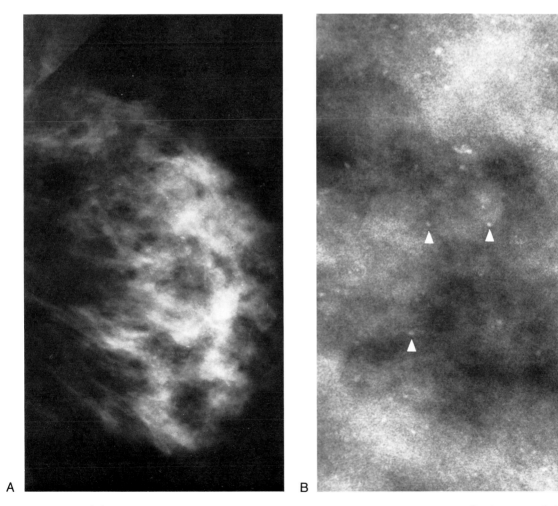

A

B

Fig. 10-10. (A) Mediolateral oblique view in a 50-year-old asymptomatic woman. Diffusely scattered dense punctate calcifications are seen. **(B)** Photographic enlargement of the midportion of the breast demonstrates the smooth, rounded contour and uniform size of the majority of the calcifications *(arrowheads)*.

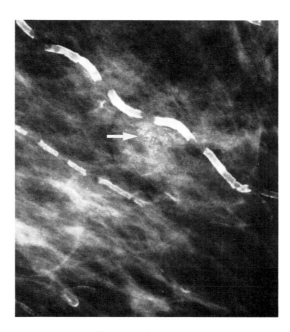

Fig. 10-11. Mediolateral oblique view, photographic enlargement, in a 71-year-old woman with a history of endometrial carcinoma. A tightly packed cluster of smooth punctate calcifications is seen *(arrow)*. Biopsy demonstrated adenosis with lobular calcifications.

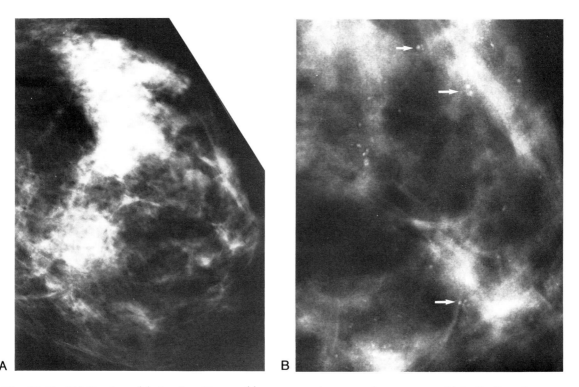

Fig. 10-12. **(A)** Craniocaudal view in a 44-year-old asymptomatic woman demonstrates widely distributed punctate microcalcifications with a tendency toward clustering. **(B)** Photographic enlargement of the anterior portion of the breast demonstrates several tight clusters *(arrows)* resulting from adenosis in scattered lobules.

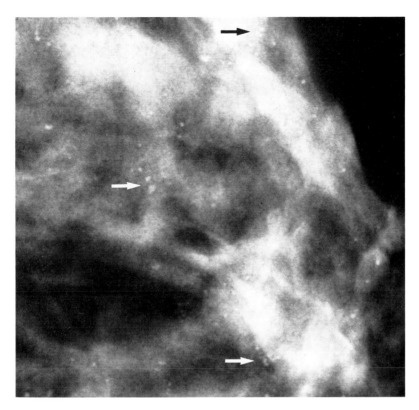

Fig. 10-13. Craniocaudal view, photographic enlargement of anterior section, in a 46-year-old woman with a clinical history of fibrocystic disease. "Pearl"-type punctate calcifications show a tendency toward clustering caused by adenosis in separate lobules *(arrows)*.

A more graphic variant of lobular calcification described in mammographic literature is termed *cystic lobular hyperplasia*. It involves a histologic process similar to adenosis but also results in a degree of cystic dilatation as well as proliferation of the lobules. When these lobules become dilated, they may develop gravity-dependent milk of calcium deposition in a "teacup" configuration (Figs. 10-14 to 10-16). Thus their appearance will change on each view, classically a meniscus on the lateral view and a faint rounded calcification with a relatively lucent center when seen en face on the craniocaudal view. Like adenosis and sclerosing adenosis, cystic lobular hyperplasia is frequently asymptomatic. It may be found associated with dense fibrosis.

Involutional calcifications are akin to those found in adenosis. They are diffuse, high-density punctate calcifications that probably had their origin in adenosis or cystic hyperplasia that calcifies as the glandular tissue atrophies. Fatty replacement ensues, leaving only

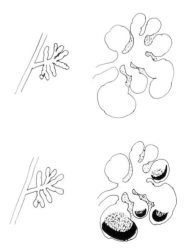

Fig. 10-14. Development of cystic lobular hyperplasia. Crescent-shaped calcifications form in the dependent portion of dilated blunt ductules. This illustration shows associated fibrosis contributing to cystic dilatation by obstructing the neck of the blunt ductules. (Adapted from Tabar and Dean,[22] with permission.)

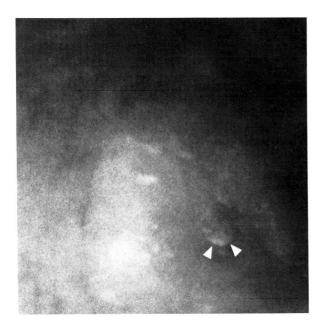

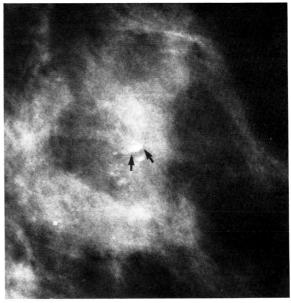

Fig. 10-15. Mediolateral oblique view with photographic enlargement of upper breast in a 42-year-old asymptomatic woman. "Teacup" gravity-dependent calcifications of cystic lobular hyperplasia are present *(arrowheads)*.

Fig. 10-16. Mediolateral oblique view with photographic enlargement of upper breast in a 47-year-old woman with a history of previous breast biopsy showing fibrocystic changes. Calcium layering dependently as "teacups" *(arrows)* in cystic lobular hyperplasia.

punctate calcifications on a fatty background (Fig. 10-17).

DUCTAL AND LOBULAR HYPERPLASTIC CHANGES

The normal ductal and terminal acinar epithelium can undergo hyperplastic changes of varying degrees. Most hyperplastic epithelial changes are not detectable either on mammography or by the palpating hand, as these early alterations cause no characteristic calcifications or mass effect. Benign lobular-type calcifications may occur with epithelial hyperplasia but are nonspecific. Ducts and blunt ductules with an epithelial lining no more than two cells deep are considered normal. Mild hyperplasia is present when the epithelium is two to four cells thick and the cells are without any nuclear or cytoplasmic features of malignancy (cellular atypia). Mild epithelial hyperplasia confers no increased risk of malignancy and is likely to be found incidentally in a biopsy specimen obtained for other reasons. Epithelial proliferation is often referred to as "normal" when the growth pattern is orderly and the cells show no atypia. The term *epitheliosis* is also used in reference to benign epithelial proliferation.

Moderate or florid hyperplasia occurs when the epithelium is greater than four cell layers thick but still has no features of cellular atypia. It confers a slightly increased risk of breast carcinoma (1.5 to 2 times) (see box). The growth pattern of the cellular hyperplasia may be solid or papillary. If the growth pattern assumes a papillary configuration, the term *papillomatosis* is often used to describe the entity. This benign proliferation of epithe-

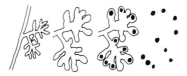

Fig. 10-17. Development of involutional calcifications. Punctate calcifications in blunt ducts remain as the glandular tissue atrophies. (Adapted from Tabar and Dean,[22] with permission.)

lial cells may partially fill small and medium-sized ducts. Again, these changes are usually asymptomatic and radiographically occult, discovered incidentally on histologic examination of breast tissue.

PAPILLOMA WITH FIBROVASCULAR CORE

The isolated single-stalk papilloma is a separate entity from papillomatosis. It is classically found in a main duct not far from the areola, as opposed to the previously described epithelial hyperplastic changes, which tend to occur in and near the smaller terminal ducts. The isolated papilloma is composed histologically of a fibrovascular core and covered by one or two layers of cells. These consist of a luminal columnar or cuboidal cell with a deeper layer similar to the small myoepithelial cell. Apocrine metaplasia of the luminal cells may occur as well. Unlike the asymptomatic entity of papillomatosis, the papilloma may cause symptoms of bleeding from the nipple or a palpable para-areolar mass. Mammographically, this lesion is not usually evident unless calcification has occurred. In this situation, a rounded calcification of ductal caliber is seen, often with a "raspberry" configuration. Occasionally the papilloma will present on the mammogram as a small mass lesion or as a dilated duct. Multiple distinct papillomas can be found in one breast. When clinical symptoms suggest the presence of a papilloma, galactography can confirm the presence of an intraductal mass. Papillomas have also been demonstrated on ultrasound examination.

ATYPICAL HYPERPLASIA—DUCTAL AND LOBULAR

Hyperplasia of either the ductal or lobular epithelium may ultimately be composed of cells that demonstrate the nuclear and cytoplasmic features of malignancy (cellular atypia). These "borderline" lesions, however, do not have enough of the features of carcinoma in situ to make this diagnosis unequivocally. Such atypical hyperplasia does not produce a clinically evident mass, and there are no specific indications of these lesions mammographically. With any of the types of lobular proliferation, lobular-type calcifications may be seen but are quite nonspecific. The con-

sensus of the American College of Pathologists is that atypical hyperplasia of either lobular or ductal origin confers a moderately increased (five times) risk of breast carcinoma (see box).

CARCINOMA IN SITU

Carcinoma in situ, either ductal or lobular, straddles the line between the benign hyperplasias associated with fibrocystic change and with invasive neoplasm. Women with such a histologic diagnosis in a breast biopsy have a high risk of developing invasive breast carcinoma (8 to 10 times comparable with nonbiopsied women), if no further therapy is undertaken.

CONTROVERSIAL LESIONS OF UNCERTAIN FUTURE RISKS

Sclerosing ductal hyperplasia is a controversial lesion that has evoked increased interest in recent years as a result of the widespread screening of asymptomatic women. A prevalence of 0.9/1,000 is quoted by Tabar and Dean.[22] The lesion can be found described in the literature under several different names, including sclerosing duct hyperplasia, radial scar, and indurative mastopathy. The lesion is asymptomatic and nonpalpable. It is manifest on mammographic examination as a focus of long, thin spicules with intervening radiolucent streaks and demonstrates no solid central tumor mass. Additionally, its configuration changes with different mammographic projections (Fig. 10-18). Although the lesion is benign and the diagnosis can be strongly suggested on mammography, its strong resemblance to carcinoma warrants biopsy in virtually all cases. Histologically, the lesion consists of ductal elements associated with stellate hyalinizing fibrosis and elastosis. Assessment of the future risk of developing invasive breast carcinoma is based on the nature of the epithelial component.

JUVENILE PAPILLOMATOSIS (SWISS CHEESE DISEASE)

Juvenile papillomatosis mammographically consists of multiple, small, sharply outlined densities in a chainlike configuration. These papillomas tend to pro-

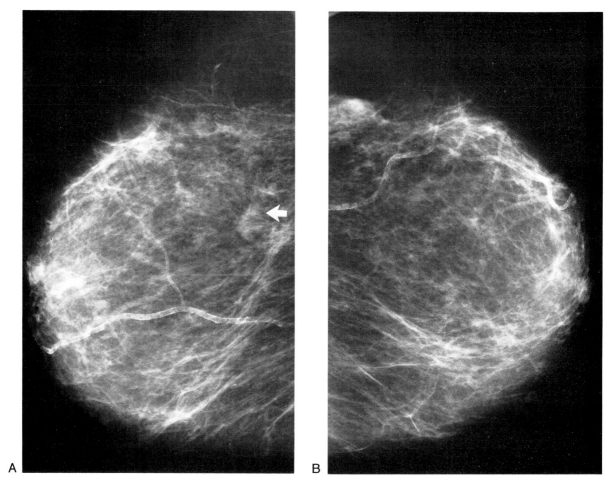

A   B

Fig. 10-18. (A & B) Left and right mediolateral oblique views of a 64-year-old woman who underwent screening mammography. The spiculated lesion in the posterior left breast *(arrows)* appears slightly different on the two projections. (Courtesy of Renato Travelli, M.D., LaCrosse, WI.) *(Figure continues.)*

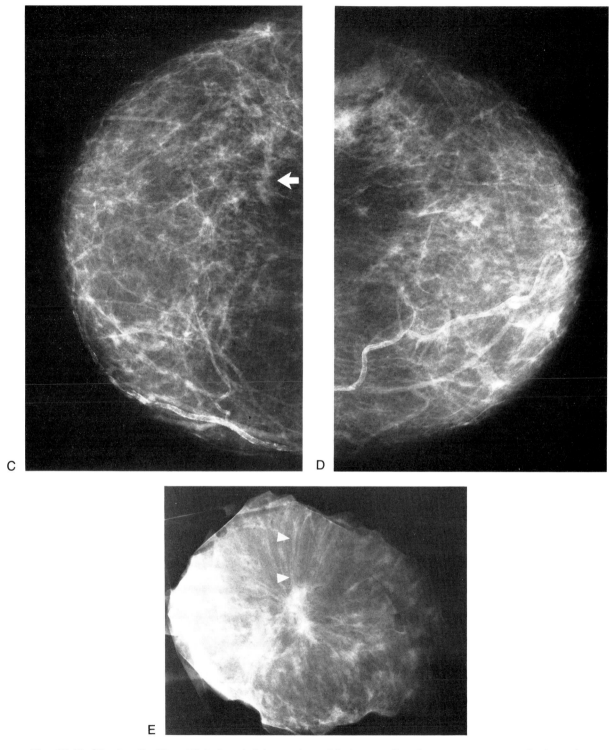

Fig. 10-18 *(Continued)*. **(C & D)** Left and right craniocaudal views. Stellate lesion is seen posteriorly *(arrows)*. **(E)** Specimen radiography of the surgically resected specimen. The radiograph demonstrates an ill-defined central mass and long radiating projections *(arrowheads)*. Histology showed sclerosing ductal hyperplasia (radial scar).

duce fluid, causing the appearance of widened ducts between the nodules. The lesion is found in the TDLU, unlike the solitary papilloma, which is found in major lactiferous ducts. The changes of juvenile papillomatosis tend to be associated with apocrine and nonapocrine hyperplasia, sclerosing adenosis, and ductal stasis. Juvenile papillomatosis is primarily a disease of the adolescent. Although the lesion shows a tendency to recur after excision, risk of future development of invasive breast carcinoma is as yet unknown.

SUMMARY

The relationship of so-called fibrocystic change to the risk of subsequent malignancy has been long debated and has been of great historical interest. Reports as early as 1940 stated that those with chronic cystic mastitis had a three- to fourfold increased risk of developing breast carcinoma. In the 1960s severe ductal epithelial hyperplasia was believed to be the specific premalignant histologic change, while the nonproliferative lesions (i.e., epithelial apocrine metaplasia, fibrosis, cysts, and sclerosing adenosis) were not felt to confer additional risk. In the 1970s specific types of atypical proliferative lobulo-alveolar lesions were described as composing a continuum to ductal carcinoma in situ and lobular carcinoma in situ.

While controversy continues over the implications of these diverse histologic changes, the most formalized opinion concerning the prognostic value of these lesions is available from the Cancer Committee of the College of American Pathologists. A summary of the consensus meeting of 1985 is included to give some indication of relative risk of developing invasive carcinoma for specific histologic changes that are traditionally included under the title of fibrocystic change (see box). The listing does not suggest, however, that a patient with the clinical manifestations of fibrocystic change should undergo biopsy without clear-cut physical or mammographic findings that warrant histologic examination.

Because of the lack of specific risk data for the *radial scar*, it is not included in this listing and is categorized by the characteristics of the epithelial components.

The question is, of course, which of these lesions associated with increased risk will progress to invasive carcinoma and which will regress or remain unchanged. There are additional unanswered questions concerning the effect that the hormonal environment has on these premalignant lesions or malignancy "markers."

How do these changes of both clinical and histologic fibrocystic change affect mammographic diagnosis? The mammographer becomes involved with fibrocystic change when a symptomatic patient arrives for mammographic evaluation with the question: "Do I have cancer?" The mammographer may then be presented with a radiographically dense image caused by the presence of fibrosis and cysts and compounded by scattered, confusing microcalcifications. An identical image may be generated from a completely asymptomatic patient undergoing mammography for screening purposes. The role of the mammographer is to separate whenever possible benign changes, including increased density and calcifications, from those alterations that truly warrant histologic examination. A knowledge of breast microanatomy and histopathology with help in this differentiation, although admittedly overlap between benign and malignant appearances does occur.

In summary, the term *fibrocystic change* or *disease* encompasses a wide variety of histologic, clinical, and radiographic entities. The terminology is poor in that it is so widely inclusive that it ultimately loses any definitive meaning. However, some of the specific histologic lesions included under the umbrella of fibrocystic change do seem to grant a moderately increased risk of breast carcinoma. These lesions may be totally invisible on mammography.

Certain fibrocystic changes are likely to produce symptoms in the affected woman. For unknown reasons some women are more likely to produce cysts, frequently causing pain and palpable masses. Changes of fibrosis and adenosis, compounded by cyclic physiologic changes involving fluid shifts also can cause pain, fullness, and tenderness often labeled clinically as fibrocystic change. Finally, the fibrocystic changes that cause increased tissue density from fibrosis, adenosis, or cyst formation will complicate the job of the mammographer in attempting to differentiate a carcinoma from the background density. Lobular calcifications can also stretch the diagnostic ability of the mammographer in differentiating them from malignant calcifications. Often the distinction cannot be clearly made when calcifications of an indeterminate character are found, and either biopsy or close follow-up may be necessary. In preference to using the term fibrocystic disease, more specific descriptions of the problem at hand should be employed, whether the findings be of a clinical, histologic, or mammographic nature.

SUGGESTED READINGS

1. Angeli A, Dogliotti L, Orlandi F, Beccati D: Mammary cysts: pathophysiology and biochemistry. Int J Rad Appl Instrum [B] 14:397, 1987

2. Azzopardi JG: Problems in Breast Pathology. WB Saunders, Philadelphia, 1980

3. Bussolati G, Cattani MG, Gugliotta P et al: Morphologic and functional aspects of apocrine metaplasia in dysplastic and neoplastic breast tissue. Ann NY Acad Sci 464:262, 1986

4. Cardeft RD, Wellings SR, Faulkin LJ: Biology of breast preneoplasia. Cancer 39:2734, 1977

5. Clark RM: Abandoning fibrocystic disease of the breast (letter). Can Med Assoc J 134:985, 1986

6. Deschamp M, Hislop TG, Band PR, et al: Study of benign breast disease in a population screened for breast cancer. Cancer Detect Prev 9:151–156, 1986

7. Devitt JE: Clinical benign disorders of the breast and carcinoma of the breast. Surg Gynecol Obstet 152:437, 1981

8. Devitt JE: Abandoning fibrocystic disease of the breast: timely end of an era. Can Med Assoc J 134:217, 1986

9. Drukker BH, deMendonca WC: Fibrocystic change and fibrocystic disease of the breast. Obstet Gynecol Clin North Am 14:685, 1987

10. Egan RL, McSweeney MB, Sewell CW: Intramammary calcifications without an associated mass in benign and malignant disease. Radiology 137:1, 1980

11. Haagensen CD: Disease of the Breast. 2nd Ed. WB Saunders, Philadelphia, 1986

12. Humphrey LJ: Fibrocystic disease and breast cancer. p. 61. In Fieg SA, McLelland R (eds): Breast Carcinoma: Current Diagnosis and Treatment. Year Book Medical Publishers, Chicago, 1983

13. Hutter RVP: Goodbye to "fibrocystic disease." N Engl J Med 312:179, 1985

14. Love SM, Gelman RS, Silen W: Fibrocystic "disease" of the breast—a nondisease? N Engl J Med 307:1010, 1982

15. Mansel RE: Benign breast disease and cancer risk: new perspectives. Ann NY Acad Sci 464:350, 1986

16. Nielsen NS, Nielsen BB: Mammographic features of sclerosing adenosis presenting as a tumor. Clin Radiol 37:371, 1986

17. Page DL, Dupont WD: Are breast cysts a premalignant marker? Eur J Cancer Clin Oncol 22:635, 1986

18. Rickert RR, Lakisher L, Hutter RVP: Indurative mastopathy: a benign sclerosing lesion of breast with elastosis which may simulate carcinoma. Cancer 47:471, 1981

19. Robbins SL, Cotran RS, Kumar: Pathologic Basis of Disease. 3rd Ed. WB Saunders, Philadelphia, 1984

20. Rosen PP, Cantrell B, Mullen DL, Depalo A et al: Juvenile papillomatosis (swiss cheese disease) of the breast. Am J Surg Pathol 4:3, 1980

21. Rubin E, Visscher DW, Alexander RW et al: Proliferative disease and atypia in biopsies performed for nonpalpable lesions detected mammographically. Cancer 61:2077, 1988

22. Tabar L, Dean PB: Teaching Atlas of Mammography. Thieme-Stratton, New York, 1983

23. Van Bogaert LJ: Taxonomy and grading of the various components of fibrocystic disease. Breast Diseases-Senologia 2:6, 1987

24. Wellings SR: Development of human breast cancer: advances in cancer research. Adv Cancer Res 31:287, 1980

25. Wellings SR, Jensen HM, Marcum RG: An atlas of subgross pathology of the human breast with special reference to possible precancerous lesions. J Natl Cancer Inst 55:231, 1975

26. Wellings SR, Wolfe JN: Correlative studies of the histological and radiographic appearance of the breast parenchyma. Radiology 129:299, 1978

11

Benign Masses

Mary Ellen Peters

Since the majority of breast masses are benign, recognizing them is important to prevent needless biopsies. A typical benign mass is round, ovoid or lobulated in shape, and has well-defined borders unless they are obscured by overlying fibroglandular tissues. An associated "halo sign," a fine rim of radiolucency, may entirely or partially surround it. One theory suggests that the halo represents compressed fat and another that it is the result of the mach effect. The halo sign is more commonly seen associated with benign masses. However, some malignant masses that mimic benign lesions, such as medullary, mucoid (colloid), and papillary carcinomas, can have a halo sign, and it may even be seen with the usual (not otherwise specified) invasive ductal carcinoma.

The presence of fat (radiolucency) within a mass indicates in most instances that it is benign. The two possible exceptions are a liposarcoma and a cystosarcoma phyllodes that contains liposarcomatous elements.

The calcifications associated with benign masses are usually relatively large and have a curvilinear, eggshell, popcorn, rosette, or globular appearance. It is unusual for benign masses to be associated with small microcalcifications.

FIBROADENOMAS

Fibroadenomas arise from lobules and are composed of both fibrous and glandular elements. Many consider them to be an extreme form of lobular hyperplasia. Although fibroadenomas can present at any age, they are usually found before the age of 30, and are the most common reason for breast biopsies in women during their 30s and early 40s. Malignancy has been reported to develop within them; this is a distinctly unusual occurrence, however. This rare malignancy is usually in the form of a lobular carcinoma in situ. Although most fibroadenomas are not clinically evident, they may present as firm, mobile masses that can be tender or painful.

Radiographically, fibroadenomas are round, ovoid, or lobulated masses that are usually entirely or partially well defined (Figs. 11-1 and 11-2). A halo is often present, bordering part or all of the mass (Figs. 11-3 and 11-4). Fibroadenomas are generally solitary, although they are multiple in 20 percent of cases and can be bilateral (Fig. 11-5). As a result of a propensity to myxomatous degeneration, fibroadenomas can calcify, especially in the postmenopausal age group. The soft

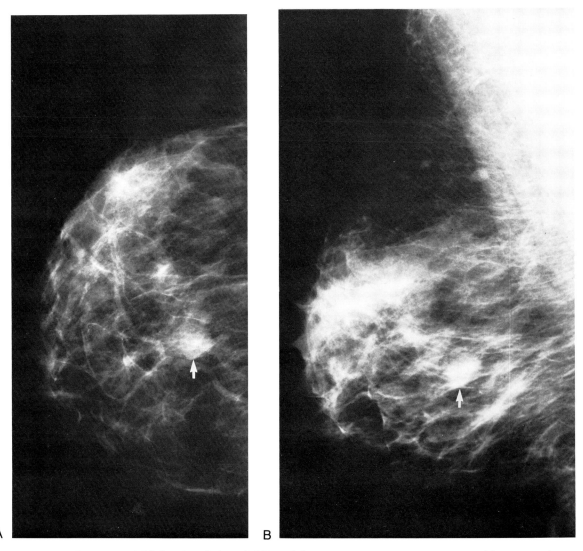

Fig. 11-1. Left craniocaudal **(A)** and mediolateral oblique **(B)** views in an asymptomatic 42-year-old woman. The study demonstrates an ovoid, homogeneous mass *(arrow)* of low density. The margins are partially ill defined. The most likely etiologies in this age group are a fibroadenoma and a cyst. Histology: fibroadenoma.

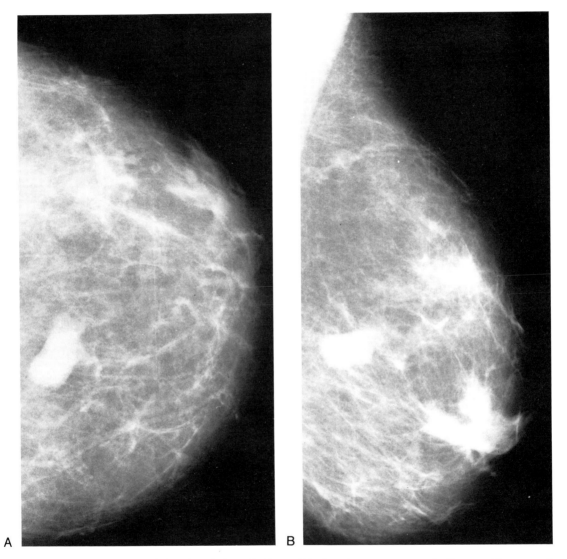

Fig. 11-2. Right craniocaudal **(A)** and mediolateral oblique **(B)** views in an asymptomatic 40-year-old woman. A 2.5-cm homogeneous mass is located in the superomedial quadrant that was proven to be a fibroadenoma on histology. The margins of the fibroadenoma are not totally well defined because of surrounding fibroglandular tissue.

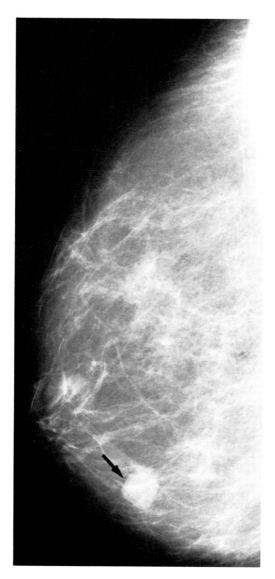

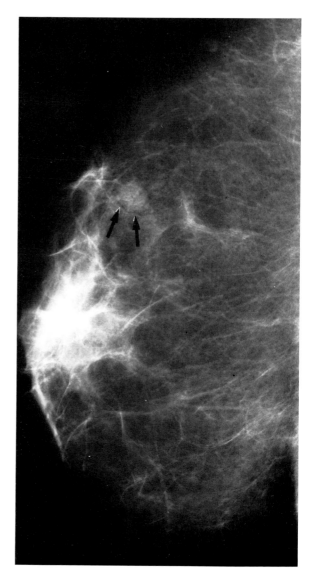

Fig. 11-3. Craniocaudal view in an asymptomatic 50-year-old woman. A halo sign *(arrow)* partially surrounds the round, low-density mass. Histology: fibroadenoma

Fig. 11-4. Craniocaudal view in an asymptomatic 41-year-old woman. The study demonstrates a round, slightly lobulated mass that has an associated halo sign *(arrows)*. Histology: fibroadenoma.

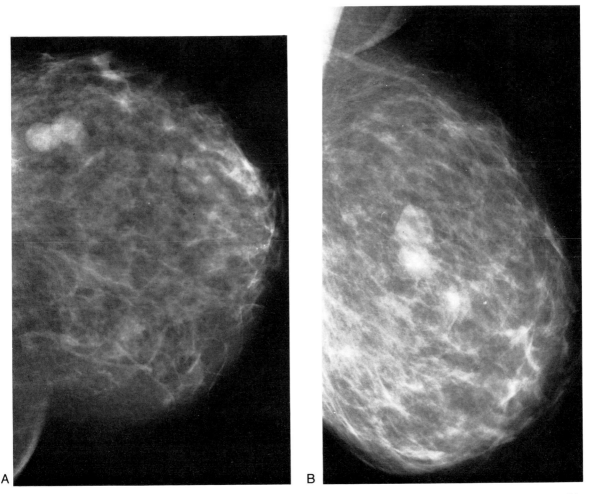

Fig. 11-5. Screening right craniocaudal **(A)** and mediolateral oblique **(B)** views in an asymptomatic 27-year-old woman with a family history of breast cancer. Two closely approximated, ovoid masses with fairly well-defined borders are located in the superolateral quadrant. The most likely etiology in this age group is fibroadenoma. Histology: two fibroadenomas.

tissue component often regresses as the fibroadenoma degenerates, until calcification, typically coarse, "popcorn"-appearing, or shell-like, is all that is visible (Figs. 11-6 to 11-9). Fibroadenomas can contain microcalcifications, grow, appear as indistinct masses, or appear as a new mass, making it impossible to differentiate them from a malignant lesion (Fig. 11-10).

Giant or Juvenile Fibroadenoma

Giant, or juvenile, fibroadenoma is a more cellular variant of the ordinary fibroadenoma and is most commonly seen in the 10 to 20-year-old age group. This type of fibroadenoma can rapidly increase in size and become very large. Radiographically, they appear as

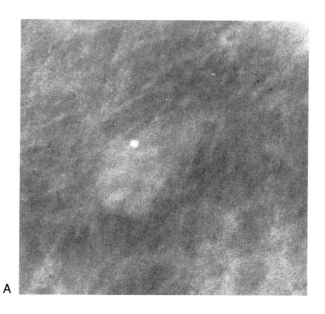

A

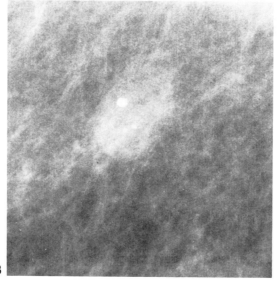

B

Fig. 11-6. *(Figure continues.)*

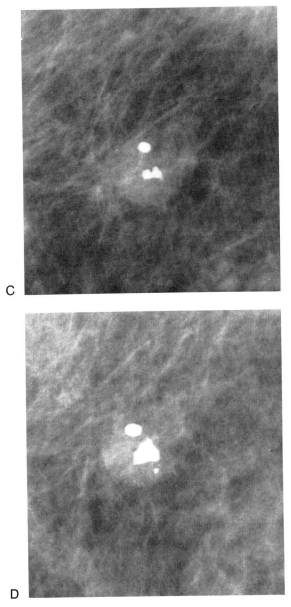

Fig. 11-6. (A–D) A series of enlargements from screening right craniocaudal views performed over a 5-year period. The initial study **(A)**, performed at age 67, demonstrates a partially well-defined mass containing a relatively large, benign-appearing calcification. Because of the benign appearance of the calcification, the mass was considered to be a fibroadenoma. The subsequent studies demonstrate progressive calcification of the mass, confirming the impression of a fibroadenoma. The final study **(D)** shows that a large portion of the soft tissue component has been replaced by calcification.

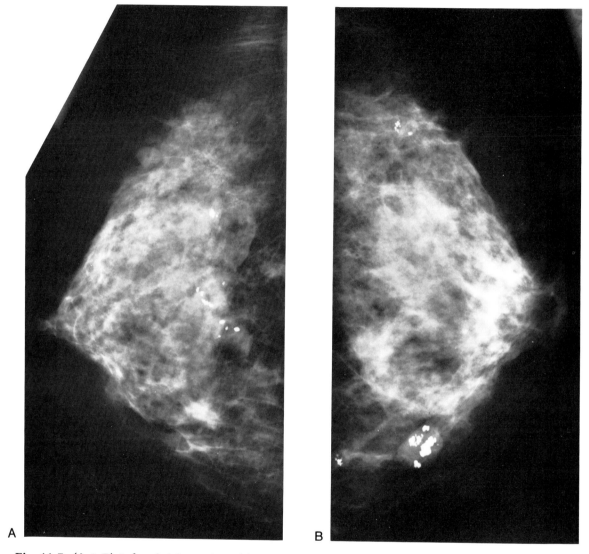

Fig. 11-7. (A & B) Left and right craniocaudal views in an asymptomatic 43-year-old woman. Groups of large coarse calcifications, some of which are associated with soft tissue masses, can be seen in both breasts. The findings are pathognomonic of bilateral calcified fibroadenomas.

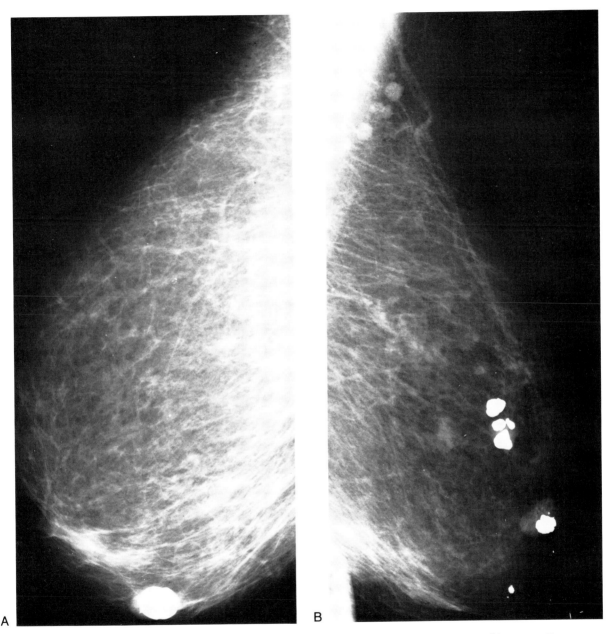

A

B

Fig. 11-8. (A & B) Left and right mediolateral oblique views in an asymptomatic 79-year-old woman. Large, smooth calcifications can be seen bilaterally. A rim of soft tissue can be seen surrounding some of the calcifications. Diagnosis: degenerated fibroadenoma.

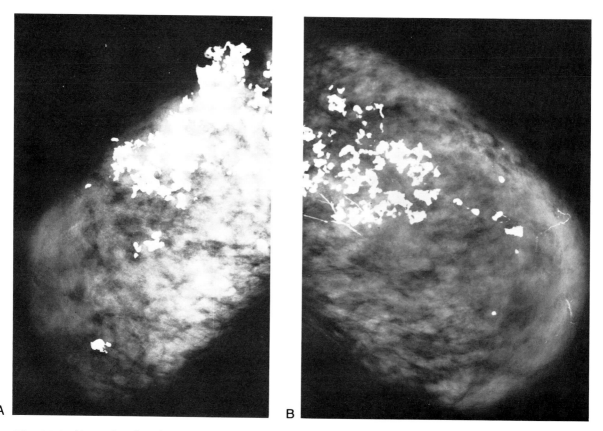

Fig. 11-9. (A & B) Left and right mediolateral oblique views in a 91-year-old woman with bilateral palpable nodules. Numerous large calcifications are present bilaterally. No soft tissue masses can be identified. The palpable masses conformed to the areas of calcifications. Diagnosis: numerous calcified fibroadenoma. Secretory and vascular calcifications, which are discussed in Chapter 12, are also present.

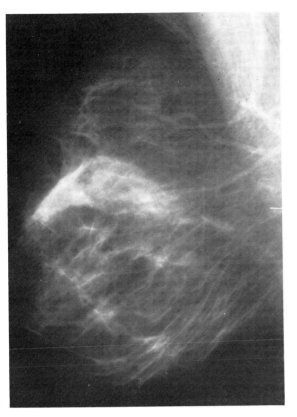 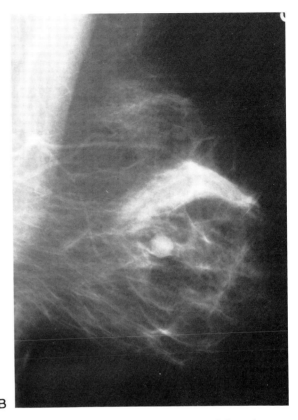

A   B

Fig. 11-10. **(A)** Right mediolateral oblique view in an asymptomatic 54-year-old woman. Normal. **(B)** Right mediolateral oblique views from a screening study 2 years later. An ovoid, well-defined, homogeneous mass of low density has developed. Although the characteristics are benign, a carcinoma must be suspected in this age group. Histology: fibroadenoma.

well-defined masses that may be associated with large, dilated veins. Although they can be multiple, juvenile fibroadenomas are most commonly solitary. Ultrasound is the preferred diagnostic modality in the younger patient if further diagnostic work-up is necessary. Most often it is not essential, because needle aspiration or excision is the most direct diagnostic approach.

TUBULAR ADENOMA AND LACTATING ADENOMA

Tubular adenoma (or pure mammary adenoma) is an uncommon benign tumor that histologically consists of epithelially lined tubular structures. Pathologically, it is a well-defined tumor, although it does not have a true capsule. We have observed one tubular adenoma that presented as a lobulated mass in a 60-year-old woman (Fig. 11-11).

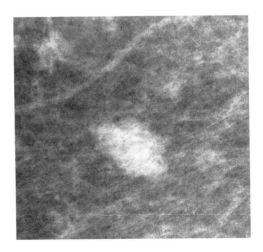

Fig. 11-11. Enlargement from a craniocaudal view in an asymptomatic 60-year-old woman. Although the borders of this lobulated mass are fairly well defined, suggesting a benign mass, a knobby carcinoma must be of strong consideration in this age group. Histology: tubular adenoma.

The lactating adenoma is considered by some to be a variant of the tubular adenoma, but others believe it is the result of the hormonal effects of pregnancy on an ordinary fibroadenoma. It can grow rapidly and become very large until lactation ceases, when it tends to regress. The diagnosis is usually made clinically.

LIPOFIBROADENOMAS

Lipofibroadenomas are infrequently seen benign breast tumors composed of both fat and glandular elements. Microscopy demonstrates areas of ducts and lobules in a stroma with varying amounts of fibrous tissue, capillary vessels, and smooth muscle interspersed with areas of adipose tissue. Unless the entire mass is examined, the pathologist probably will not be able to identify it as a lipofibroadenoma.

Most lipofibroadenomas (75 percent) are palpable and are described as firm, nontender, mobile masses. The median age at presentation is in the midforties, but they have been described from ages 15 to 88 years.

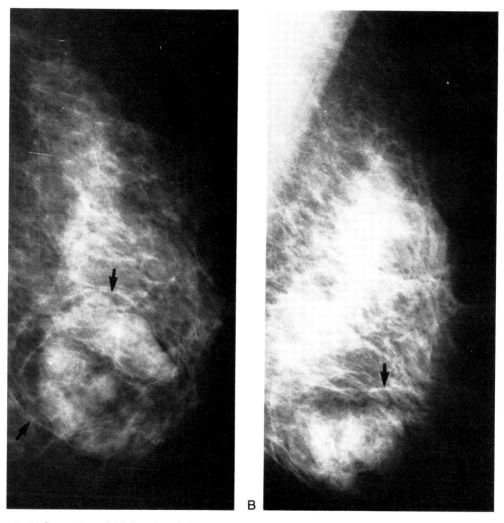

A   B

Fig. 11-12. Right craniocaudal **(A)** and mediolateral oblique **(B)** views in an asymptomatic 53-year-old woman. A mass measuring 7 cm in diameter is located in the inferomedial quadrant. The mass appears to be surrounded by a "capsule" *(arrows)*. The central portion of the mass is radiolucent-radiodense, with perimeter of the tumor being primarily radiolucent. Histology: lipofibroadenoma.

Because of its mixed fat and glandular elements, Wolfe[26] has likened its radiographic appearance to a cauliflower. The tumor circumference is usually radiolucent, while its central portion is mixed radiolucent-radiodense. Often a "capsule" surrounds the tumor. This is a pseudocapsule and represents displaced normal surrounding trabeculae. Lipofibroadenomas commonly measure 3 to 5 cm, although they can become very large, measuring up to 10 cm (Figs. 11-12 and 11-13). Large coarse calcifications can develop within them, but this is infrequently observed.

Two other entities that one should consider in the differential diagnosis of lipofibroadenoma are cystosarcoma phyllodes with liposarcomatous elements and liposarcoma. All three are infrequently seen tumors.

TENSION CYSTS

Tension cysts are generally seen after the age of 30 and are uncommon after menopause. They develop as the result of an obstructed apocrine cyst. Because the epithelial lining of the apocrine cyst cannot absorb fluid at the same rate as it is secreted and the outflow tract is blocked, tension occurs within the cyst, and it enlarges. Etiologies for the obstruction include benign epithelial hyperplasia of ductules and ducts, apocrine proliferation, kinking of an extralobular duct, fibrous obliteration of small ducts, and papillomas. Although the etiology of obstruction in the vast majority of cases is benign, carcinomas can be the cause of the occlusion.

On the mammogram, tension cysts present as round-to-oval homogeneous densities that are most often solitary, but are frequently multiple and bilateral. They may be of high or low density. At times, well-defined margins are evident, and a halo sign may be seen. More often, a portion of the margin is obscured by surrounding fibroglandular tissues (Figs. 11-14 to 11-17). Indistinct margins can also be caused by inflammatory changes produced by cyst contents leaking into the parenchyma.

Tension cysts are variable in size, measuring from a few millimeters to several centimeters in diameter. In a relatively short period of time, they can become very large or disappear completely. Their apparent size on mammograms is dependent upon the forcefulness of the compression used during mammography, information that may be useful to differentiate a cyst from a solid mass. Compression is also known to cause the cyst to rupture and disappear.

The capsule of a cyst can calcify, although not commonly, producing eggshell, semilunar, or ring-shaped calcifications. This type of calcification may be seen

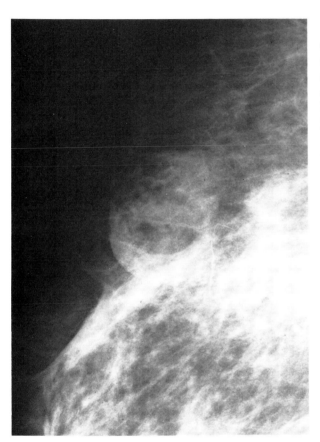

Fig. 11-13. Enlargement from a mediolateral oblique view in an asymptomatic 59-year-old woman. The margins of this 4-cm radiodense-radiolucent mass are well defined, except in one area where the fat within the mass blends with the fatty replaced fibroglandular tissues. Unlike Fig. 11-12, the perimeter of the mass is primarily radiodense, and no "capsule" can be identified. The differential diagnosis includes lipofibroadenoma, cystosarcoma with liposarcomatous elements, and a liposarcoma. The most likely diagnosis is lipofibroadenoma, since the mass is not palpable. Also, sarcomas and cystosarcoma phyllodes are usually denser and often appear lobulated. Histology: lipofibroadenoma.

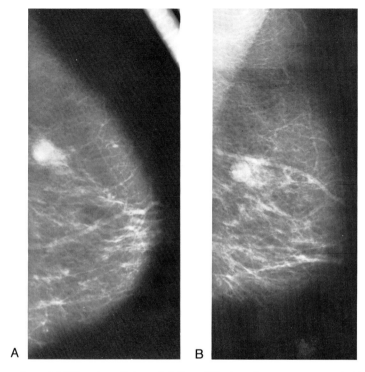

A   B

Fig. 11-14. Right craniocaudal **(A)** and mediolateral oblique **(B)** views in an asymptomatic 69-year-old woman. A 12-mm mass is present in the superolateral quadrant. On the oblique view the margins are well defined, and a halo sign partially surrounds the mass. The margins are less well defined on the craniocaudal view. An ultrasound examination demonstrated a cyst. The ill-defined margins on the craniocaudal view are the result of surrounding fibroglandular tissue.

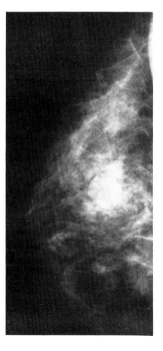

Fig. 11-15. Craniocaudal view in an asymptomatic 49-year-old woman. The study demonstrates a round, homogeneous mass with an associated halo sign. Cyst and fibroadenoma are the two most likely etiologies, although a carcinoma mimicking a benign mass must also be of consideration. An ultrasound examination proved it to be a cyst.

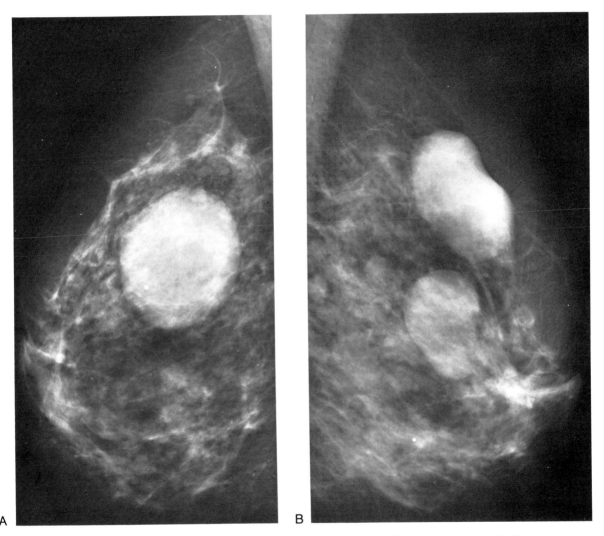

A   B

Fig. 11-16. (A & B) Left and right mediolateral oblique views in a 49-year-old woman with two palpable masses on the right and one on the left. Two large, homogeneous masses are seen on the right and one on the left, as well as bilateral smaller masses. (A calcification is superimposed over the large left mass.) Halos partially surround the masses. In the presence of multiple, bilateral, well-defined masses, the most likely diagnosis in this age group is cysts, which was proven by ultrasound.

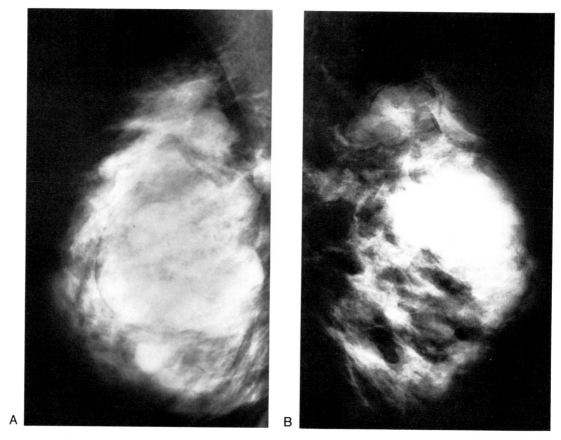

Fig. 11-17. (A & B) Left and right mediolateral oblique views in a 40-year-old woman with bilateral palpable masses. Round masses of varying size can be seen in both breasts. Some of the masses are associated with a halo sign. Ultrasound demonstrated multiple, bilateral cysts.

after aspiration and probably results from hemorrhage (Fig. 11-18). Tabar and Dean[25] have written that calcification may be seen in the wall of the cyst associated with a papillary carcinoma, but this is a rare occurrence.

The presence of a solitary cyst should raise the possibility of an underlying carcinoma causing obstruction of a duct. In spite of the fact that an associated malignancy is infrequent, radiologists should search for an accompanying group of microcalcifications or an ill-defined mass signifying the presence of a carcinoma particularly in the postmenopausal age group. Intracystic carcinomas are also rare, but should be a consideration in the presence of a solitary cyst.

If the suspected mammographic cyst is not palpable for diagnostic aspiration, ultrasound may be of benefit (see Ch. 20).

LIPOMAS

Lipomas are a common benign tumor of the breast. These slow-growing tumors usually present in older women and are of no clinical significance. Occasionally a woman will complain of an enlarged breast as the result of the presence of a lipoma.

Mammographically, lipomas present as an area of lucency with a surrounding thin capsule and are more

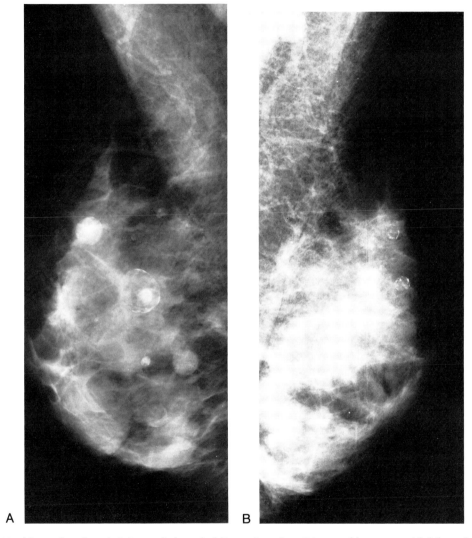

Fig. 11-18. (A & B) Left and right mediolateral oblique views in a 56-year-old woman with bilateral palpable masses and a history of multiple cyst aspirations. Ring and shell-like calcifications can be seen bilaterally resulting from bleeding into cysts at the time of aspiration. Several noncalcified cysts are also present.

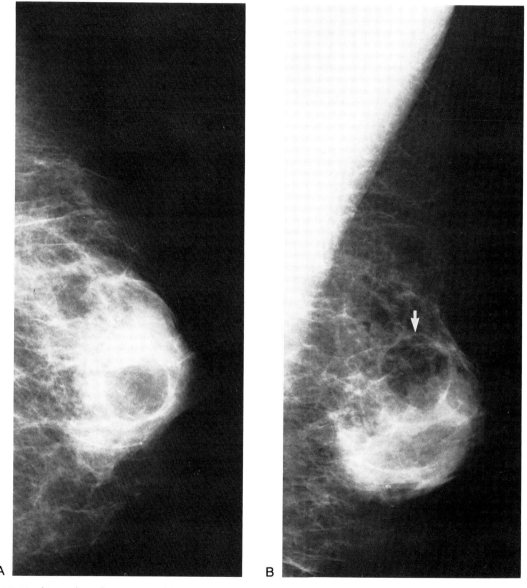

A   B

Fig. 11-19. (A & B) Right craniocaudal and mediolateral oblique views in an asymptomatic 54-year-old woman. The study demonstrates a well-delineated, 3-cm area of lucency with a surrounding capsule *(arrow)*. The findings are typical of a lipoma.

easily detected in the dense fibroglandular breast than in the fatty replaced breast (Figs. 11-19 and 11-20). They vary in size and can reach large proportions. Infarction of a lipoma is uncommon but can result in coarse or plaquelike calcifications. Fatty lobules, which are partially surrounded by trabeculae and Cooper's ligaments should not be confused with lipomas.

GALACTOCELES

Galactoceles are milk-containing cysts caused by inspissated milk obstructing a duct. They occur in women who abruptly stop breast feeding. This diagnosis is usually made on the basis of clinical history and needle aspiration, obviating the need for a mammogram.

The fibroglandular tissues are very dense during lactation; therefore mammography is of limited benefit. If mammography is performed, a galactocele may be seen as a round mass of variable density. Since milk contains lipid, the mass may be entirely lucent or may be of water- and fat-density. Examinations performed with a horizontal beam may show a fat-fluid level. Commonly, galactoceles are multiple and measure less than 3 cm in diameter. Capsular calcification can occur, producing a ring or eggshell appearance.

PAPILLOMAS

Papillomas are the most common cause of bloody or serous nipple discharge. Solitary papillomas usually develop within the retroareolar ducts, and multiple papillomas usually occur in the peripheral ducts. Most papillomas are not detectable on the mammogram. When visible, they may present as a solitary, round mass in the retroareolar area, a large solitary retroareolar duct, or clustered, small, round, peripheral densities. The masses usually are of low density (Figs. 11-21 and 11-22). Calcification of papillomas can occur, producing a crescent, rosette, or eggshell appearance.

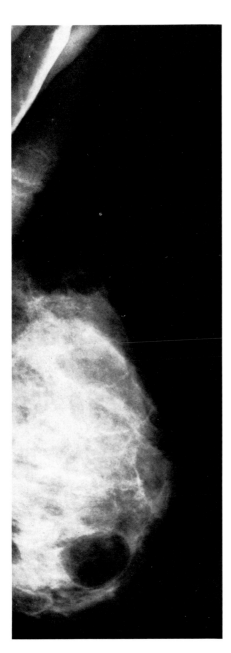

Fig. 11-20. Mediolateral oblique view in an asymptomatic 46-year-old woman. An area of lucency surrounded by a thin capsule is present inferiorly. Diagnosis: lipoma.

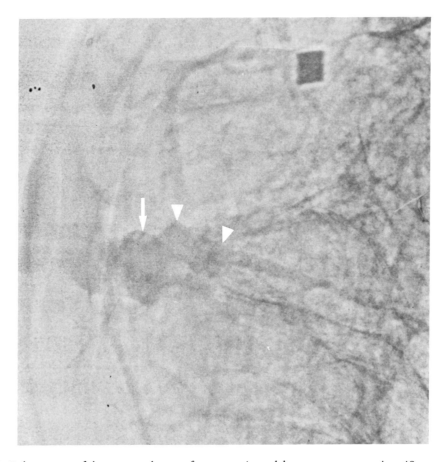

Fig. 11-21. Enlargement of the retroareolar area from a craniocaudal xeromammogram in a 48-year-old woman with bloody nipple discharge. The study demonstrates a round mass *(arrow)*, the borders of which are partially well defined, and a dilated duct *(arrowheads)* adjacent to the dorsal aspect of the mass. Papilloma and carcinoma should be of consideration. Histology: papilloma.

FIBROMATOSIS

Fibromatosis, an infiltrating fibroblastic proliferation, is a rare tumor of the breast. It does not metastasize, but can be locally aggressive and recur after resection. The breast involvement is usually not primary. Most often it is the result of extension of fibromatosis from the pectoralis fascia. Most cases have occurred in women in their late forties, although it has been reported from ages 8 to 80 years.

Both the clinical and the mammographic presentation of fibromatosis can simulate malignancy. Clinically, a mass that can be associated with skin or nipple retraction may be palpated. The mammogram generally demonstrates an ill-defined or spiculated mass with no associated calcifications.

GRANULAR CELL MYOBLASTOMA

Granular cell myoblastomas are rare benign tumors of the breast that can arise within the skin or within the parenchyma. Those that originate in the parenchyma can be mistaken for malignancy both clinically and mammographically and sometimes on pathologic examination. Radiographically, they appear as round masses with tentacle-like projections.

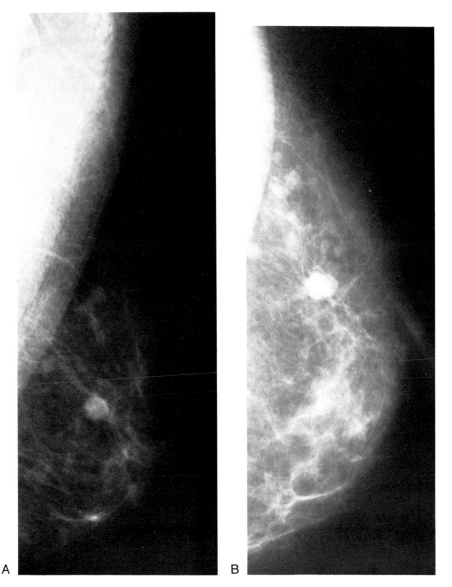

A   B

Fig. 11-22. Right mediolateral oblique **(A)** and craniocaudal **(B)** views in an asymptomatic 69-year-old woman. Multiple round masses are located in the superolateral quadrant. Diagnostic considerations include papillomas, cysts, metastases, and fibroadenomas. The possibility that the largest mass represents a carcinoma should be a strong consideration. Histology: multiple papillomas.

CYSTOSARCOMA PHYLLODES

The majority of cystosarcoma phyllodes tumors are benign, with 20 percent malignant. This tumor is discussed in Chapter 14.

SUGGESTED READINGS

1. Azzopardi JG: Problems in Breast Pathology. WB Saunders, Philadelphia, 1979
2. Cederlund CG, Gustavsson S, Linell F et al: Fibromatosis

of the breast mimicking carcinoma at mammography. Br J Radiol 57:98, 1984

3. Crothers JG, Butler NF, Fortt RW et al: Fibroadenolipoma of the breast. Br J Radiol 58:191, 1985

4. Dewhurst J: Breast disorders in children.and adolescents. Pediatr Clin North Am 28:287, 1981

5. Fayemi AO, Braun EV, Remy R: Fibromatosis of the breast. Am J Surg Pathol 3:501, 1979

6. Fisher ER, Palekar AS, Redmond C et al: Pathologic findings from the national surgical adjuvant breast project (protocol no. 4) VI. Invasive papillary cancer. AJCP 73:313, 1980

7. Gomez A, Mata JM, Donoso L et al: Galactocele: three distinctive radiographic appearances. Radiology 158:43, 1986

8. Gump FE, Sterschein MJ, Wolff M: Fibromatosis of the breast. Surg Gynecol Obstet 153:57, 1981

9. Haagensen CD: Diseases of the Breast. 3rd Ed. WB Saunders, Philadelphia, 1986

10. Hertel BF, Zaloudek C, Kempson RI: Breast adenomas. Cancer 37:2891, 1976

11. Hessler C, Schnyder P, Ozzello L: Hamartoma of the breast: diagnostic observation of 16 cases. Radiology 126:95, 1978

12. Homer MJ: Mammographic Evaluation of Breast Masses. p. 1. In: Campbell RE (ed): Contemporary Diagnostic Radiology. Vol. 2, Williams & Wilkins, Baltimore 1979

13. Homer MJ: Imaging features and management of characteristically benign and probable benign breast lesions. Radiol Clin North Am 25:939, 1987

14. Kalisher L, Long JA, Peyster RG: Extra-abdominal desmoid of the axillary tail mimicking breast carcinoma. AJR 126:903, 1976

15. Lanyi M: Diagnosis and Differential Diagnosis of Breast Calcifications. Springer-Verlag, New York, 1986

16. Martin JE: Atlas of Mammography: Histologic and Mammographic Correlations. Williams & Wilkins, Baltimore, 1982

17. Millis RR: Atlas of Breast Pathology. MTP Press Limited, Lancaster, England, 1984

18. Murad TM, Swaid S, Pritchett P: Malignant and benign papillary lesions of the breast. Hum Pathol 8:379, 1977

19. Orsi CJ, Feldhaus L, Sonnenfeld M: Unusual lesions of the breast. Radiol Clin North Am 21:67, 1983

20. Paulus DD: Benign diseases of the breast. Radiol Clin North Am 21:27, 1983

21. Pennes DR, Homer MJ: Disappearing breast masses caused by compression during mammography. Radiology 165:327, 1987

22. Rosen Y, Papasozomenos SC, Gardner B: Fibromatosis of the breast. Cancer 41:1409, 1978

23. Shepstone BJ, Wells CA, Berry AR et al: Mammographic appearance and histopathological description of a muscular hamartoma of the breast. Br J Radiol 58:459, 1985

24. Sickles EA: Breast calcifications: mammographic evaluation. Radiology 160:289, 1986

25. Tabar L, Dean PB: Teaching Atlas of Mammography. Thieme-Stratton, New York, 1983

26. Wolfe JN: Xeroradiography of the Breast. 2nd Ed. Charles C Thomas, Springfield, 1983

12
Other Benign Processes

Dawn R. Voegeli

FAT NECROSIS

Fat necrosis of the breast most commonly results from blunt trauma, biopsy, or cosmetic surgery. It can also follow breast infection or radiation therapy. Although 30 to 50 percent of patients give no history of trauma, it is likely that they have overlooked some remote incident.

The injury causes necrosis, with death and dissolution of fat cells. Healing occurs by fibrosis, which begins at the periphery of the lesion, and a connective tissue capsule may be formed. The oily substance within the lesion and the connective tissue capsule often calcify.

Many patients with fat necrosis are asymptomatic, but most will present with a painful, tender breast mass. The lesion is often superficial and can be quite hard and fixed. Because of fibrous proliferation around the mass, it is often larger clinically than it is radiographically. Skin thickening and retraction are present in approximately 50 percent of cases. The lesion can thus mimic carcinoma. Signs of inflammation may be present, and ecchymosis is present in 20 to 30 percent of cases.

The radiographic appearance of fat necrosis is extremely variable and can simulate carcinoma. A poorly defined and even stellate mass with hazy borders may be present (Fig. 12-1). In other cases the mass may be encapsulated, with mixed fat and water density (Figs. 12-2 and 12-3). A totally lucent mass with a connective tissue capsule ("oil cyst") is also common (Figs. 12-4 and 12-5). The fibrous capsule often calcifies (Figs. 12-6 and 12-7).

The calcifications associated with these masses are also quite varied in appearance (Fig. 12-8). There may be small rod-like calcifications irregularly scattered or grouped within the mass (Figs. 12-9 and 12-10). Dense spherical calcifications 2 to 3 mm in diameter may also be present, with no associated mass (Fig. 12-11). Serial radiographs demonstrate that the lesions generally become more densely calcified over time (Fig. 12-12).

Postbiopsy fat necrosis should be reassessed periodically with physical examination and radiographs to ensure that the suspicious lesion initially prompting biopsy has actually been removed. If the initial lesion was malignant, follow-up studies are necessary to exclude recurrence.

163

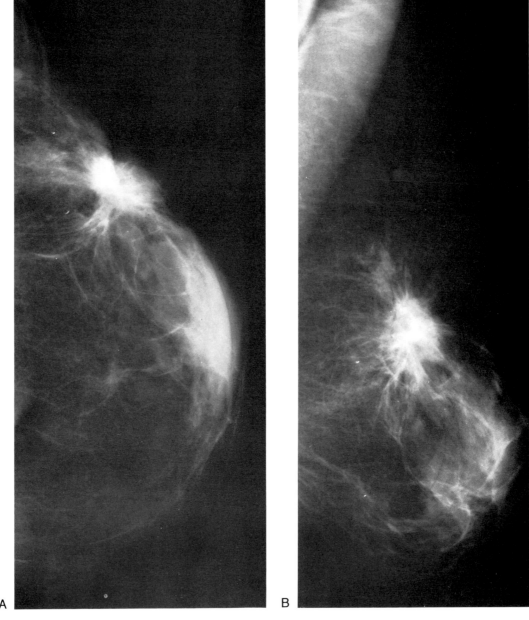

Fig. 12-1. Craniocaudal (**A**) and mediolateral oblique (**B**) views in a 77-year-old woman 3 months following biopsy of the right breast. A dense, spiculated mass associated with architectural distortion and skin retraction and thickening is present. Histology: fat necrosis.

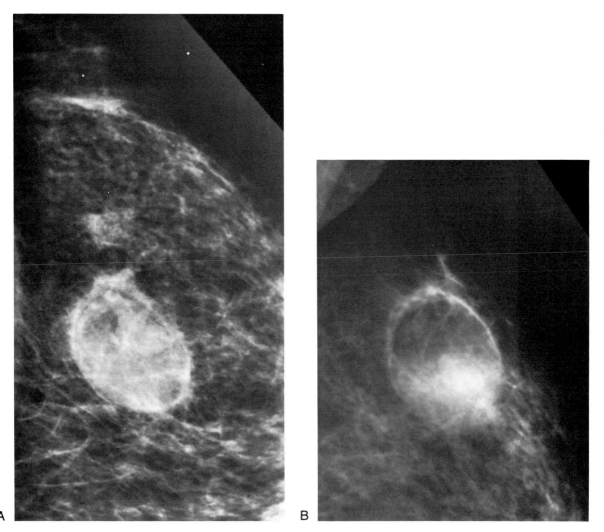

A   B

Fig. 12-2. Enlargements of craniocaudal **(A)** and mediolateral oblique **(B)** views in this 68-year-old woman 3 months after a benign biopsy. An encapsulated mass of mixed fat and water density is present. Histology: fat necrosis.

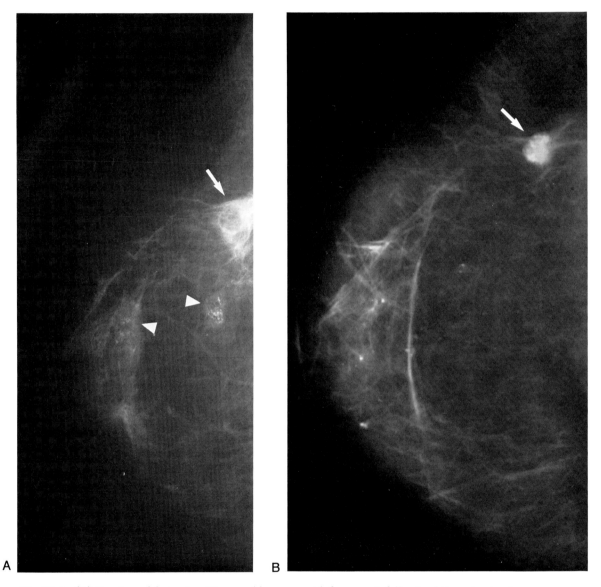

Fig. 12-3. **(A)** Craniocaudal view in a 63-year-old woman with fat necrosis following bilateral reduction mammoplasty. A mass of mixed fat and water density is present *(arrow)*. Other areas of poorly defined density are associated with tiny rod-like calcifications *(arrowheads)*. **(B)** Craniocaudal view 3 years later shows mixed density mass is now denser and partially calcified *(arrow)*. The other areas of density and calcifications have largely resolved.

Fig. 12-4. A totally lucent mass with a connective tissue capsule *(arrows)* represents fat necrosis in this 32-year-old woman who had been kicked in this breast by a horse.

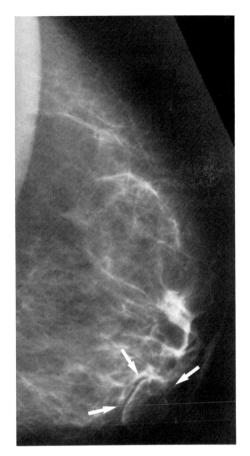

Fig. 12-5. Enlargement demonstrates an uncalcified oil cyst in this 71-year-old woman with no history of trauma *(arrow)*.

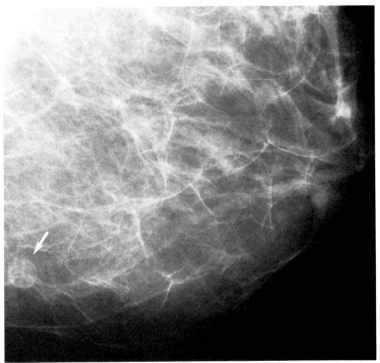

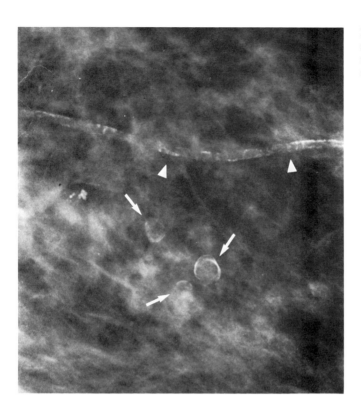

Fig. 12-6. Multiple partially calcified oil cysts are present in this woman with no history of trauma *(arrows)*. Note vascular calcification *(arrowheads)*.

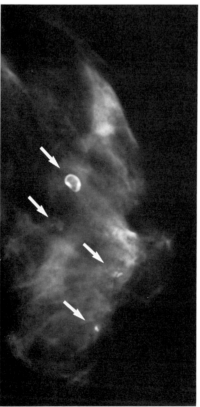

Fig. 12-7. Craniocaudal view in a 53-year-old woman who underwent reduction mammoplasty shows several areas of calcification representing fat necrosis *(arrows)*. These areas have been stable for 5 years.

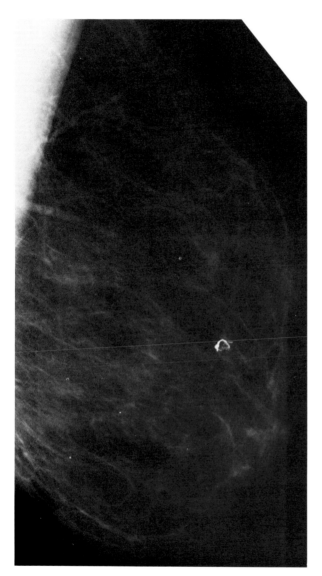

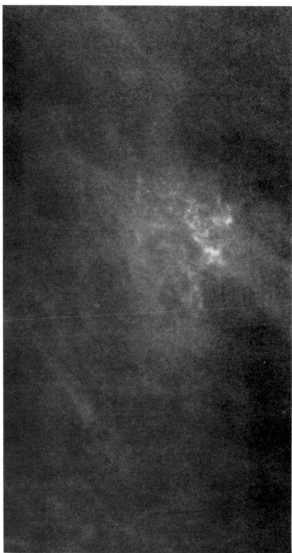

Fig. 12-8. Irregular calcification in an area of previous biopsy represents fat necrosis in this 50-year-old woman.

Fig. 12-9. Enlargement in a 45-year-old woman who had a breast biopsy 19 months previously. An ill-defined density associated with irregular microcalcifications of varying sizes is present and suggests malignancy. Histology: fat necrosis.

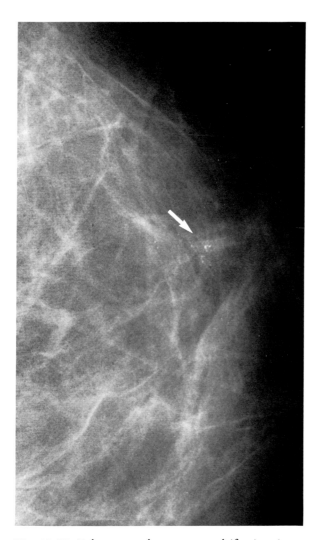

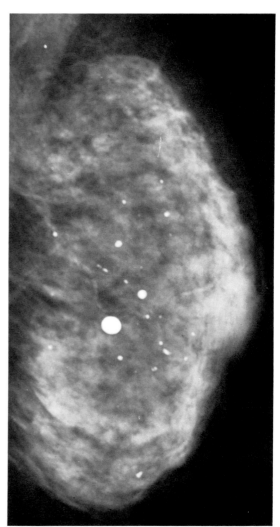

Fig. 12-10. Enlargement demonstrates calcifications in an area of previous abscess, probably representing fat necrosis *(arrow)*.

Fig. 12-11. Dense spherical calcifications of fat necrosis are present in this patient who had a previous biopsy.

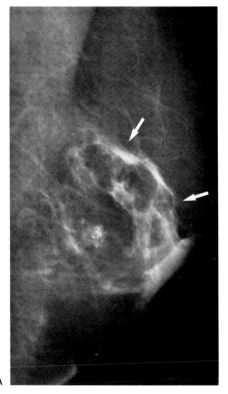

A

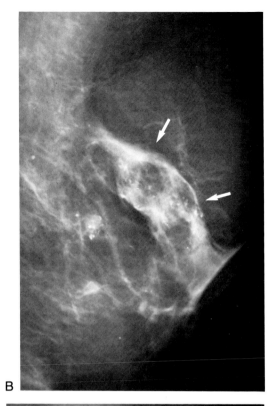

B

Fig. 12-12. (A–C) Serial mediolateral oblique views over a period of 1 year in a 63-year-old woman who had undergone reduction mammoplasty. There is progressive calcification of an area of mixed density fat necrosis *(arrows)*.

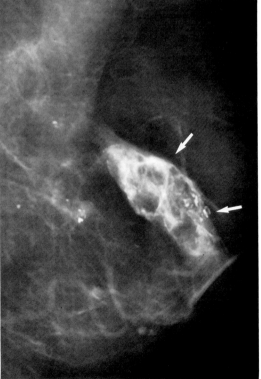

C

HEMATOMA

Blunt or surgical trauma is the most common cause of breast hematoma. Patients who are anticoagulated or who have clotting abnormalities may develop hematomas after seemingly insignificant trauma.

The combination of hemorrhage and edema results in an ill-defined mass or a diffuse area of increased density on the mammogram. Localized skin thickening is often present. Although the findings simulate carcinoma, the history of trauma suggests a conservative approach. Within 4 to 6 weeks the abnormality will decrease

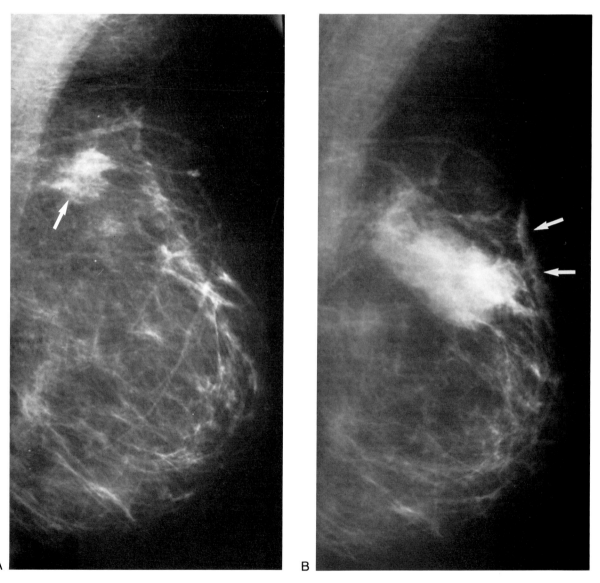

A   B

Fig. 12-13. (A) Mediolateral oblique view in a 46-year-old woman who had had a left mastectomy for breast carcinoma. A new ill-defined density is present superiorly *(arrow)*. The patient underwent biopsy. Histology: normal breast tissue. **(B)** Two weeks later a firm mass was palpable at the biopsy site and a mediolateral oblique view shows a dense hematoma in this area. Skin thickening is present *(arrows)*. *(Figure continues.)*

markedly in size or even disappear (Fig. 12-13). Occasionally a hematoma may organize and persist as an irregular or more sharply defined mass. Fat necrosis or scar formation may be late findings.

If mammography and needle aspiration of a palpable mass are planned, it is best to perform the mammogram first. This is because needle aspiration may lead to hematoma formation, and a subsequent mammogram could be falsely interpreted as positive for carcinoma (Fig. 12-14). Alternatively, a large hematoma could obscure important mammographic details.

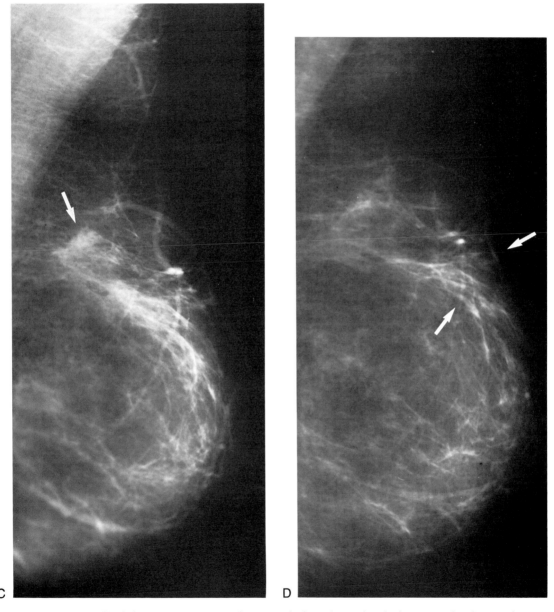

C   D

Fig. 12-13 *(Continued).* **(C)** Repeat mammography 2 months later shows that the hematoma has decreased in size. An area of residual density superiorly may represent part of the original abnormality *(arrow).* **(D)** Three months later there has been almost complete resolution of the hematoma. Minimal architectural distortion remains *(arrows),* as well as the area of residual density superiorly.

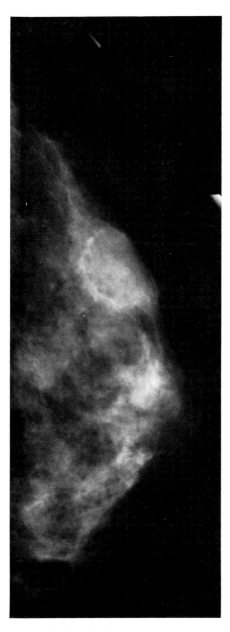

Fig. 12-14. Mediolateral oblique view in a patient who had needle aspiration of a palpable mass prior to mammography. There is a dense, ill-defined mass present superiorly. Clinically, a hematoma is now present. It is not possible to determine whether the mammographic mass is due entirely to hematoma, or if an underlying carcinoma is present.

As with fat necrosis, hematomas occurring after breast biopsy should be followed clinically and mammographically to ensure that the original abnormality was completely removed.

ACUTE MASTITIS AND ABSCESS

Acute mastitis occurs almost exclusively during lactation. The typical clinical features include fever and chills, painful breast swelling, redness and hyperemia of the skin, and an increased white blood cell count with a left shift. Painful axillary lymphadenopathy may be present, and multiple abscesses may develop within the breast. This clinical picture in a lactating woman is diagnostic, and mammography is rarely performed. The usual causative organism is *Staphylococcus aureus,* and therapy consists of 10 to 14 days of antibiotics.

Mastitis and abscess formation in older patients is uncommon, and usually results from infection of sweat or sebaceous glands. Patients may present with a low-grade fever and a painful, tender mass. Lesions are most commonly superficial. They may involve the nipple and areola, and skin thickening and retraction are often present (Fig. 12-15). If diffuse changes are present, the physical findings mimic inflammatory carcinoma of the breast.

Mammography is more commonly performed in these older patients. Unfortunately, the mammographic findings may also simulate carcinoma. Radiographs demonstrate a poorly defined area of increased density. A prominent venous pattern, thickening and retraction of the nipple and skin, and axillary lymphadenopathy may be present (Fig. 12-16). A more localized and poorly defined mass may represent an abscess (Fig. 12-17).

Patients may be treated conservatively with a trial of antibiotics if there is a clinical suspicion of infection. If an advanced carcinoma were actually present, delay of treatment for 1 to 2 weeks would probably make no difference in the patient's prognosis.

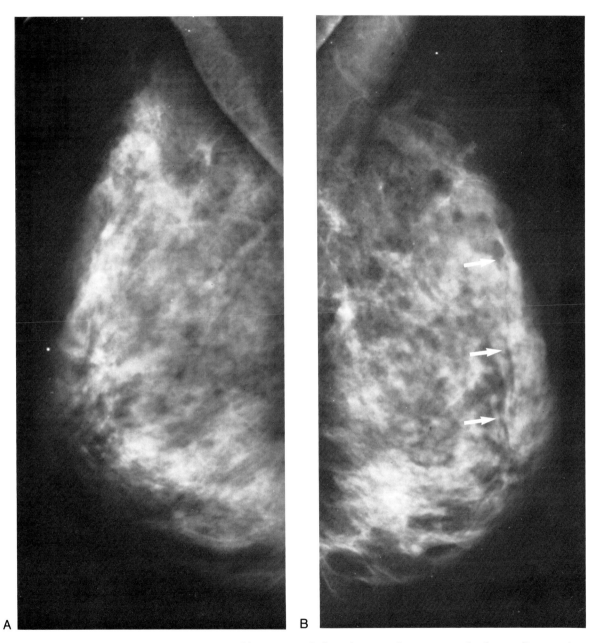

A   B

Fig. 12-15. Localized mastitis in a 42-year-old woman with dense breasts. There is a superficial area of increased density associated with skin thickening **(B & D,** *arrows*). Comparison views of the contralateral breast are included **(A & C).** *(Figure continues.)*

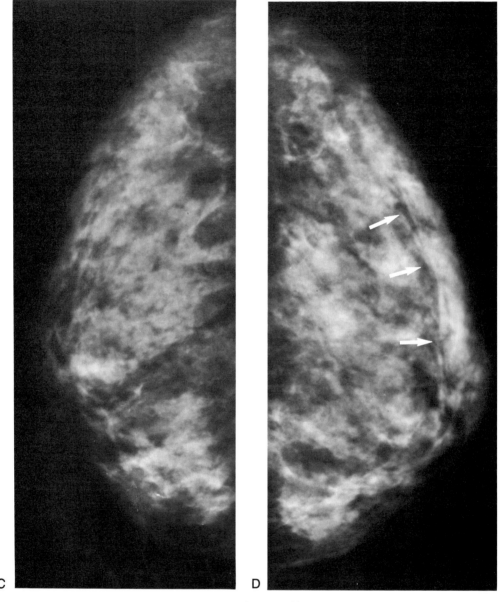

C   D

Fig. 12-15 *(Continued).*

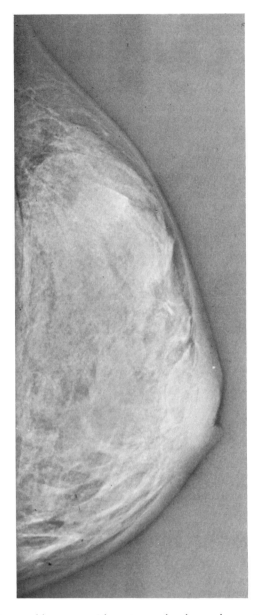

Fig. 12-16. Xerogram in a 37-year-old woman with a retroareolar abscess demonstrates thickening and retraction of the nipple and areola. The abscess itself is difficult to define.

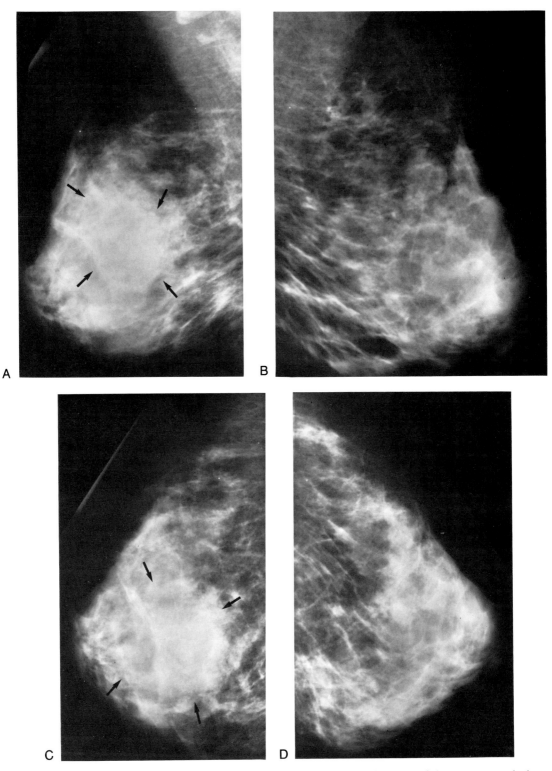

Fig. 12-17. A poorly defined area of increased density is present in the left breast of this woman with dense fibroglandular tissue (**A & C,** *arrows*). Comparison views of the right breast (**B & D**) help to define the asymmetry.

CHRONIC ABSCESS

In the presence of a chronic abscess, the mammogram demonstrates a masslike density with architectural distortion. The abscess may be encapsulated, with somewhat smooth borders. Skin and nipple thickening and retraction may be present. Such an appearance, coupled with a less dramatic response to antibiotic therapy, causes this lesion to be easily confused with carcinoma.

"SECRETORY DISEASE"

Inspissated lactiferous material can be retained within dilated mammary ducts. The material may calcify, producing large, dense, smooth calcifications. The calcifications tend to be multiple and bilateral and are oriented toward the nipple. They may be needlelike or spherical (Figs. 12-18 and 12-19).

Retained lactiferous material may also extravasate periductally, causing a chemical mastitis. The resulting chronic inflammatory reaction results in plasma cell infiltration, hence the term "plasma cell mastitis." Necrosis, periductal fibrosis, and intraductal or periductal calcifications result. The condition usually occurs in older women.

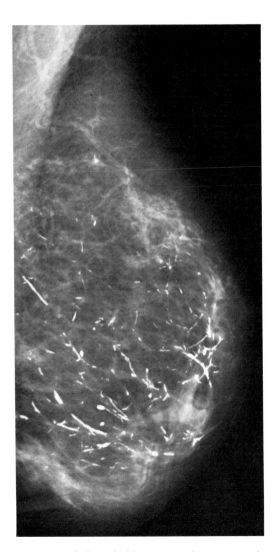

Fig. 12-18. Mediolateral oblique view demonstrates large, dense, needlelike intraductal secretory calcifications. Note their orientation toward the nipple.

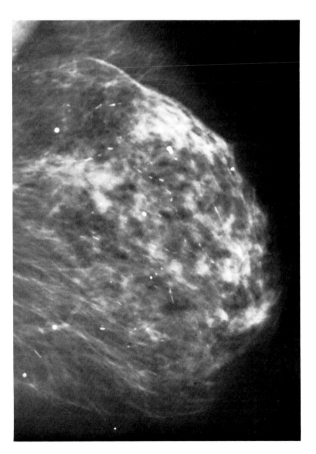

Fig. 12-19. Mediolateral oblique view demonstrates both spherical and needlelike secretory calcifications. The calcifications are large, dense, and smooth in appearance.

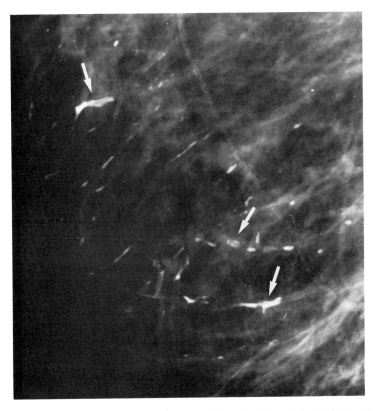

Fig. 12-20. Enlargement demonstrates typical calcifications of periductal mastitis. Both intraductal and periductal *(arrows)* needlelike calcifications are present.

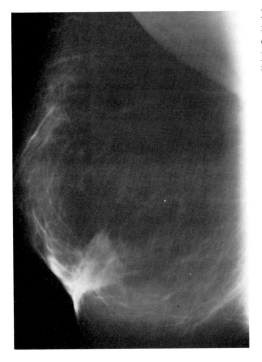

Fig. 12-21. Mediolateral oblique view shows a retroareolar triangle of increased density associated with nipple retraction in this patient with plasma cell mastitis. Typical calcifications are absent.

The typical calcifications seen in periductal mastitis are large, smooth, and dense. They are either needlelike or spherical and have hollow centers if they are periductal in location (Fig. 12-20). They are most often multiple and bilateral and are oriented toward the nipple. The needlelike calcifications may exhibit a branching pattern. The spherical calcifications may actually represent fat necrosis.

Although plasma cell mastitis can occur anywhere in the breast, it is classically located in the subareolar area and causes clinically palpable subareolar thickening. Serous or milky nipple discharge may occur, and nipple retraction frequently develops over the course of several years. No clinical signs of inflammation are present. Mammography typically demonstrates a triangular area of increased subareolar density, with its apex directed toward the nipple. Areolar thickening and retraction may be present, as well as the classic coarse, radiating calcifications described above (Fig. 12-21).

ARTERIAL CALCIFICATION

Arterial calcification is associated with advanced age and may be more common in the breasts of patients with diabetes or hypertension. It appears as parallel discontinuous bands following a sinuous course (Fig. 12-22). Although well-developed arterial calcification is easily identified, the early stages with only sparse calcifications can simulate malignancy. Additional oblique and magnification views may be helpful for clarification (Fig. 12-23).

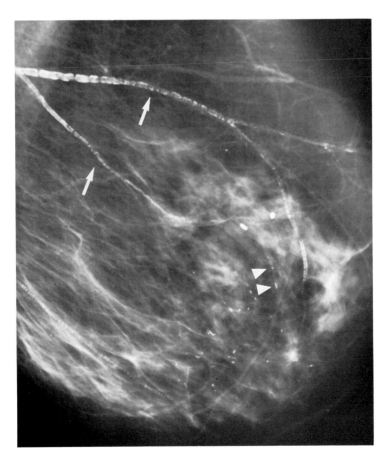

Fig. 12-22. Well-developed vascular calcifications appear as parallel discontinuous bands *(arrows)*. Early vascular calcifications are more isolated *(arrowheads)*. Scattered secretory calcifications are also present.

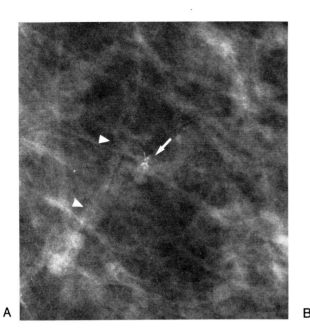

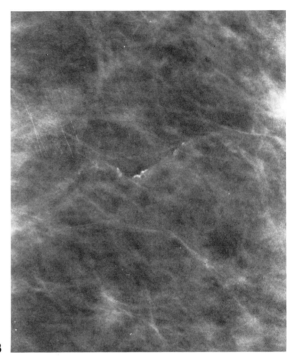

A

B

Fig. 12-23. (A) Enlargement of a craniocaudal view reveals suspicious-appearing calcifications *(arrow)* adjacent to several blood vessels *(arrowheads)*. **(B)** Enlargement of the mediolateral oblique view demonstrates that these are actually early vascular calcifications.

SUGGESTED READINGS

1. Adair FE, Munzer JT: Fat necrosis of the female breast. Am J Surg 74:117, 1947
2. Baber CE, Libshitz HI: Bilateral fat necrosis of the breast following reduction mammoplasties. AJR 128:508, 1977
3. Bassett LW, Gold RH, Cove HC: Mammographic spectrum of traumatic fat necrosis: the fallibility of "pathognomonic" signs of carcinoma. AJR 130:119, 1978
4. Bassett LW, Gold RH, Mirra JM: Nonneoplastic breast calcifications in lipid cysts: development after excision and primary irradiation. AJR 138:335, 1982
5. Coren GS, Libshitz HI, Patchefsky AS: Fat necrosis of the breast: mammographic and thermographic findings. Br J Radiol 47:758, 1974
6. Haagensen CD: Diseases of the Breast. 2nd Ed. WB Saunders, Philadelphia, 1971
7. Hoeffken W, Lányi M: Mammography. WB Saunders, Philadelphia, 1977
8. Orson LW, Cigtay OS: Fat necrosis of the breast: characteristic xeromammographic appearance. Radiology 146:35, 1983
9. Paulus DD: Benign diseases of the breast. Radiol Clin North Am 21:27, 1983
10. Schmitt EL, Threatt B: Mammographic intra-arterial calcifications. J Assoc Can Radiol 35:14, 1984
11. Sickles EA: Breast calcifications: mammographic evaluation. Radiology 160:289, 1986
12. Vanel D, Bergiron C, Contesso G, Kobotek G, Piékarski JD, Markovitz P: Étude radio-clinico-pathologique de 29 cystosteatonécroses mammaries primitives. J Radiol 62:7, 1981

13

Mammographic Signs of Malignancy

Dawn R. Voegeli

The usual breast carcinoma arises from the epithelium of the mammary duct. It begins as cellular hyperplasia and progresses to atypia and the eventual formation of an intraductal mass. This mass then becomes invasive by penetrating the basement membrane of the duct. From there, the tumor metastasizes to axillary lymph nodes and to distant sites by way of the lymphatic system. Associated with growth of the carcinoma is a proliferation of the adjacent connective tissue elements of the breast. The various stages of tumor development and associated connective tissue hyperplasia lead to a wide range of mammographic signs of malignancy. Depending on the stage of development, the signs may be easily recognizable (e.g., a spiculated mass) or very subtle (e.g., a vague asymmetric density). The density of the surrounding fibroglandular tissue is also important, in that normal tissue may obscure these signs.

The survival rate of patients with breast carcinoma is inversely related to tumor size and to the number of axillary lymph nodes that are found to contain malignant cells. This fact has led to an increase in routine mammographic screening of asymptomatic women in hopes of detecting carcinomas at their earliest possible, and even curable, stages. It has been shown that mammographic screening does not detect more cancers;

rather, the same tumors are diagnosed at earlier stages. The term "minimal carcinoma" can be used to describe some of these early cancers. As originally defined by Gallager and Martin,[3] it includes (1) noninvasive intraductal carcinoma, (2) lobular carcinoma in situ, and (3) invasive carcinoma forming a mass with a diameter no greater than 0.5 cm in diameter. These criteria have been modified in the National Cancer Institute definition, which includes any carcinoma no more than 1.0 cm in size. Only 5.5 percent of minimal carcinomas are associated with positive axillary lymph nodes. This category of tumors may include up to 95 percent of curable lesions, and the 10-year survival of patients in this group is reported to be 95 percent.

The radiologist must recognize not only the obvious primary and secondary signs of more advanced cancers, but also the subtle changes associated with early carcinomas. As many as 20 percent of breast carcinomas are diagnosed by these early signs. Unfortunately, the specificity of these subtle signs is less than that of the classical signs. If we attempt to detect curable cancer, we must accept a significant number of false-positive biopsies, as illustrated by the fact that many screening programs have only a 10 to 30 percent true positive rate for the detection of carcinoma.

PRIMARY SIGNS
OF CARCINOMA

The primary signs of carcinoma as detected by mammography are those due to the tumor itself. They include masses and calcifications.

Masses

The masses caused by breast carcinoma vary significantly in appearance. They tend to be very dense and are most often classified into one of three categories: stellate, knobby, or circumscribed.

Stellate lesions tend to have an intermediate growth rate and are associated with a significant degree of fibrous proliferation. Because of this connective tissue hyperplasia, the clinical size of a mass is often greater than the size as measured by mammography. Stellate cancers are infiltrative in nature and are often associated with secondary signs of malignancy such as skin thickening, retraction, and architectural distortion. Malignant calcifications are also commonly present (see next

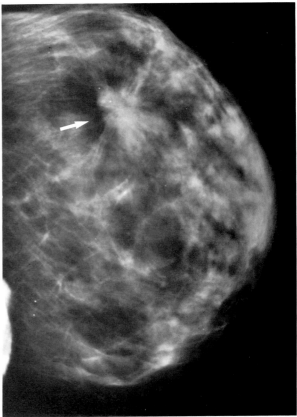

Fig. 13-2. Craniocaudal view demonstrating an infiltrating ductal carcinoma that has formed a stellate mass *(arrow)*.

section). A stellate lesion is composed of a central mass whose borders are made up of radiating spicules of various lengths (Figs. 13-1 and 13-2). The central mass is dense and should not have lucencies within it. The spicules are dense, fine, and radiate in all directions, especially toward the nipple. Malignant cells are often found growing out along the spicules, and "satellite" masses often form along their course (Fig. 13-3).

Stellate masses are usually the easiest type of cancer to recognize on mammography, although they may be obscured by surrounding dense fibroglandular tissue (Fig. 13-4). Overlap of normal breast tissue may mimic a stellate lesion. Further evaluation with oblique, coned down compression and magnification films will usually reveal that the density is due to overlap (Figs. 13-5 and 13-6).

Knobby or nodular masses tend to be more cellular and rapidly growing and are less often associated with con-

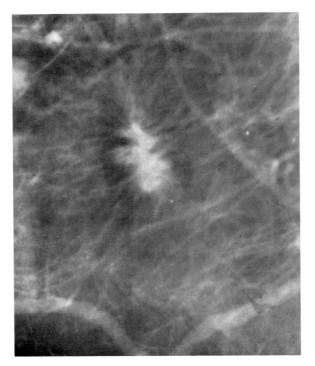

Fig. 13-1. This typical stellate carcinoma is composed of a dense central tumor mass and radiating spicules of various lengths. Histology: infiltrating ductal carcinoma.

Fig. 13-3. Enlargement of an infiltrating ductal carcinoma that has formed many "satellite" masses *(arrows)*. Note the fine calcifications scattered throughout the lesion.

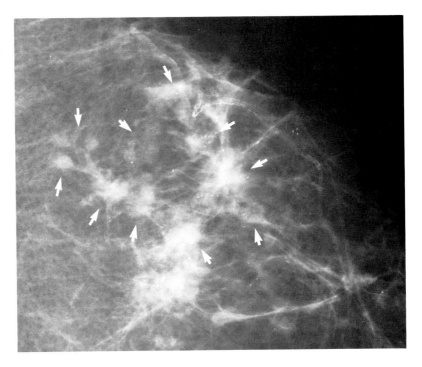

Fig. 13-4. Mediolateral view demonstrating a stellate mass in the superior portion of the breast *(arrows)*. This infiltrating ductal carcinoma is partially obscured by overlapping dense fibroglandular tissue.

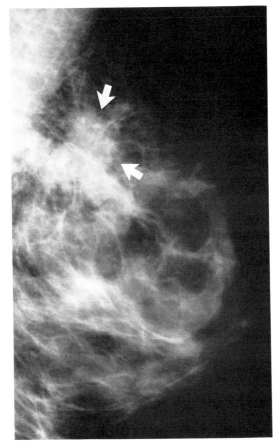

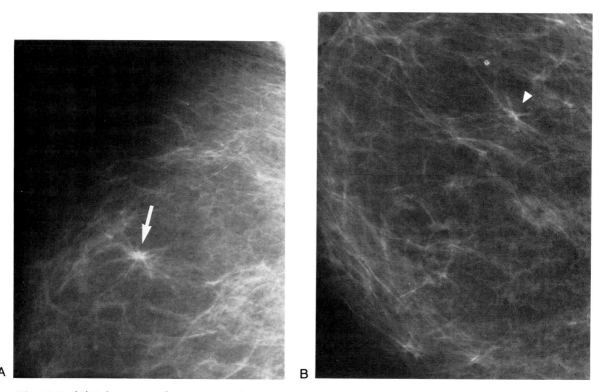

Fig. 13-5. (A) Enlargement of an apparent stellate mass on the mediolateral oblique view *(arrow)*. **(B)** An additional film with slightly different obliquity demonstrates that the apparent stellate mass is not volumetric in nature and is caused by overlap of normal structures *(arrowhead)*.

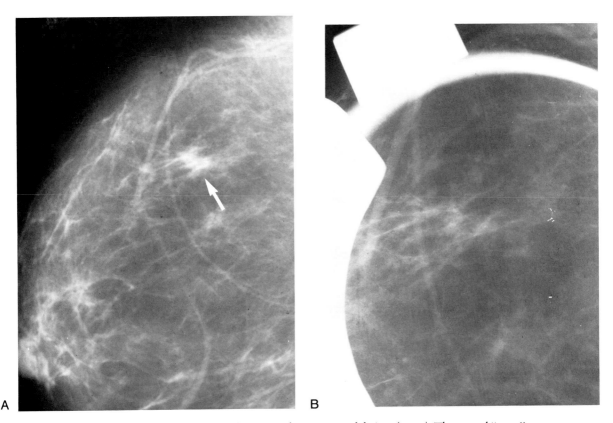

A B

Fig. 13-6. (A) There is an apparent stellate density on this craniocaudal view *(arrow)*. The central "mass" appears to have lucencies within it. **(B)** A coned down compression view with magnification demonstrates that no mass is present.

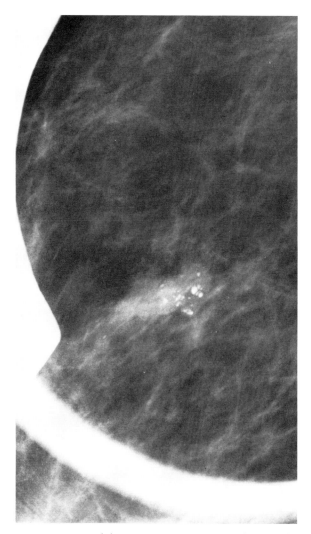

Fig. 13-7. Coned down compression view with magnification shows a knobby carcinoma. Note the poorly defined borders and associated microcalcifications.

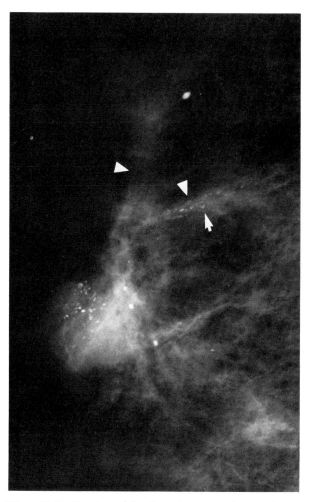

Fig. 13-8. Craniocaudal view demonstrating a dense, knobby tumor. This infiltrating ductal carcinoma has extensions radiating out into the surrounding breast tissue *(arrowheads)*. Malignant-type calcifications are present within the mass and its extensions *(arrow)*.

nective tissue changes. The tumor is composed of multiple tiny masses, which overlap to form a dense, knobby lesion with indistinct borders (Fig. 13-7). The mass may eventually form radiating spicules and may be associated with skin thickening and retraction (Fig. 13-8). Malignant calcifications may also be present.

Well-circumscribed masses are expanding lesions that displace adjacent breast tissue and tend to cause fewer secondary changes. The tumor may be round, oval, or lobulated in shape, and its borders are completely or partially well defined (Fig. 13-9). There may even be an associated "halo" sign, which is a rim of radiolucency surrounding part or all of the mass. Previously thought to be pathognomonic of a benign lesion, the halo sign has since been described in association with well-circumscribed malignancies. Although 98 percent of circumscribed masses are benign, some types of carcinoma

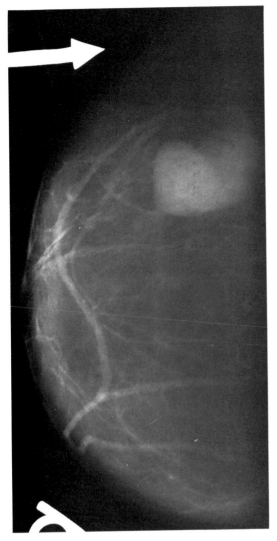

Fig. 13-9. This well-circumscribed and lobulated mass is an intracystic papillary carcinoma.

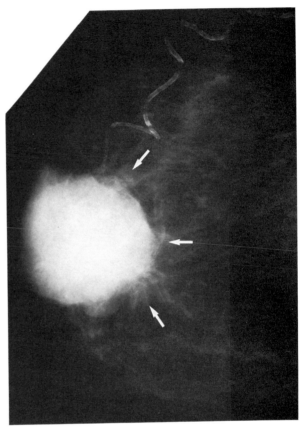

Fig. 13-10. Craniocaudal view demonstrating a large, dense retroareolar infiltrating ductal carcinoma with mostly well-defined borders. Other segments of the border are poorly defined and even spiculated *(arrows)*.

typically present in this fashion, including medullary, mucinous, and papillary carcinoma of the breast, as well as sarcomas, metastases, lymphoma, leukemia, and myeloma. These tumors are discussed in detail in Chapter 14. A segment of indistinct border, slight skin thickening or retraction, or a few radiating connective tissue spicules may be the only sign of malignancy, and one must search carefully for these signs (Fig. 13-10). Additional oblique or coned down compression views

may be very helpful in this regard, and ultrasound can be useful in determining whether a mass is cystic or solid.

Many masses are mixed in appearance (e.g., partially well-defined and partially stellate), as illustrated in Figure 13-11. In addition, many of them do not fit clearly into any of these groups, but present only as irregular or poorly defined masses (Fig. 13-12). Sickles reported

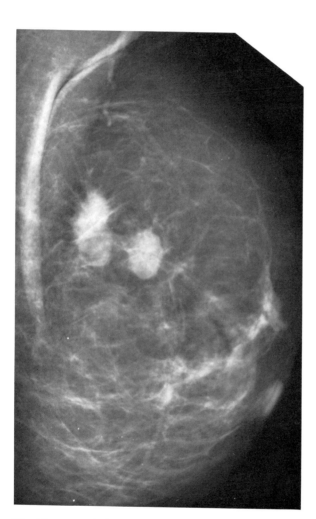

Fig. 13-11. Mediolateral oblique view of an unusual bilobed infiltrating ductal carcinoma that is partially well defined and partially stellate in outline.

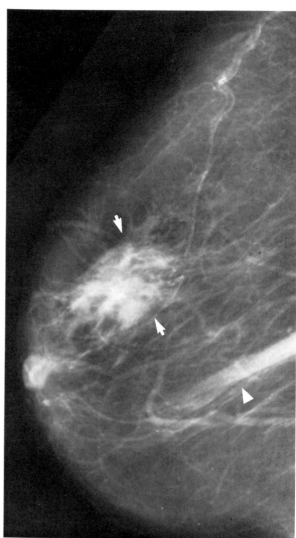

Fig. 13-12. Mediolateral oblique view demonstrating an irregular, poorly defined infiltrating ductal carcinoma *(arrows)*. A skin fold is seen inferiorly *(arrowhead)*.

that only 16 percent of the masses in his series of 300 nonpalpable carcinomas fit into one of the "classic" categories.

Calcifications

Although up to 80 percent of breast carcinomas have calcifications on histologic examination, radiographically visible calcifications are present in only 55 percent. Approximately two-thirds of these cases will demonstrate calcifications associated with a mass, while the remainder will have only calcifications. In other words, approximately 20 percent of breast carcinomas will present only with calcifications. Whether these calcifications are caused by mineralization of necrotic debris or are secretory products of increased cellular activity is unknown. The most typical characteristic of malignant calcifications is their extreme variability. They vary in distribution, size, form, density, and number (Fig. 13-13). The calcifications tend

to form in clusters. The number of calcifications within a cluster is extremely variable, and multiple clusters may be present. They may be present alone, or found within or near a mass. The distribution of calcifications is usually random, although they can follow the course of a mammary duct.

Malignant calcifications are generally smaller than typical benign calcifications. They range in size from 0.08 to 5 mm but are usually 0.2 mm or less in size. A diagnostic feature is that the calcifications within a single cluster will vary in size.

Calcifications also vary greatly in shape, both in general and within a single cluster. They may be linear, branching, round, lacelike, angular, punctate, or granular. Their borders are irregular in contour. The density of malignant calcifications is also variable. They tend to be less dense than typical benign calcifications and will vary in density within a single cluster.

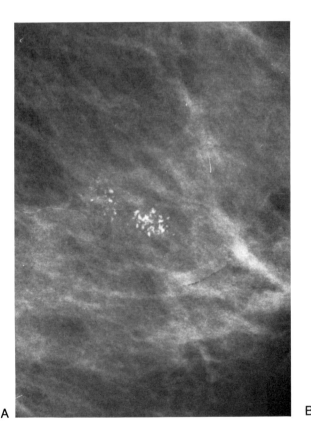

A

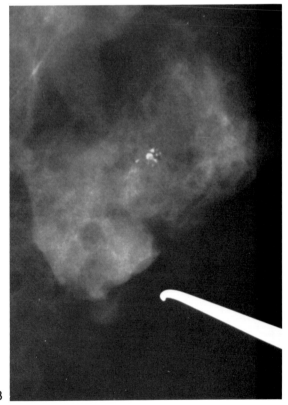

B

Fig. 13-13. (A–F) Enlargements of malignant calcifications in five different patients. The calcifications vary in size, shape, and density within each cluster, and also from case to case. *(Figure continues.)*

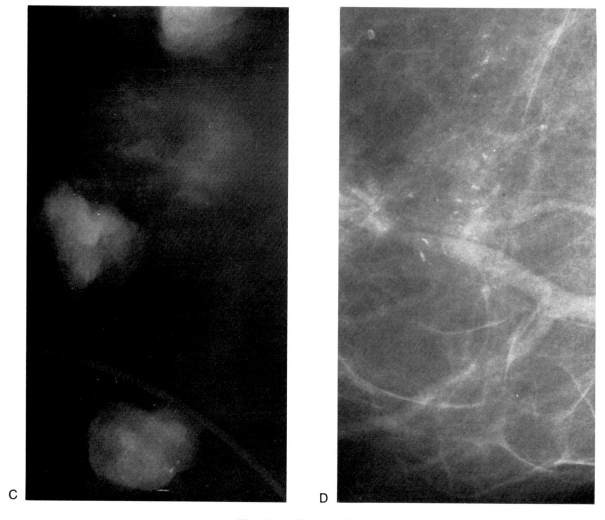

Fig. 13-13 *(Continued)*.

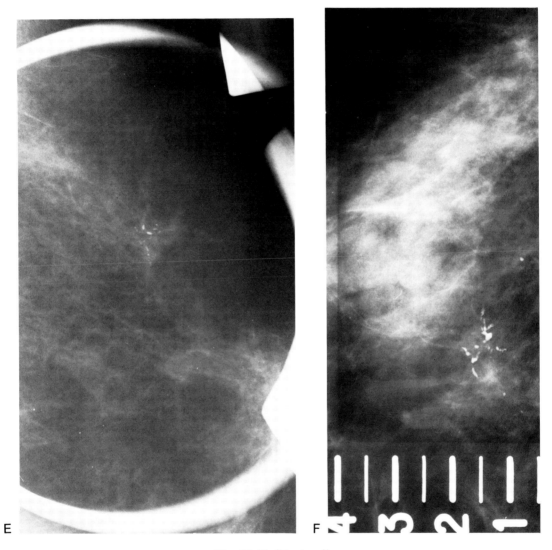

Fig. 13-13 *(Continued).*

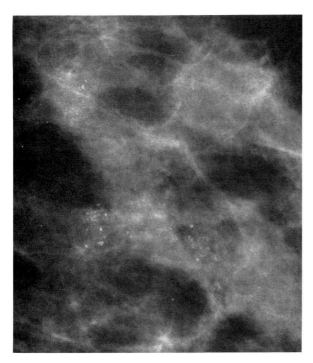

Fig. 13-14. Multiple clusters of calcifications are the only sign of malignancy in this comedocarcinoma. The tumor was mostly intraductal but did show a few areas of infiltration.

Comedocarcinoma is a type of breast cancer that grows extensively within the mammary ducts, filling them with plugs of yellow pastelike material. The bulk of the tumor is intraductal, but invasive foci may be present. Usually there are no clinical signs of carcinoma and no masses are found on mammography. The mammogram instead demonstrates malignant-appearing calcifications forming casts within dilated mammary ducts. The calcifications will vary in size, shape, and density but are classically irregular linear and branching forms. Only a single duct may be involved, or the tumor may be more extensive and may fill multiple ducts within a defined area of the breast (Figs. 13-14 and 13-15).

In spite of the discussion above, reliable differentiation of benign from malignant calcifications is not always possible. In fact, only up to 25 percent of biopsies performed because of suspicious calcifications may actually be malignant. The problem arises because many benign conditions form calcifications that mimic malignancy. Adenosis, papillomatosis, fat necrosis, and

early calcifications in fibroadenomas and arteries may be misleading. The use of microfocal spot magnification can greatly improve diagnostic accuracy in the evaluation of calcifications. It results in sharper, more detailed images and greater spatial resolution. Individual calcifications are more clearly seen, and additional calcifications can often be detected. Although magnification may rarely reveal a small carcinoma that would not otherwise have been detected, its main use is to provide a definitive benign or malignant diagnosis in patients whose conventional mammograms are equivocal. Use of this technique should result in fewer biopsies of benign lesions.

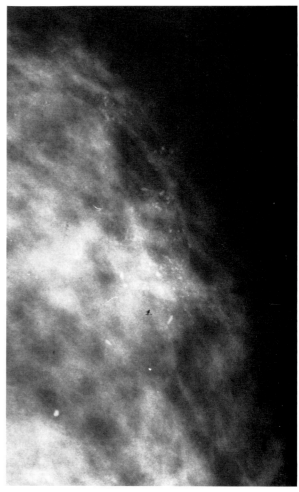

Fig. 13-15. Classic malignant calcifications are scattered throughout a confined area of the breast in this example of comedocarcinoma. The cancer was entirely intraductal.

SECONDARY SIGNS OF MALIGNANCY

The secondary signs of carcinoma are changes within the breast that occur as a result of the tumor. They include architectural distortion, skin thickening and retraction, nipple and areolar thickening and retraction, abnormal ductal patterns, increased vascularity, and lymphadenopathy.

Architectural Distortion

The desmoplastic reaction associated with carcinoma results in a localized change in the appearance of the breast parenchyma. An increase in stromal and periductal collagen causes a retractive phenomenon that has a varied appearance depending on its location. It may result in an abnormal arrangement of the mammary ducts and Cooper's ligaments. It may cause distortion or infolding of the normal interfaces between the breast parenchyma and subcutaneous or retromammary fat (Figs. 13-16 to 13-19). This localized architectural distortion should be visible in two different projections. It may be the only visible sign of carcinoma, especially in very dense breasts. Additional magnification, coned down compression, and oblique views may be helpful in better defining the abnormal area.

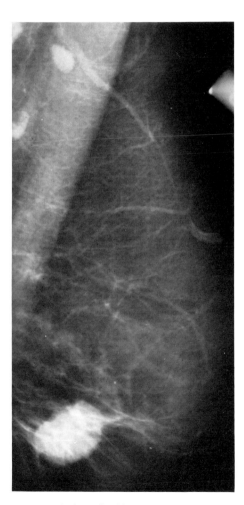

Fig. 13-16. Mediolateral oblique view demonstrating a well-defined mass with surrounding architectural distortion. Histology: infiltrating ductal carcinoma.

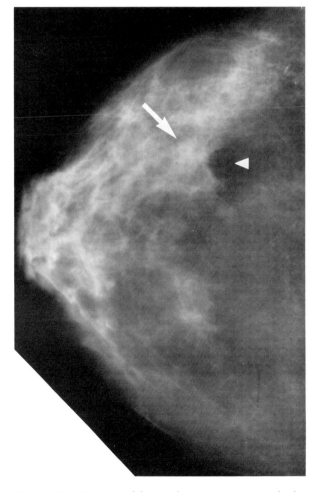

Fig. 13-17. Craniocaudal view demonstrating a poorly defined carcinoma *(arrow)* with associated "tenting" or retraction of the glandular tissue posteriorly *(arrowhead)*.

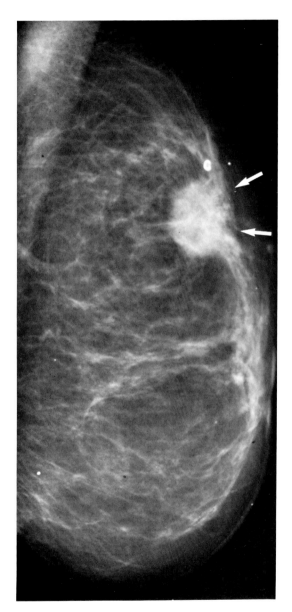

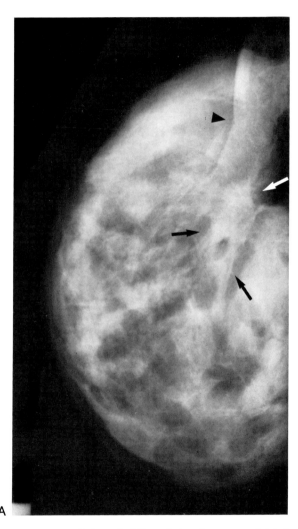

A

Fig. 13-18. Mediolateral oblique view demonstrating a poorly defined mass which distorts the normal interface between the breast parenchyma and the subcutaneous fat *(arrows)*. Although difficult to appreciate on this reproduction, localized skin thickening is present over this infiltrating ductal carcinoma.

Fig. 13-19. Mediolateral oblique **(A)** and craniocaudal **(B)** views demonstrate architectural distortion *(arrows)* and skin thickening and retraction *(arrowheads)*. The underlying stellate mass is difficult to identify. Histology: infiltrating ductal carcinoma with all axillary lymph nodes free of metastases *(Figure continues)*.

Skin Thickening and Retraction

Skin retraction is due to the fibrosis and shortening of Cooper's ligaments, which is incited by the carcinoma. This phenomenon is the same as that discussed in the section on architectural distortion. The skin loses its normal convex border and becomes flat or even concave. The retraction must be seen in tangent to be appreciated on the mammogram and is often not appreciated clinically. Spicules of connective tissue and tumor may be visible between the cancer and the skin. The presence of skin retraction suggests a locally advanced carcinoma.

The normal mammary skin thickness ranges from 1.5 to 3.0 mm and should be symmetric bilaterally. The skin is usually thicker in the inframammary area. Localized skin thickening is usually located near the tumor and indicates a locally advanced cancer (Fig. 13-20). It must be seen in tangent to be appreciated and is often detected on the mammogram before it is appreciated clinically. It may call attention to an otherwise poorly seen mass.

Diffuse skin thickening occurs with "inflammatory carcinoma" and is a result of diffuse lymphangitic metastases. This type of carcinoma is discussed in detail in Chapter 14.

Nipple and Areolar Changes

Nipple retraction is worrisome if it is unilateral and of recent onset. It is caused by thickening and foreshortening of the retroareolar ducts in response to a retroareolar carcinoma (Fig. 13-21). It may also be caused by a more distant tumor that has spread to the retroareolar area. The ducts between the tumor and nipple-areolar complex are often prominent (Fig. 13-22). Associated thickening of the areola may be present. Paget's disease of the breast is an uncommon type of breast carcinoma that mainly involves the nipple and areola and is discussed in detail in Chapter 14.

Abnormal Ductal Patterns

Carcinoma may cause shortening, distortion, or dilatation of the mammary ducts, presenting as localized prominence and tortuosity of multiple ducts, or as a

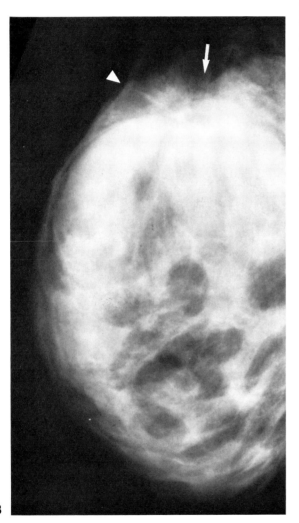

B

Fig. 13-19 *(Continued)*.

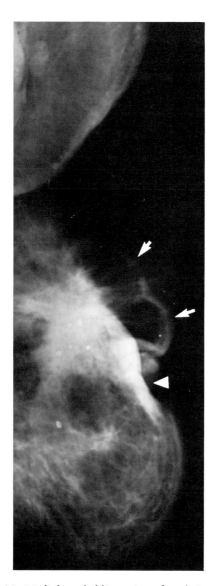

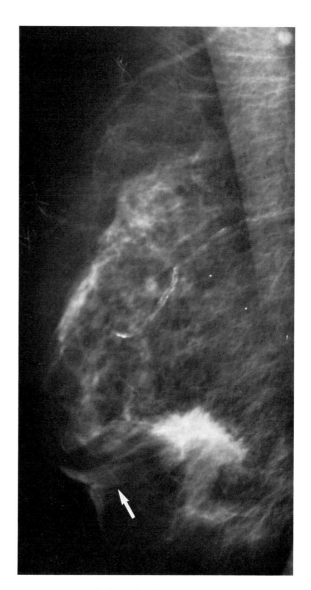

Fig. 13-20. Mediolateral oblique view of an obviously invasive stellate carcinoma, associated with marked skin thickening and retraction *(arrows)*, as well as nipple retraction *(arrowhead)*. Skin thickening is also present in the axillary fold, where the anterior borders of metastatic lymph nodes are visualized.

Fig. 13-21. Mediolateral oblique view demonstrating a poorly defined infiltrating ductal carcinoma in the retroareolar area. There is prominence of the ducts between the tumor and the nipple *(arrow)* and associated nipple retraction.

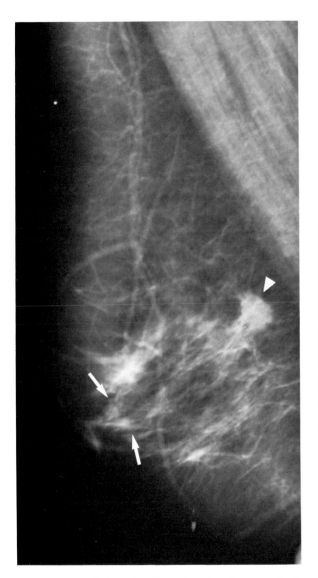

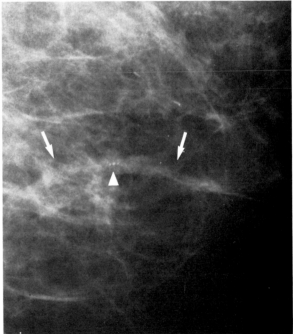

Fig. 13-22. Mediolateral oblique view showing a poorly defined mass *(arrowhead)*. Although the tumor is quite posterior in location, there is mild nipple retraction (a new finding clinically). Note that there is prominence of the ducts between the tumor and the nipple *(arrows)*. Histology: infiltrating ductal carcinoma.

Fig. 13-23. Enlargement demonstrating a single dilated duct extending for several centimeters into the retroareolar area *(arrows)*. A few calcifications are noted along the course of the duct *(arrowhead)*. Histology: papillomatosis and intraductal carcinoma.

solitary dilated duct. Any dilated duct extending 2 cm or more into the breast is considered abnormal (Fig. 13-23).

Asymmetric ductal dilatation indicates that something is growing within the duct and causing it to expand. As an isolated sign, this finding is nonspecific and may be caused by hyperplasia, a papilloma, debris, or a carci-

noma (Fig. 13-24). The dilated duct may even be empty (Fig. 13-25). Most often the cause of asymmetric ductal ectasia is benign.

Symmetrical ductal ectasia is a benign condition of unknown etiology commonly seen in the breasts of postmenopausal women and should not be confused with malignancy. The symmetric nature of the abnormality

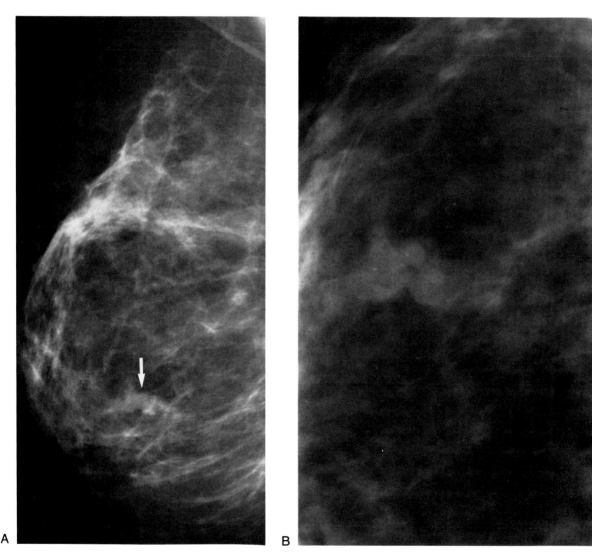

A   B

Fig. 13-24. (A) Mediolateral oblique view demonstrating a dilated and tortuous duct in the retroareolar area *(arrow)*. **(B)** An enlargement better demonstrates the dilated duct and associated fine microcalcifications. Histology: epithelial hyperplasia and a papilloma.

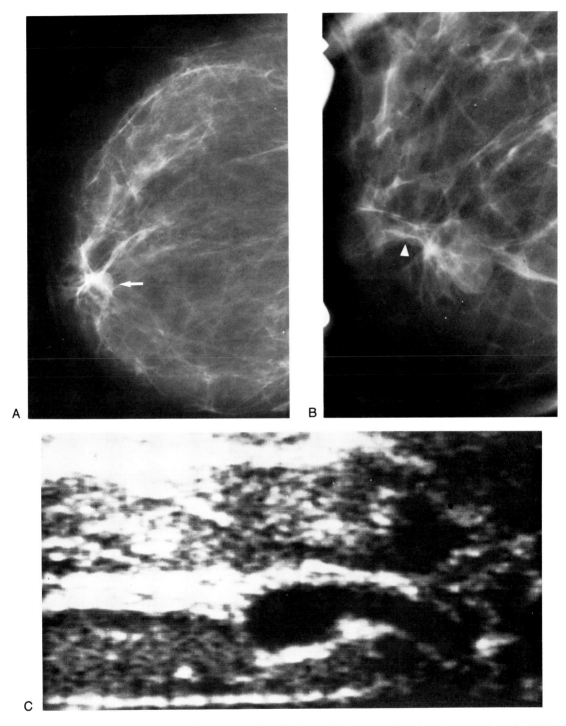

Fig. 13-25. **(A)** Craniocaudal view showing a well-defined round density in the subareolar area *(arrow)*. **(B)** An enlargement demonstrates a connection between the nipple and the mass *(arrowhead)* and suggests that it may represent a dilated duct. **(C)** Ultrasound demonstrates the dilated and empty duct coursing toward the nipple.

is the key finding (Figs. 13-26 to 13-28). It is characterized by dilatation of the subareolar collecting ducts, with periductal fibrosis and inflammation. Spontaneous intermittent nipple discharge is often present. Pathologic examination demonstrates that the ducts are usually empty, although they may contain debris.

Increased Vascularity

Carcinoma may be associated with an increase in the size and number of veins within the breast. A vein may be considered enlarged if its diameter is 1.5 times that of the normal veins. This sign is of limited significance.

Large veins may be seen in the absence of any abnormality or may be associated with inflammatory conditions. The size of the veins can also be changed with the degree of compression used in performing the mammogram.

Lymphadenopathy

An increase in number, density, or size of the axillary lymph nodes should be considered suspicious for metastatic carcinoma. The abnormal nodes are usually ovoid, lack a normal fatty hilum, and are closely packed (Fig. 13-29). They may rarely contain malignant mi-

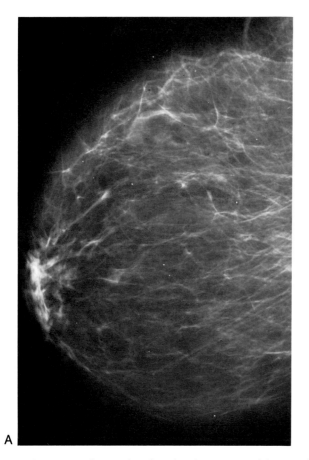 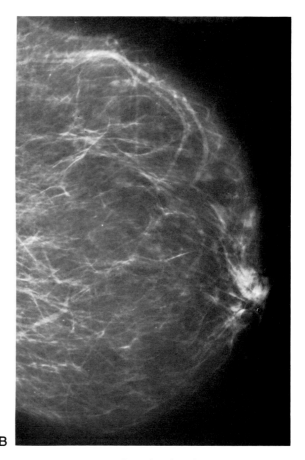

A   B

Fig. 13-26. (A & B) Left and right craniocaudal views demonstrate symmetric subareolar ductal ectasia in this asymptomatic postmenopausal woman. This finding is of no clinical significance.

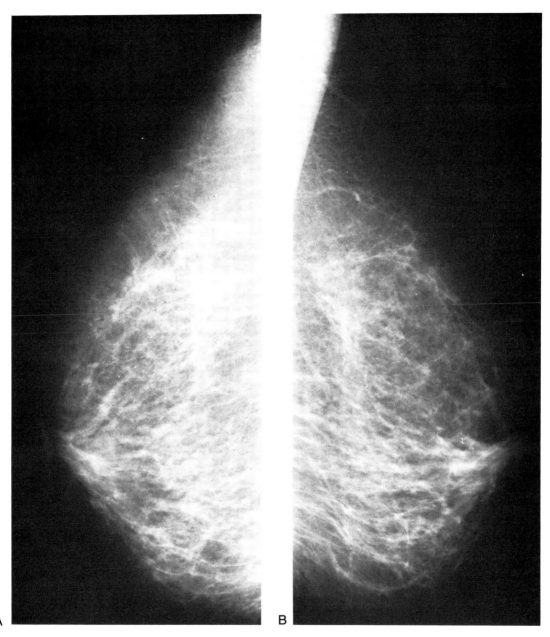

A   B

Fig. 13-27. (A & B) Left and right mediolateral oblique views reveal subareolar ductal ectasia in this postmenopausal woman. She complained of bilateral green-colored nipple discharge.

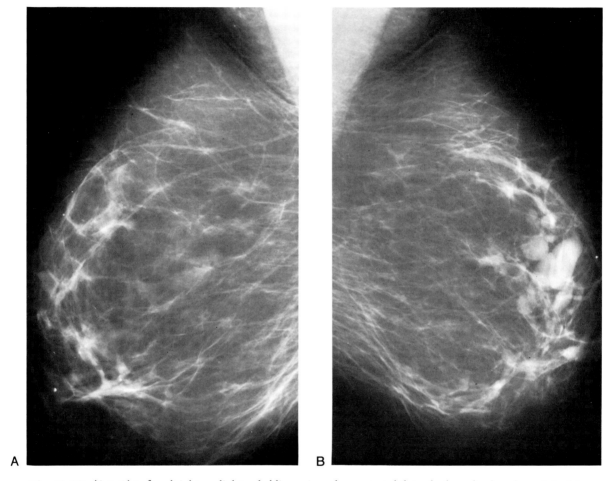

A B

Fig. 13-28. **(A & B)** Left and right mediolateral oblique views demonstrate bilateral subareolar ductal ectasia in this asymptomatic postmenopausal woman. The changes are more severe on the right side **(B),** with formation of areas of cystic dilatation.

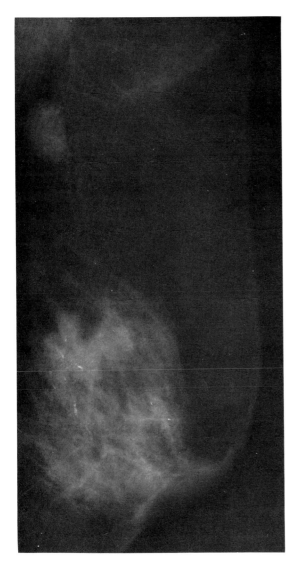

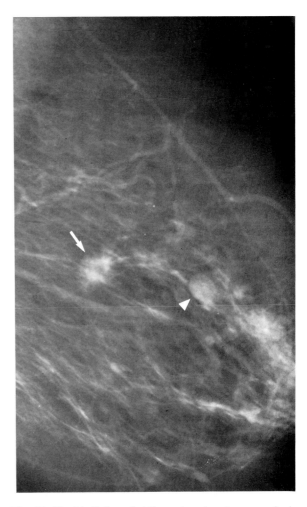

Fig. 13-29. Mediolateral oblique view demonstrating a spiculated mass that contains malignant calcifications. Nipple retraction is present as well. An abnormally dense axillary lymph node without a fatty hilum is present and was shown to contain metastatic carcinoma.

Fig. 13-30. Mediolateral oblique view showing a poorly defined carcinoma deep in the breast *(arrow)* and an additional well-defined mass anteriorly *(arrowhead)*. The well-defined mass is an intramammary lymph node that contains metastatic carcinoma.

crocalcifications. The underlying breast carcinoma is usually evident on mammography. If a tumor cannot be identified, other causes of lymphadenopathy should be considered. This topic is considered in detail in Chapter 9.

Breast carcinoma may rarely metastasize to intramammary lymph nodes, which appear as well-circumscribed, dense, round, or ovoid masses. They contain no lucent center or hilum and are usually greater than 1 cm in diameter (Fig. 13-30).

SUBTLE SIGNS OF CARCINOMA

The subtle or indirect signs of carcinoma include a developing density, an asymmetric density, minimal

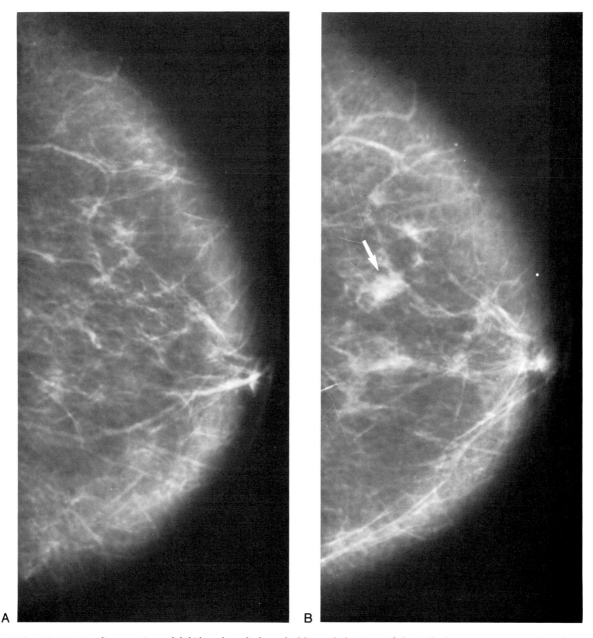

Fig. 13-31. Baseline craniocaudal **(A)** and mediolateral oblique **(C)** views of the right breast are compared with films done 18 months later **(B & D),** revealing a small, poorly defined neodensity *(arrows)*. *(Figure continues.)*

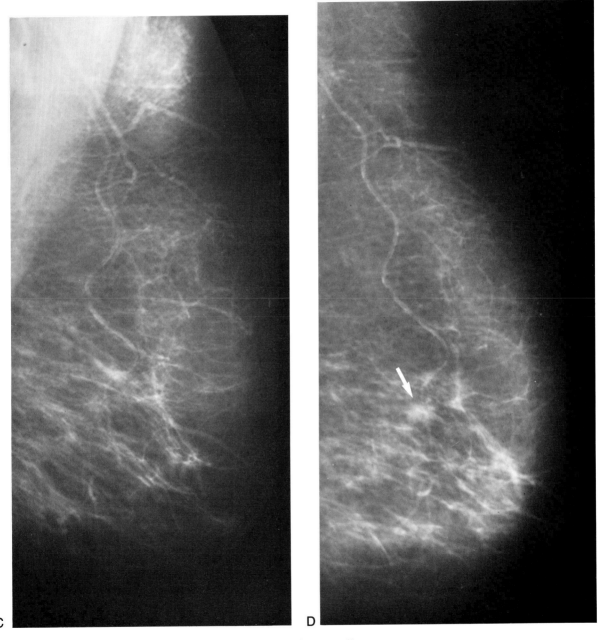

C   D

Fig. 13-31 *(Continued)*.

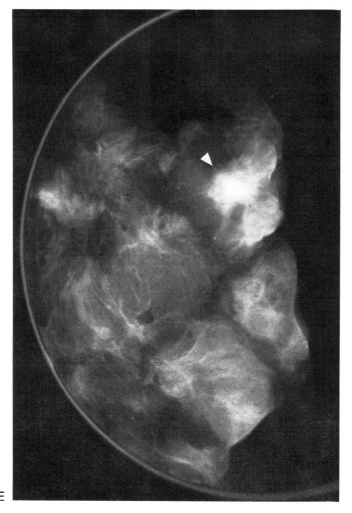

E

Fig. 13-31 *(Continued)*. A specimen radiograph **(E)** better demonstrates this mass *(arrowhead)*. Histology: infiltrating ductal carcinoma with one of eight axillary lymph nodes positive for carcinoma.

architectural distortion, a single dilated duct, and clustered microcalcifications. All but the first two of these signs have been described above as primary or secondary signs of malignancy. They may also be considered as subtle signs of carcinoma when they present early on, before the formation of an obvious invasive mass. Up to 20 percent of carcinomas are detected by these indirect signs. Their recognition is important because they are the signs of early or minimal breast carcinoma.

Developing Density

The appearance of a new, focal density on serial mammograms suggests an interval carcinoma. This is especially true in older patients whose breasts are basically involuting structures. Cysts and inflammatory changes may also cause new densities in the breasts of these older women. In premenopausal women, the appearance of the breast may change with fluctuating hormone levels. A new density should be evaluated in light of the patient's stage in the menstrual cycle, and short-term follow-up may be indicated.

Baseline mammograms are very important, because these developing densities have no characteristic mammographic features. Without the previous films, they would often be dismissed as the overlap of normal tissues (Figs. 13-31 to 13-33).

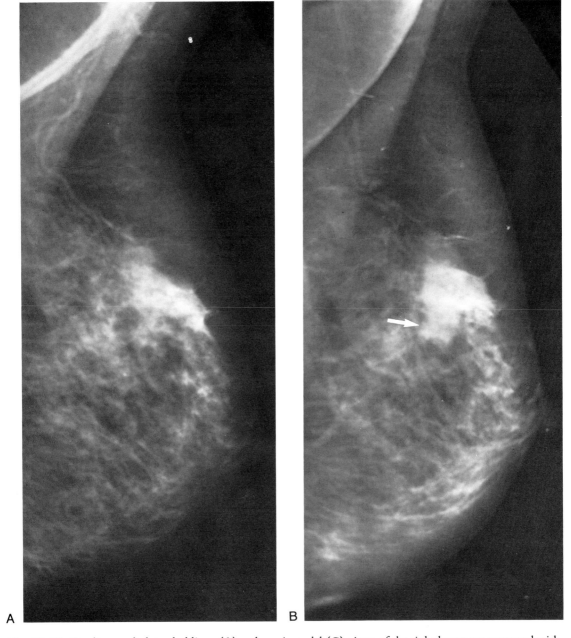

Fig. 13-32. Baseline mediolateral oblique **(A)** and craniocaudal **(C)** views of the right breast are compared with films done 19 months later, when the patient had developed new palpable thickening in the upper outer quadrant of this breast. The follow-up views **(B & D)** demonstrate an area of increased density *(arrows)*. There is associated architectural distortion noted posteriorly **(D)**. *(Figure continues.)*

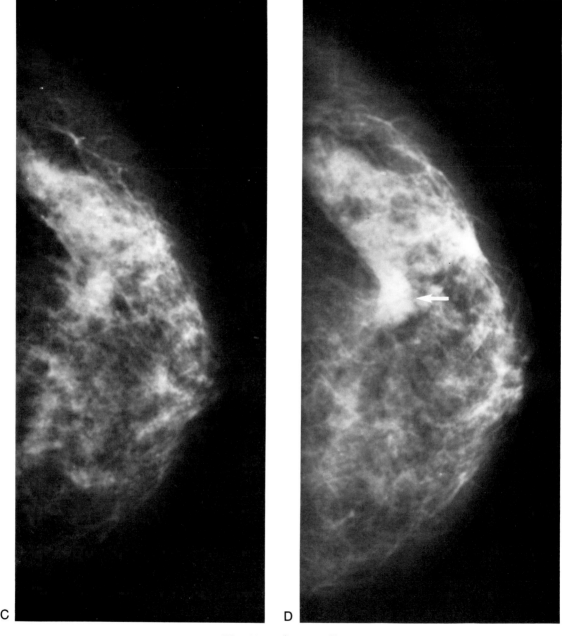

C

D

Fig. 13-32 *(Continued)*.

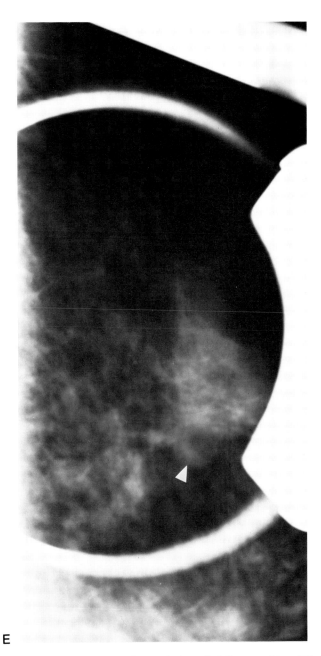

E

Fig. 13-32 *(Continued)*. A magnification view in the mediolateral oblique position **(E)** demonstrates the mass *(arrowhead)*. Histology: infiltrating ductal carcinoma.

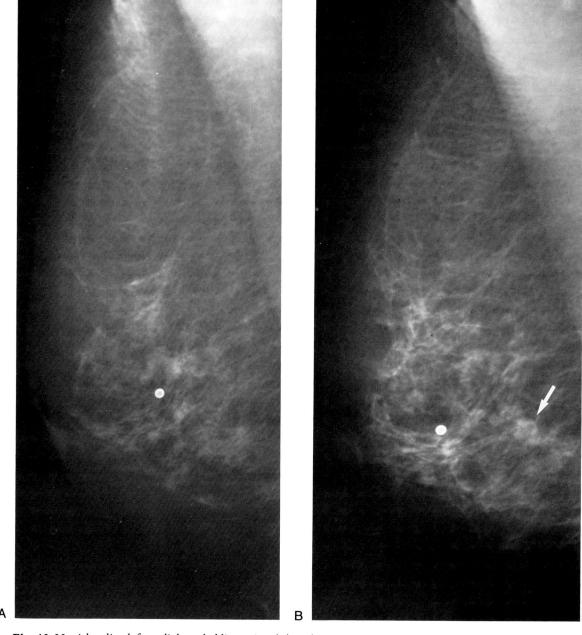

A   B

Fig. 13-33. A baseline left mediolateral oblique view **(A)** in this 66-year-old woman who had had a right mastectomy for carcinoma is compared with a follow-up mediolateral oblique view 15 months later **(B).** The follow-up film demonstrates a subtle neodensity *(arrow)*. Histology: infiltrating ductal carcinoma.

Asymmetric Density

It is important to compare the breasts to each other carefully. Any area of asymmetry should be evaluated with additional views, because a vague increase in density may be the only sign of an early carcinoma. A suspicious area of asymmetry should be volumetric in two projections and should not have lucencies (fat) running through it (Figs. 13-34 to 13-36). A density that is identified on only one view, or multiple areas of asymmetric density, should be followed with serial mammography and physical examination. An asymmetric density associated with a palpable abnormality is especially worrisome, and biopsy should be strongly considered.

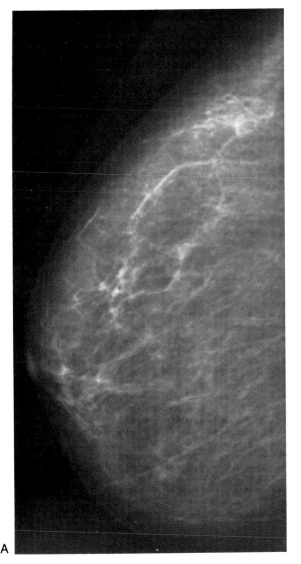

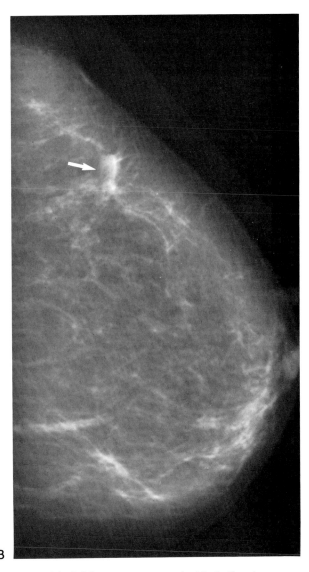

A   B

Fig. 13-34. Mediolateral oblique **(A)** and craniocaudal **(C)** views of the left breast are compared with similar views of the right breast **(B & D)**. There is a poorly defined area of asymmetric density in the superolateral quadrant of the right breast *(arrows)*. Histology: early infiltrating carcinoma with all axillary lymph nodes negative for tumor. *(Figure continues.)*

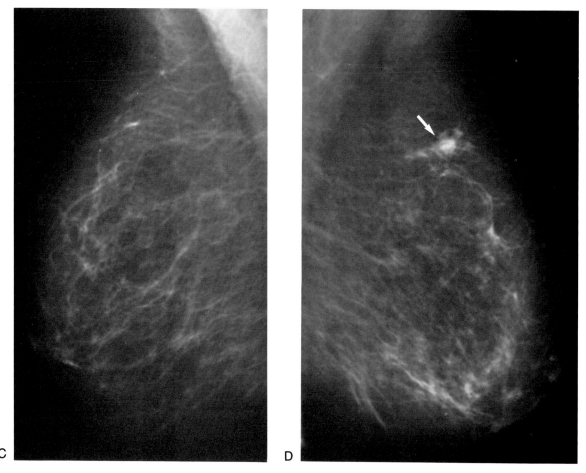

C   D

Fig. 13-34 *(Continued)*.

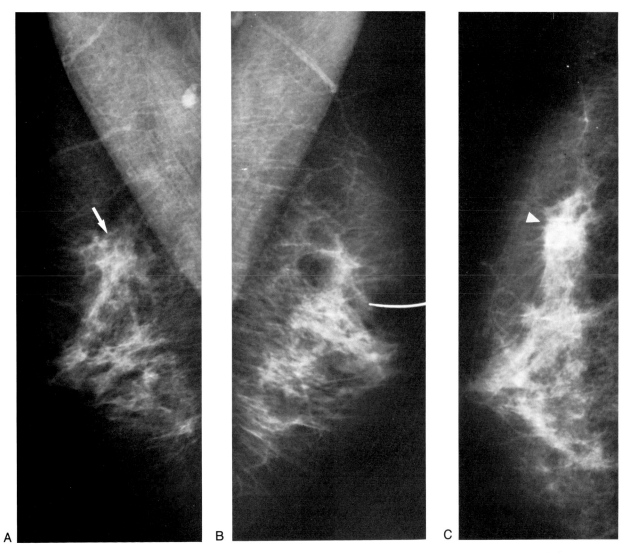

Fig. 13-35. Comparison of a mediolateral oblique view of the left breast **(A)** with a similar view of the right breast **(B)** reveals an area of asymmetric increased density superiorly on the left *(arrow)*. A craniocaudal view of the left breast **(C)** demonstrates the density in the lateral portion of the breast *(arrowhead)*. Histology: infiltrating lobular carcinoma.

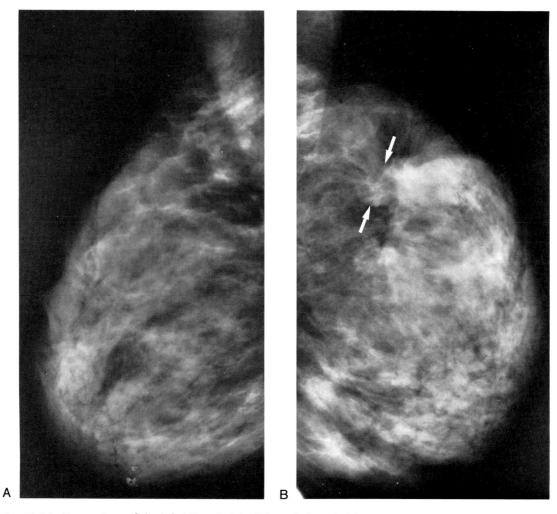

A   B

Fig. 13-36. Comparison of the left **(A)** and right **(B)** mediolateral oblique views in this 49-year-old woman demonstrates an area of asymmetric increased density and architectural distortion on the right *(arrows)*. It is difficult to identify the borders of the mass. Histology: infiltrating ductal carcinoma with all axillary lymph nodes free of metastases.

SUGGESTED READINGS

1. Bedwani R, Vana J, Rosner D, Schmitz RL, Murphy GP: Management and survival of female patients with "minimal" breast cancer: as observed in the long-term and short-term surveys of the American College of Surgeons. Cancer 47:2769, 1981
2. Egan RL, McSweeney MB, Sewell CW: Intramammary calcifications without an associated mass in benign and malignant diseases. Radiology 137:1, 1980
3. Gallager HS, Martin JE: An orientation to the concept of minimal breast cancer. Cancer 28:1505, 1971
4. Homer MJ: Mammary skin thickening. Contemp Diagn Radiol 4:1, 1981
5. Homer MJ: Nonpalpable breast abnormalities: a realistic view of the accuracy of mammography in detecting malignancies. Radiology 153:831, 1984
6. Martin JE: Atlas of Mammography: Histologic and Mammographic Correlations. Williams & Wilkins, Baltimore, 1982
7. Martin JE, Moskowitz M, Milbrath JR: Breast cancer missed by mammography. AJR 132:737, 1979
8. Moskowitz M: Mammographic screening: significance of minimal breast cancers. AJR 136:735, 1981
9. Moskowitz M: The predictive value of certain mammographic signs in screening for breast cancer. Cancer 51:1007, 1983
10. Powell RW, McSweeney MB, Wilson CE: X-ray calci-

fications as the only basis for breast biopsy. Ann Surg 197:555, 1983

11. Sickles EA: Further experience with microfocal spot magnification mammography in the assessment of clustered breast microcalcifications. Radiology 137:9, 1980

12. Sickles EA: Mammographic detectability of breast microcalcifications. AJR 139:913, 1982

13. Sickles EA: Mammographic features of "early" breast cancer. AJR 143:461, 1984

14. Sickles EA: Mammographic features of 300 consecutive nonpalpable breast cancers. AJR 146:661, 1988

15. Swann CA, Kopans DB, Koerner FC, McCarthy KA, White G, Hall DA: The halo sign and malignant breast lesions. AJR 149:1145, 1987

16. Wilhelm MC, de Paredes ES, Pope T, Wanebo HJ: The changing mammogram: a primary indication for needle localization biopsy. Arch Surg 121:1311, 1986

14

Uncommon Malignancies of the Breast

Mary Ellen Peters

INFLAMMATORY CARCINOMA

Inflammatory carcinoma accounts for 1 to 2 percent of all breast malignancies. The term inflammatory carcinoma implies dermal lymphatic carcinomatosis. The histopathologic type of carcinoma present is variable. In Robbins' series, the median age of occurrence was 55 years.[2] The prognosis in all age groups is dismal. In the premenopausal age group, the survival is approximately 2 years, and for postmenopausal women it is 3 years. The clinical findings can develop rapidly within the involved breast, which becomes larger and firmer as the result of edema. The patient often complains of pain and tenderness, and the breast appears erythematous and is warm to touch.

Mammography demonstrates that the involved breast is larger and denser than the contralateral breast. It may be so dense that the internal architecture of the breast cannot be visualized. Diffuse skin thickening is seen, and the trabeculae often appear thickened. No mass can be delineated on the mammogram. Associated axillary adenopathy is frequently seen (Figs. 14-1 and 14-2).

TUBULAR CARCINOMA

Tubular carcinomas are relatively rare and when not accompanied by other forms of breast carcinoma have a

good prognosis. However, they are frequently found in association with other types of carcinoma, and the prognosis is then dictated by the associated type. Radiographically, they cannot be differentiated from the usual (not otherwise specified) invasive ductal carcinoma (Fig. 14-3).

MEDULLARY CARCINOMA

Medullary carcinomas comprise 4 percent of all malignant tumors of the breast. Because they are well demarcated and have a soft consistency, they can be mistaken for benign tumors both radiographically and clinically. The majority of these tumors have a good prognosis. In Riolfi's series, two-thirds occurred in the postmenopausal age group.[2]

Radiographically, they present as round or lobulated masses that tend to be peripheral in location and of high density. The margins can be sharp and a halo sign may be evident. At time, the masses are poorly marginated. They do not contain calcification (Figs. 14-4 to 14-6).

PAPILLARY CARCINOMA

Papillary carcinomas are of three types: intraductal, intracystic, and invasive. They are slow-growing and

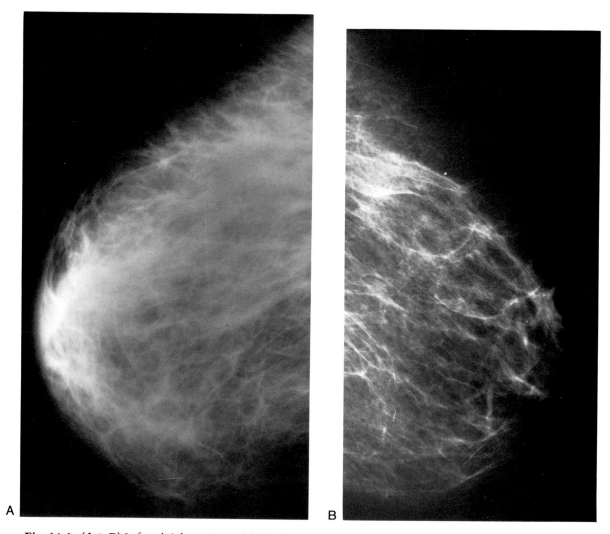

A

B

Fig. 14-1. (A & B) Left and right craniocaudal views in a 38-year-old woman with an enlarged, erythematous left breast. The left breast is dense, as the result of skin and trabecular thickening. (The radiographs demonstrated the skin thickening well. As in many cases of properly exposed screen-film studies, it is necessary to evaluate the skin with bright light.) Differential diagnosis includes inflammatory carcinoma, obstruction of a lymphatic chain that drains the breast, metastatic disease from a contralateral carcinoma, and lymphoma. Histology: inflammatory carcinoma.

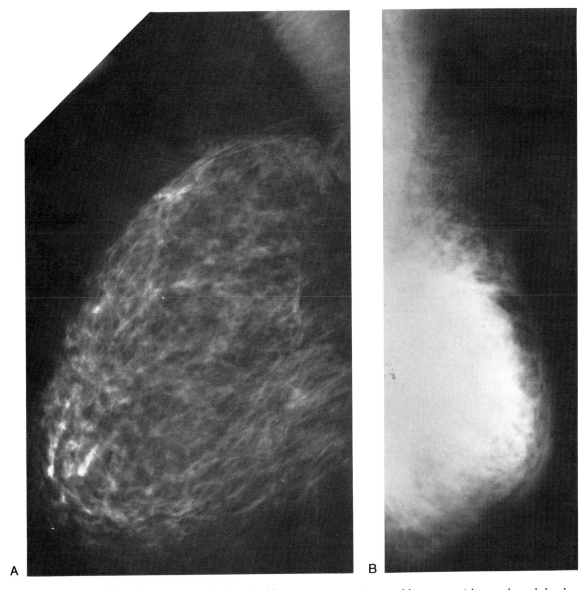

A   B

Fig. 14-2. (A & B) Left and right mediolateral oblique views in a 36-year-old woman with an enlarged, hard, erythematous right breast. The right breast appears dense, and the skin is diffusely thickened. It appears smaller than the left, since adequate compression could not be attained. Because of the marked increased density, an underlying mass cannot be excluded. Therefore a large abscess or an advanced carcinoma associated with a large mass should be considered in addition to an inflammatory carcinoma. Histology: inflammatory carcinoma.

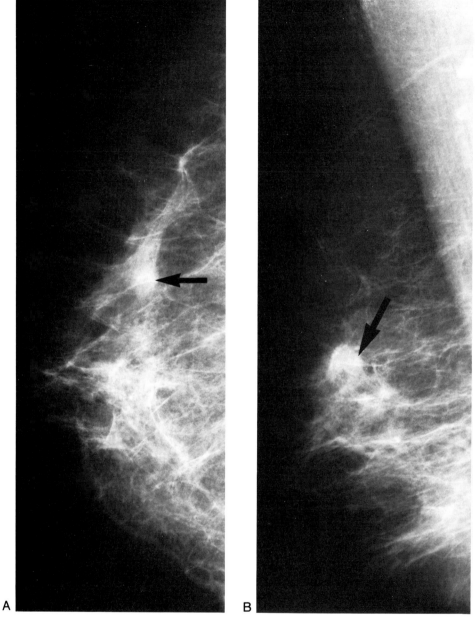

Fig. 14-3. Left craniocaudal (**A**) and mediolateral oblique (**B**) views in an asymptomatic 60-year-old woman. The study demonstrates an ill-defined mass *(arrow)* that cannot be distinguished from the usual invasive ductal carcinoma. Histology: pure tubular carcinoma.

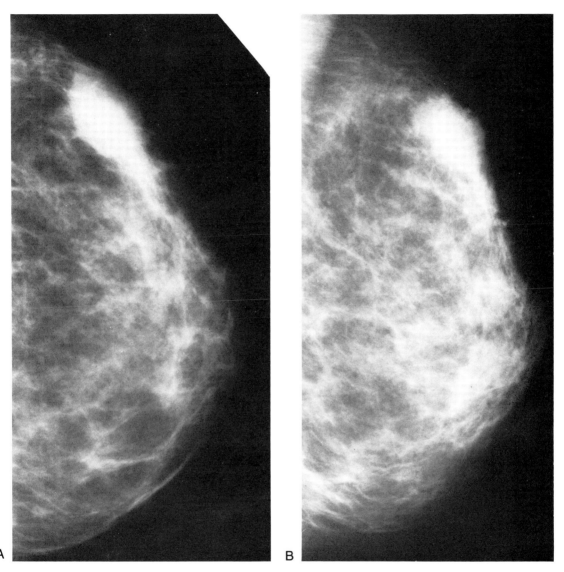

Fig. 14-4. Right craniocaudal (**A**) and mediolateral oblique (**B**) views in a 37-year-old woman with a palpable mass. An ovoid mass can be seen in the superolateral quadrant. Segments of the margins are ill defined. A screening study had been negative 5 months previously. The most common masses in this age group are fibroadenoma and cyst. Histology: medullary carcinoma. (Courtesy of Dr. Kenneth Billings, Marshfield Clinic, Marshfield, WI.)

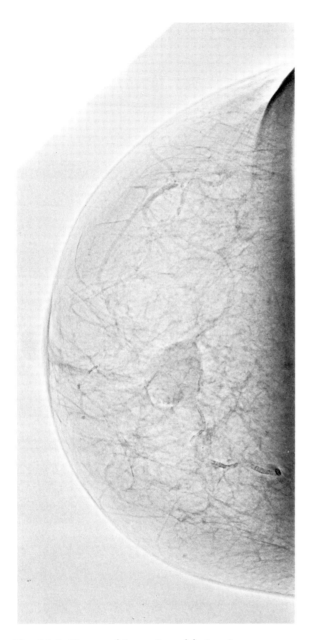

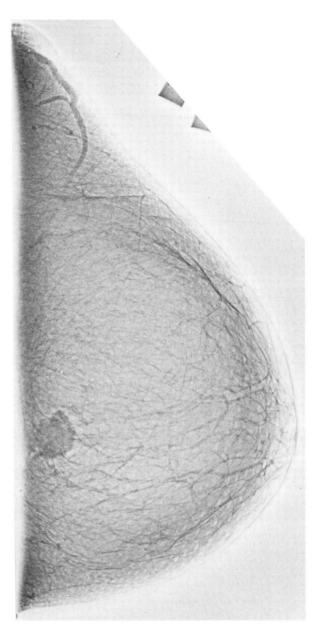

Fig. 14-5. Xerographic craniocaudal view in an asymptomatic 60-year-old woman. The study demonstrates a solitary, round mass. Only small segments of the mass are ill defined. A solitary mass in the postmenopausal age group should always suggest carcinoma. Histology: medullary carcinoma. (Courtesy of Dr. Kenneth Billings, Marshfield Clinic, Marshfield, WI.)

Fig. 14-6. Xerographic craniocaudal view in an asymptomatic 57-year-old woman. A solitary, lobulated, ill-defined mass is seen. Histology: medullary carcinoma. (Courtesy of Dr. Kenneth Billings, Marshfield Clinic, Marshfield, WI.)

have a favorable prognosis. Usually they occur in the postmenopausal age group. Approximately 1 percent of all usual (not otherwise specified) invasive ductal carcinomas are associated with papillary carcinomas.

Commonly, papillary carcinomas are of low density and mimic benign tumors on the mammogram. Their contour may be round, lobulated, dumbbell-shaped, or bilobed (Figs. 14-7 to 14-10). Often they are well marginated, but they may be ill defined as the result of overlying fibroglandular tissues, invasion, or an associated ductal carcinoma (Fig. 14-11). Calcification can be seen within the wall of an intracystic papillary carcinoma.

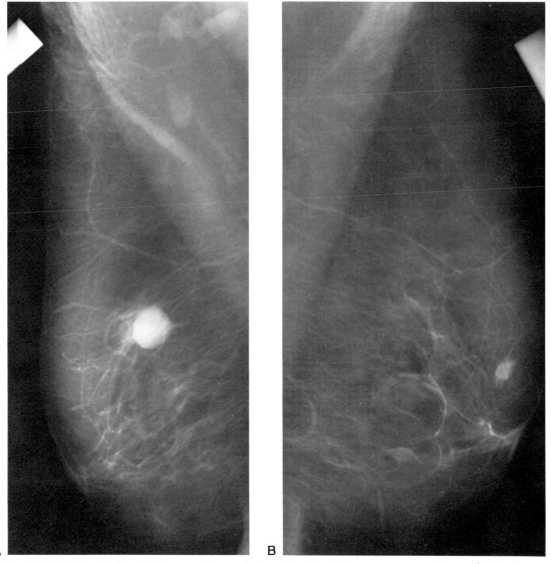

A   B

Fig. 14-7. (A & B) Left and right mediolateral oblique views in a 64-year-old woman with a left palpable mass. Bilateral round masses are present. The left mass is well marginated; the right is less well defined. Both are of low density. Histology: bilateral, intracystic papillary carcinoma.

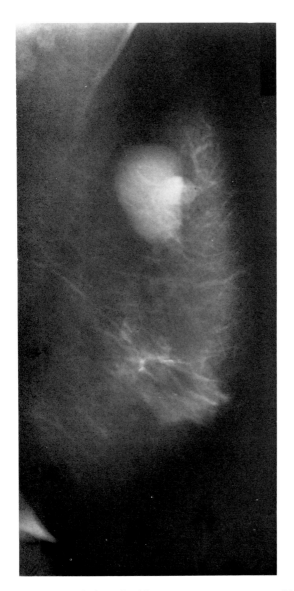

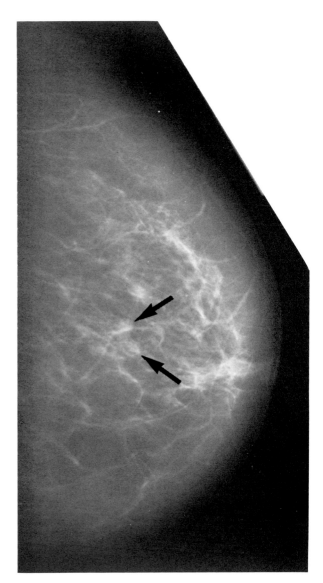

Fig. 14-8. Mediolateral oblique view in a 55-year-old woman with a palpable mass. The study demonstrates a large, low-density, lobulated mass with distinct margins. Histology: intracystic papillary carcinoma.

Fig. 14-9. Craniocaudal view from a screening study in a 59-year-old woman. A small, bilobed mass *(arrows)* is present. The margins are quite well defined. Histology: intraductal papillary carcinoma.

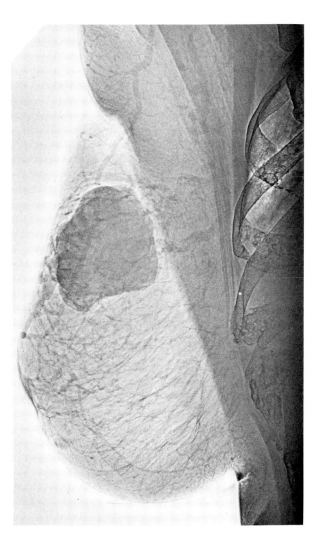

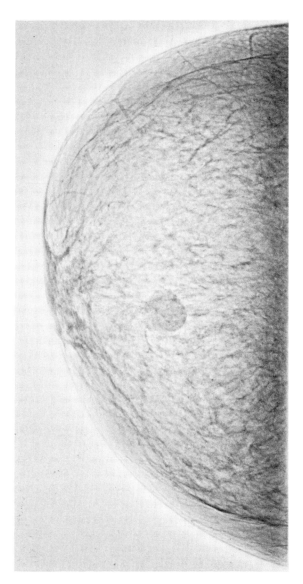

Fig. 14-10. Xerographic lateral view in a 75-year-old woman who was known to have a palpable mass for 10 years. The large, well-defined, lobulated mass is a proven noninvasive papillary carcinoma.

Fig. 14-11. Xerographic craniocaudal view in a 66-year-old woman with a palpable mass. The posterior margin of the mass is well defined. Anteriorly, it is ill defined. Pathology demonstrated an intracystic papillary carcinoma associated with a usual invasive ductal carcinoma, which accounts for the ill-defined anterior margin.

MUCOID (COLLOID) CARCINOMA

Three percent of all breast malignancies are mucoid (colloid) carcinomas. Other terms applied to this tumor are gelatinous carcinoma, mucin-producing carcinoma, and mucinous carcinoma. The average age of occurrence was 68.6 years in Silverberg's series,[2] but McDivitt[2] found the median age no different than that for the usual ductal carcinoma (54.3 years). The prognosis of this tumor is good.

On the mammogram, mucoid carcinomas appear as round or lobulated masses of low density. They may be well circumscribed and have an associated halo sign, or the margins may be blurred. Like medullary carcinomas, they are commonly peripheral in location (Fig. 14-12).

CARCINOID TUMORS

Carcinoid tumors of the breast may be primary or secondary. In Cubilla and Woodruff's series, the primary form was not associated with the carcinoid syndrome.[2] The median age of occurrence in their series was 54 years. On gross pathologic examination, the tumors have been reported to be well circumscribed. Mixed tumors with both mucoid and carcinoid elements may occur. We have seen one such tumor that appeared as a lobulated mass (Fig. 14-13).

LOBULAR CARCINOMA

Lobular carcinoma in situ does not produce mammographic findings. It is usually found coincidentally on a biopsy. Invasive lobular carcinoma does produce iden-

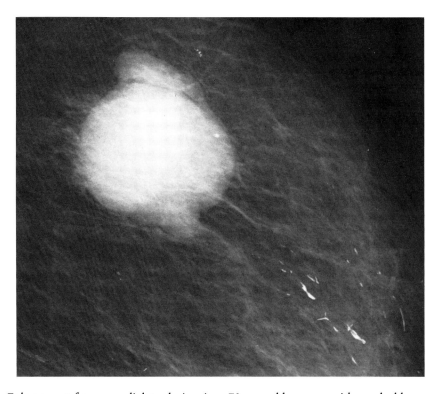

Fig. 14-12. Enlargement from a mediolateral view in a 70-year-old woman with a palpable mass. The study demonstrates a large, lobulated mass of low density. A halo sign partially surrounds it. The calcifications are superimposed and are not in the mass. Histology: mucoid carcinoma. Note the secretory calcifications.

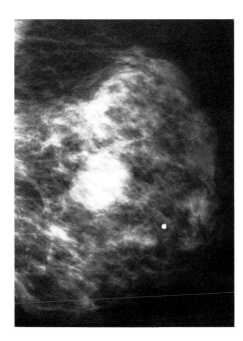

Fig. 14-13. Mediolateral oblique view in a 63-year-old woman with a palpable mass. A 3-cm mildly lobulated mass of relative low density is seen. Histology: a mixed mucoid-carcinoid carcinoma.

Fig. 14-14. Right craniocaudal **(A)** and mediolateral oblique **(B)** views in a 54-year-old woman with a palpable mass. The study demonstrates an ill-defined mass in the superolateral quadrant that cannot be distinguished from the usual invasive ductal carcinoma. Histopathology: invasive lobular carcinoma.

tifiable radiographic changes. The findings are indistinguishable from the usual invasive ductal carcinoma with the exception that lobular carcinoma is less often associated with calcifications (Fig. 14-14).

SARCOMAS

Sarcomas of the breast are classified into two main types, depending upon the presence or absence of epithelial elements. Those with epithelial elements are categorized as cystosarcoma phyllodes and those without epithelial elements are categorized as stromal sarcomas.

Cystosarcoma Phyllodes

Cystosarcoma phyllodes is a fibroepithelial tumor. The term cystosarcoma is a misnomer, since 80 percent are benign. The benign form can have tentaclelike projections extending out into the breast parenchyma that can lead to recurrence after surgery. Malignant forms are differentiated from benign by the presence of increased

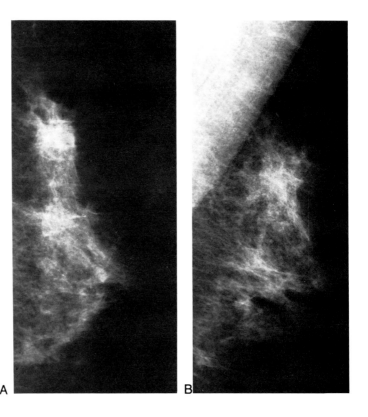

A   B

mitotic activity, overgrowth of stroma, an infiltrating edge, and marked atypia. The most common malignant form is fibrosarcoma, followed by liposarcoma, chondrosarcoma, osteosarcoma, and myosarcoma.

The benign form presents at an average age of 45 years; the malignant form usually presents 3 to 5 years later. The tumors are generally large at the time of presentation, measuring 4 to 6 cm in diameter. Some may grow as large as 30 to 40 cm. Rapid growth can occur in both forms, and with very large tumors the skin acquires a taunt, shiny appearance and may even ulcerate.

Cystosarcoma phyllodes tumors present on the mammogram as multilobulated round masses of variable size. Some mimic the appearance of a fibroadenoma. The entire circumference of the tumor may appear well defined, but often one area is indistinct as the result of invasion into the fibroglandular tissues. If liposarcomatous elements are present, areas of lucency may be seen

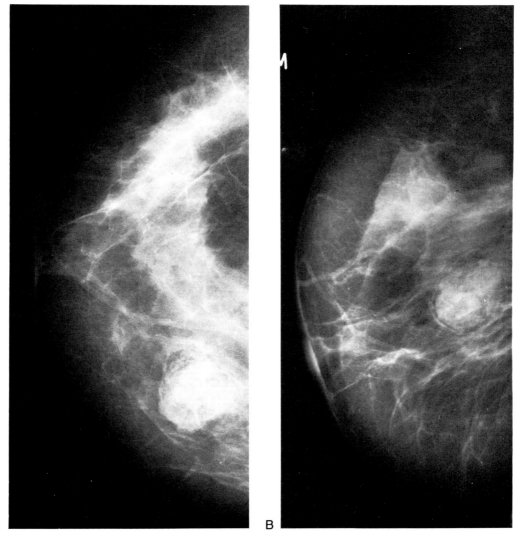

A   B

Fig. 14-15. Left craniocaudal **(A)** and mediolateral oblique **(B)** views in an asymptomatic 44-year-old woman. A mixed radiodense-radiolucent mass is present in the superomedial quadrant with what appears to be a "capsule." This was considered to be a lipofibroadenoma and a biopsy was not performed. *(Figure continues.)*

within the mass. Calcification within the tumor is infrequently observed but is usually coarse when found. Enlarged veins may be an accompanying finding (Figs. 14-15 and 14-16).

Axillary lymphadenopathy can be present; however, the adenopathy is usually secondary to reactive hyperplasia from tissue necrosis or ulceration rather than metastasis. The malignant form usually spreads via the hematogenous route.

Stromal Sarcoma

Stromal sarcomas of the breast are exceedingly rare, accounting for approximately 1 percent of all breast malignancies. The various forms of this tumor include fibrosarcoma, leiomyosarcoma, osteosarcoma, liposarcoma, and angiosarcoma. The median age for presentation approximates that for the usual ductal carcinoma except for angiosarcoma, which presents earlier.

Stromal sarcomas grow rapidly, and the palpable mass

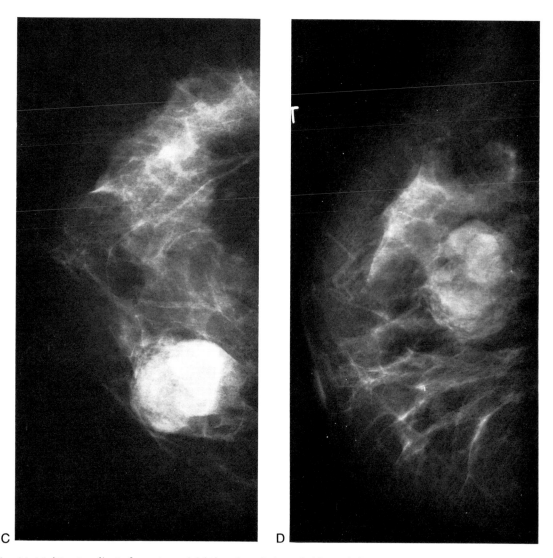

Fig. 14-15 *(Continued)*. Left craniocaudal **(C)** and mediolateral oblique **(D)** views 6 months later, at which time a mass was palpable. The mass has increased in size but continues to be of mixed density. Histology: cystosarcoma phyllodes with liposarcomatous elements.

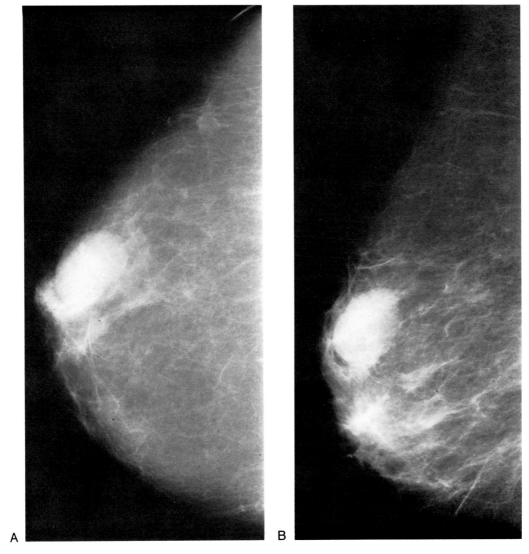

Fig. 14-16. Left craniocaudal **(A)** and mediolateral oblique **(B)** views in a 56-year-old with a palpable mass. A 3.5 cm dense, homogeneous mass is present. A halo partially surrounds the mass. Histology: malignant cystosarcoma phyllodes. (Courtesy of Dr. John Wentz, Richland Center, WI.)

corresponds closely to the radiographic size. Since sarcomas spread hematogenously, lymph node enlargement does not occur unless it is secondary to an inflammation caused by necrosis of the tumor. Radiographically, they present as large, well-defined, round, or lobulated masses that can mimic benign tumors (Fig. 14-17). These masses are often very dense, probably

reflecting the propensity for development of bone and cartilage within them. Spicules of bone extending out from the tumor have been described in osteogenic sarcoma.

Angiosarcomas are the most aggressive form of breast malignancy. They present as rapidly enlarging painless

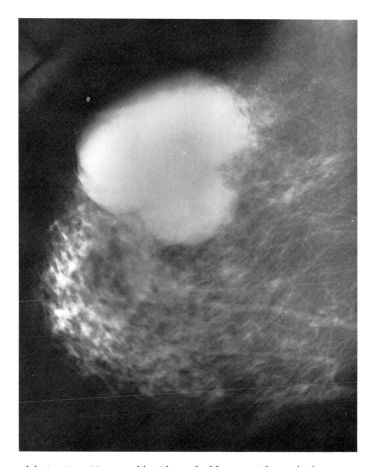

Fig. 14-17. Craniocaudal view in a 59-year-old with a palpable mass. The study demonstrates a huge, lobulated, dense mass. Portions of the borders are associated with a halo, but other segments are indistinct. Histology: fibrosarcoma.

masses that can be associated with bluish discoloration of the skin. The usual mammographic finding is a large, lobulated, poorly defined mass.

ADENOID CYSTIC CARCINOMA

Adenoid cystic carcinoma is a rare tumor of the breast. On pathologic examination, it can appear cystic and be fairly well defined. A large number of the cases reported in the pathologic literature have been subareolar or adjacent to the areola. The prognosis of this tumor is good. Because of its rarity, the mammographic findings are not well described. Martin[22] states that

adenoid cystic carcinomas have no characteristic radiographic features.

PAGET'S DISEASE OF THE NIPPLE

Paget's disease of the nipple is associated with 1 to 2 percent of breast carcinomas and is a clinical rather than a radiographic diagnosis. The histopathologic cell type of the associated tumor may be either infiltrating ductal carcinoma or in situ ductal carcinoma. Pure lobular carcinoma associated with Paget's disease is distinctly unusual. Neoplastic cells (Paget cells) infiltrate the epidermis of the nipple. Clinically, the nipple is erythema-

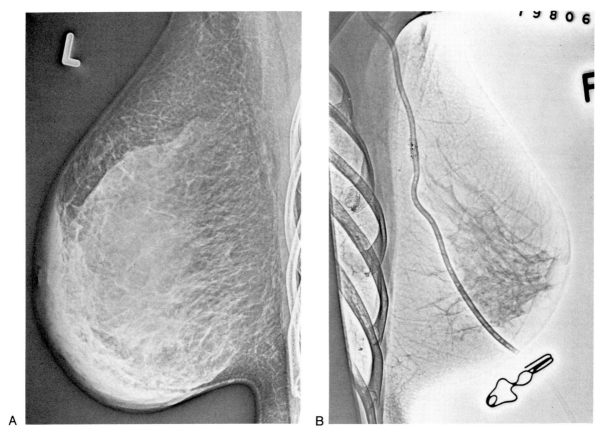

Fig. 14-18. (A & B) Left and right xerographic lateral views of a 36-year-old woman with a palpable left breast mass, associated with skin thickening. Considerations include a large carcinoma, abscess, and lymphoma. Histology: lymphoma (primary of the breast). (Courtesy of Dr. T.A.S. Matalon, Rush-Presbyterian-St. Luke's Medical Center, Chicago, IL.) *(Figure continues.)*

tous and may exhibit eczematous changes. In over one-half the patients, the carcinoma cannot be palpated.

The mammogram usually demonstrates carcinoma in the retroareolar area, although the tumor may be located anywhere in the breast. Malignant-appearing calcifications can be observed within the nipple. Thickening of the nipple is rarely identifiable.

LYMPHOMA

Lymphoma of the breast may either be primary or secondary. The primary form accounts for 0.12 to 0.53 percent of all breast malignancies; the secondary form has a slightly higher incidence. The median age of

presentation for the primary form is 60 years, and the prognosis is usually poor, as these patients commonly develop widespread disease. Any type of lymphoma can involve the breast, but non-Hodgkin's disease is the most common in both primary and secondary forms. In both the primary and secondary lymphomas, the mammographic picture is usually of round, oval, or lobulated masses varying in size from 2 to 3 cm. These can be quite well defined or be moderately spiculated (Fig. 14-18). The masses can be multiple or bilateral in the secondary form, but this is an uncommon presentation in the primary form. Lymphomas of the breast can also present as a generalized increased density with thickening of the trabeculae and skin similar to the findings seen in association with inflammatory carcinoma and with obstruction of a lymphatic chain that drains the

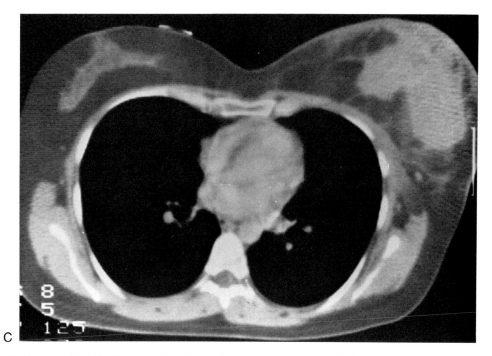

C

Fig. 14-18 *(Continued).* **(C)** CT scan of the chest. The study demonstrates the large mass and skin changes of the left breast.

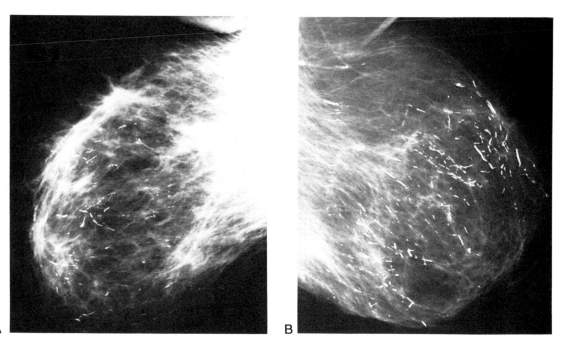

A

B

Fig. 14-19. (A & B) Left and right mediolateral oblique views in a 66-year-old woman with enlargement and increased firmness of the left breast. Diffuse thickening of the trabeculae and skin are present on the left. Diagnostic considerations include inflammatory carcinoma, obstruction of a lymphatic chain that drains the breast, metastasis from a contralateral breast carcinoma, and lymphoma. Histology: lymphoma (primary of the breast). Note the diffuse secretory calcifications.

breast (Fig. 14-19). This type of presentation more commonly occurs in the secondary form. Lymph node enlargement is seen in both primary and secondary forms.

LEUKEMIA

All types of leukemia can involve the breast. The patient may even present clinically with breast involvement antedating the diagnosis of leukemia. Involvement is usually bilateral. The patient may present with diffuse enlargement of the breasts and a mammographic picture of generalized increased density. Skin thickening may be evident. Alternatively, masses of variable size and definition may be seen. The findings regress with therapy, and the parenchymal pattern generally returns to normal.

METASTASES

The most common secondary breast tumor in women is metastases from a contralateral breast carcinoma. There are two modes of presentation. Metastases can be manifested as diffuse skin thickening, generalized increased parenchymal density, and a prominent trabecular pattern resulting from lymphatic invasion (Fig. 14-20). The second form of presentation is a mass lesion. It should be remembered, however, that a second primary breast carcinoma is more common than metastasis from a contralateral breast carcinoma.

The next most common metastasis is malignant melanoma followed by bronchogenic carcinoma, sarcoma, and ovarian carcinoma. Almost any tumor, however, can metastasize to the breast. In most series, the metastases have presented as masses that are usually well defined, but they can appear indistinct. The most common location of these masses is in the superolateral quadrant, and they tend to be superficial (Fig. 14-21). They can be bilateral and multiple, but more commonly they are solitary and unilateral. It is distinctly uncommon for these metastases to contain calcifications; ovarian carcinoma is the only reported exception.

McCrea et al.[23] have reported metastases from extramammary sites presenting as skin thickening on the mammogram. They also described one case of metastatic oat cell carcinoma causing asymmetry of the fibroglandular tissues.

OTHER RARE CARCINOMAS

Other rare breast carcinomas include signet-ring cell carcinoma, squamous cell carcinoma, spindle cell

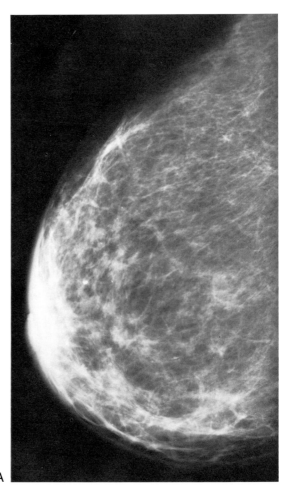

A

Fig. 14-20. Left craniocaudal **(A)**, mediolateral oblique **(B)**, and mediolateral coned compression **(C)** views in a 73-year-old woman with an enlarged, firm breast and a contralateral mastectomy for carcinoma. The skin and trabeculae are thickened. Findings suggestive of a mass are present on the oblique view *(arrow)*. The coned compression view proves the "mass" to be normal parenchyma. The differential diagnosis is similar to that of Figure 14-19 except that metastatic breast carcinoma should be the presumed diagnosis in this case. Histology: consistent with metastatic breast carcinoma. *(Figure continues.)*

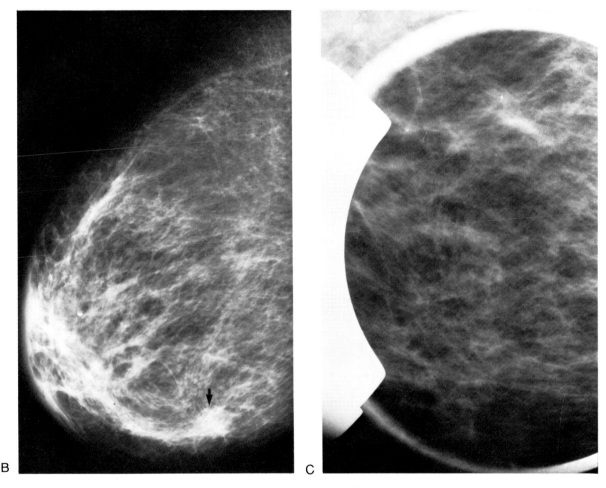

B   C

Fig. 14-20 *(Continued)*.

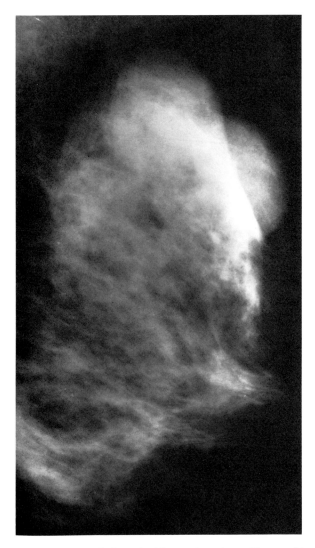

Fig. 14-21. Mediolateral oblique view in a 62-year-old woman with a palpable breast mass and a past history of a vaginal melanoma. The study demonstrates two round masses located peripherally. Histology: metastatic melanoma.

(pseudosarcomatous) carcinoma, apocrine carcinoma, and carcinosarcoma. Childhood breast carcinoma is also distinctly unusual. Secretory or juvenile carcinomas were first described in children but can also occur in adults. They are slow-growing, well-circumscribed tumors that have a good prognosis. Infiltrating ductal carcinomas have also been described in children. The most common tumor in the pediatric age group is the benign fibroadenoma.

SUGGESTED READINGS

1. Achram M, Issa S, Rizk G: Osteogenic sarcoma of the breast: some radiological aspects. Br J Radiol 58:264, 1985
2. Azzopardi JG: Problems in Breast Pathology. WB Saunders, Philadelphia, 1979
3. Bassett WB, Weiss RB: Plasmacytomas of the breast: an unusual manifestation of multiple myeloma. South Med J 72:1492, 1979
4. Berger SM, Gershon, Cohen J: Mammography of breast sarcoma. AJR 87:76, 1962
5. Bohman LG, Bassett LW, Gold RH, Voet R: Breast metastases from extramammary malignancies. Radiology 144:309, 1982
6. Carter D, Orr S, Merino M: Intracystic papillary carcinoma of the breast. Cancer 52:14, 1983
7. Chen KTK, Kirkegaard DP, Bocian JJ: Angiosarcoma of the breast. Cancer 46:368, 1980
8. Cole-Beuglet C, Sariano R, Kutz AB, Meyer JE, Kopans DB, Goldberg BB: Ultrasound, x-ray mammography, and histopathology of cystosarcoma phyllodes. Radiology 146:481, 1983
9. Dewhurst J: Breast disorders in children and adolescents. Pediatr Clin North Am 28:287, 1981
10. D'Orsi CJ, Feldhaus LE, Sonnenfeld M: Unusual lesions of the breast. Radiol Clin North Am 21:67, 1983
11. Epstein EE: Fibrosarcoma of the breast: a case report. South Afr Med J 57:288, 1980
12. Gartenhaus WS, Mir R, Pliskin A, Grunwald H, Wise L, Papantoniou A, Kahn LB: Granulocytic sarcoma of breast: aleukemic bilateral metachronus presentation and literature review. Med Pediatr Oncol 13:22, 1985
13. Grace WR, Cooperman AM: Inflammatory breast cancer. Surg Clin North Am 65:151, 1985
14. Grant EG, Holt RW, Chun B, Richardson JD, Orson LW, Cigtay OS: Angiosarcoma of the breast: sonographic, xeromammographic, and pathologic appearance. AJR 141:691, 1983
15. Haagensen CD: Diseases of the Breast. 3rd Ed. WB Saunders, Philadelphia, 1986
16. Hajdu SI, Urban JA: Cancers metastatic to the breast. Cancer 29:1691, 1972
17. Holland J, Frei E: Cancer Medicine. 2nd Ed. Lea & Febiger, Philadelphia, 1982
18. Hunter TB, Martin PC, Dietzen CD, Tyler LT: Angiosarcoma of the breast: two case reports and a review of the literature. Cancer 56:2099, 1985
19. Kushner LN: Hodgkin's disease simulating inflammatory breast carcinoma on mammography. Radiology 92:350, 1969
20. Lentle BC, Ludwig R, Camuzzini G: Breast involve-

ment in non-African Burkitt's lymphoma. J Can Assoc Radiol 31:204, 1980

21. Lumsden AB, Harrison D, Chetty U, Going JJ, Muir B: Osteogenic sarcoma—a rare primary tumor of the breast. Eur J Surg Oncol 11:183, 1985

22. Martin JE: Atlas of Mammography: Histologic and Mammographic Correlations. Williams & Wilkins, Baltimore, 1982

23. McCrea ES, Johnston C, Haney PJ: Metastases to the breast. AJR 141:685, 1983

24. McCrea ES, Johnston C, Keramti B: Cystosarcoma phyllodes. South Med J 79:543, 1986

25. McIntosh IH, Hooper AA, Millis RR, Greening WP: Metastatic carcinoma within the breast. Clin Oncol 2:393, 1976

26. McDivitt RW, Boyce W, Gersell D: Tubular carcinoma of the breast: clinical and pathological observations concerning 135 cases. Am J Surg Pathol 6:401, 1982

27. Merino MJ, Berman M, Carter D: Angiosarcoma of the breast. Am J Surg Pathol 7:53, 1983

28. Meyer JE, Kopans DB, Long JC: Mammographic appearance of lymphoma of the breast. Radiology 135:623, 1980

29. Millis RR: Atlas of Breast Pathology. MTP Press Limited, Lancaster, England, 1984

30. Millis RR, Atkinson MK, Tonge KA: The xerographic appearances of some uncommon malignant mammary neoplasms. Clin Radiol 27:463, 1976

31. Moncado R, Cooper RA, Garces M, Badrinath K: Calcified metastases from malignant ovarian neoplasm. Radiology 113:31, 1974

32. Murad TM, Swaid S, Pritchett P: Malignant and benign papillary lesions of the breast. Hum Pathol 8:379, 1977

33. Peters GN, Wolff M: Adenoid cystic carcinoma of the breast—report of 11 new cases: review of the literature and discussion of biological behavior. Cancer 52:680, 1972

34. Pope TL, Fechner RE, Wilhelm MC, Wanebo HJ, de Paredes ES: Lobular carcinoma in situ of the breast: mammographic features. Radiology 168:63, 1988

35. Pope TL, Norman A, Brenbridge, Sloop FB, Morris JR, Carpenter J: Primary histiocytic lymphoma of the breast: mammographic, sonographic, and pathologic correlation. J Clin Ultrasound 13:667, 1985

36. Rhoden SA: Radiologic seminar CCXXXIV: lymphoma of the breast: case report. J MSMA 24:331, 1983

37. Schouten JT, Weese JL, Carbone PP: Lymphoma of the breast. Ann Surg 194:749, 1981

38. Tabar L, Dean PB: Teaching Atlas of Mammography. Thieme-Stratton, New York, 1983

39. Toombs BD, Kalisher L: Metastatic disease to the breast: clinical, pathologic and radiographic features. AJR 129:673, 1977

40. Watt AC, Haggar AM, Krasickey GA: Extraosseous osteogenic sarcoma of the breast: mammographic and pathologic findings. Radiology 150:34, 1984

41. Wiseman C, Liao KT: Primary lymphoma of the breast. Cancer 29:1705, 1972

42. Wolfe JN: Xeroradiography of the Breast. 2nd Ed. Charles C Thomas, Springfield, 1983

15

The Benign Postsurgical Breast

Mary Ellen Peters

POST–BENIGN BIOPSY

With the increasing number of breast biopsies, the radiologist must be familiar with the mammographic changes that result from surgery. These changes include architectural distortion, parenchymal scarring, asymmetry of the fibroglandular tissues, parenchymal and dermal calcifications, skin thickening, and skin retraction.

Fibrosis and fat necrosis at the surgical site cause architectural distortion, manifested by disordered trabeculae, an abnormal fat-glandular interface, retraction, and linear densities (Figs. 15-1 and 15-2). Fibrosis and fat necrosis can also result in a parenchymal scar simulating a scirrhous carcinoma (Fig. 15-3). In Sickle and Herzog's series,[14] these postsurgical changes were most pronounced at 0 to 6 months and tended to regress with time. Although both the architectural distortion and parenchymal scar can simulate carcinoma, the scar mimicking the scirrhous carcinoma is the most troublesome and most often necessitates biopsy.

Wolfe[17] differentiates scars from stellate carcinomas associated with skin retraction by examining the spicules that extend out to the skin. He describes the spicules of the scar as curvilinear and thick, while those of the carcinoma are thin and straight (Fig. 15-4). On palpation, scars feel like an area of thickening, while carcinomas feel larger than the "mass" evident on the mammogram. Although these "differentiating features" can be helpful, they are not always reliable.

A biopsy should not be delayed if there is reasonable question that the changes represent a carcinoma. If postsurgical changes are thought to be more likely, the radiographic and clinical findings should be monitored. Regression of the changes or long-term (several years) stability indicate that the findings were secondary to surgery (Fig. 15-4). Progression, however, indicates the presence of a carcinoma.

Since a scar simulating a carcinoma might develop, why not obtain a baseline postoperative mammogram? The idea is impractical and economically unfeasible since in the majority of cases this is not a problem. Sickles and Herzog,[15] in reviewing their series, found that it is most cost-effective to obtain postoperative mammograms 3 months after surgery in those who either have previously developed a breast parenchymal scar requiring diagnostic biopsy, or who are known keloid-formers.

Asymmetry of the fibroglandular tissues can be the result of a biopsy. This appearance can suggest the presence of a mass in the normal contralateral breast; the

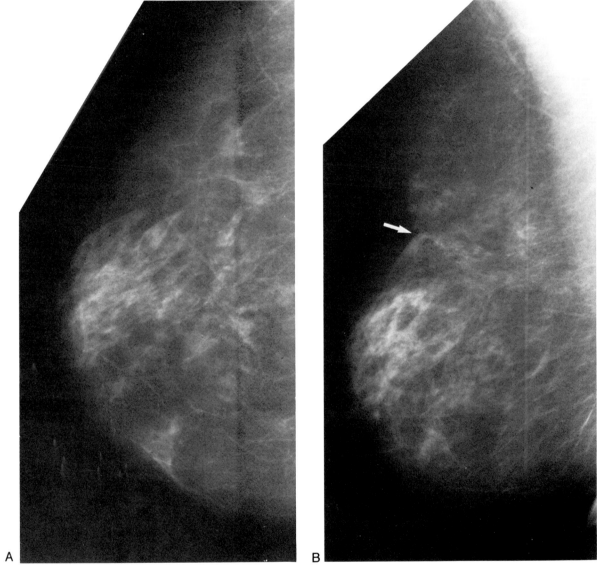

A   B

Fig. 15-1. Left craniocaudal **(A)** and mediolateral oblique **(B)** views in an asymptomatic 63-year-old woman who had a superolateral quadrant benign biopsy 3 years previously. The study demonstrates retraction *(arrow)* of the parenchyma on the mediolateral oblique view. Distortion is seen on the craniocaudal view. Follow-up studies were stable. Diagnosis: scar.

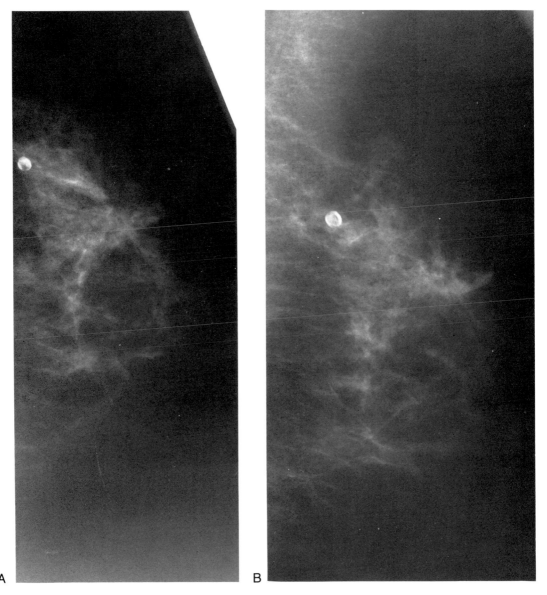

Fig. 15-2. Right craniocaudal **(A)** and mediolateral oblique **(B)** views in an asymptomatic 55-year-old woman with a history of a benign biopsy 1 year previously. The study demonstrates distortion of the parenchyma and a calcified oil cyst in the superolateral quadrant. Subsequent studies were stable. Diagnosis: scar.

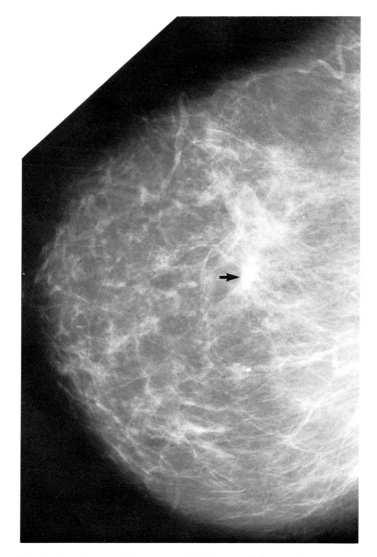

Fig. 15-3. Craniocaudal view in a 45-year-old woman with a history of a benign biopsy 2 years previously. A stellate mass *(arrow)* is present in the area of the previous biopsy. A second biopsy was performed that demonstrated fibrosis. Diagnosis: scar simulating stellate carcinoma.

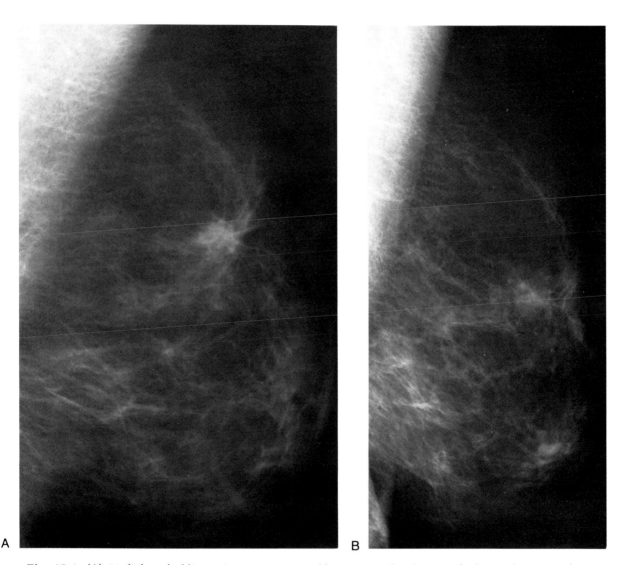

A B

Fig. 15-4. (A) Mediolateral oblique view in a 62-year-old woman with a history of a benign biopsy in the superolateral quadrant 1 year previously. The study demonstrates a mass with thick, curvilinear spicules extending out to the skin. No findings of a carcinoma were present clinically. **(B)** Follow-up 6-month mediolateral view. The mass has decreased in size. *(Figure continues.)*

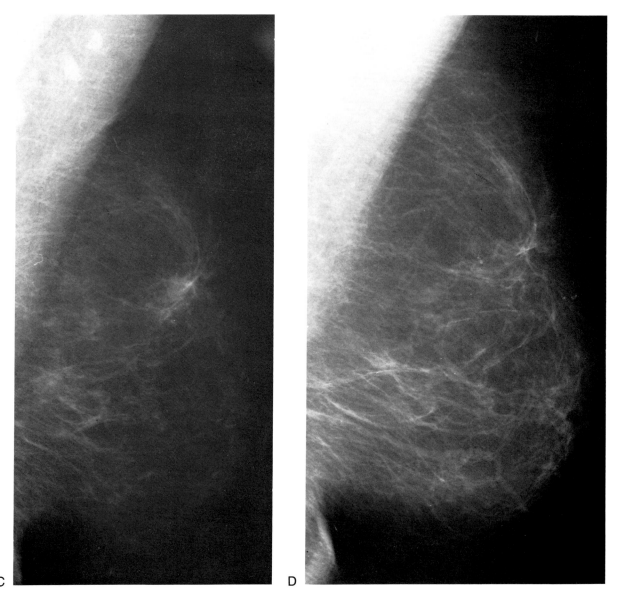

C

D

Fig. 15-4 *(Continued)*. **(C)** A second 6-month mediolateral view follow-up study. Progressive decrease in size is seen. **(D)** Mediolateral oblique view 1 year later. The scar has almost totally resolved.

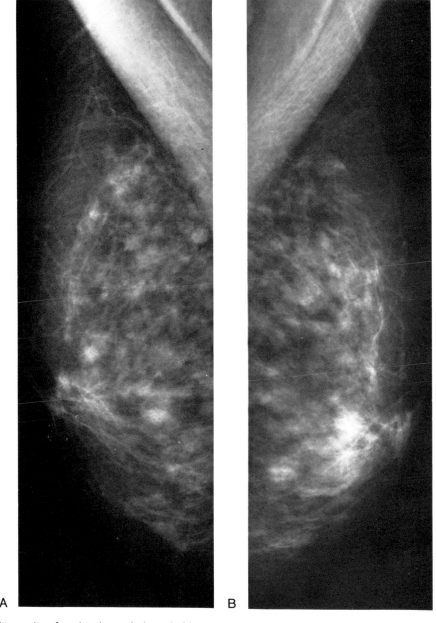

A   B

Fig. 15-5. (A & B) Left and right mediolateral oblique views in an asymptomatic 55-year-old woman who had a benign biopsy in the left inferomedial quadrant. The fibroglandular tissues are asymmetric. There is greater density inferior to the nipple on the right. The asymmetry is the result of the left biopsy. No abnormalities are present.

absence of glandular tissue in the biopsied breast creates asymmetry (Fig. 15-5). Clinical history is imperative in the interpretation of mammograms!

Calcification in the wall of an oil cyst is the most characteristic type of calcification observed in the postsur-

gical breast. Initially, an oil cyst appears as a radiolucent or mixed radiolucent-radiodense lesion varying in size from a few millimeters to 3 cm. They are the result of fats reduced to fatty acids and the formation of a surrounding fibrous capsule. The capsule frequently calcifies to produce a crescent, ring, or shell-like appearance and is termed liponecrosis macrocystica calcificans (Figs. 15-2 and 15-6).

Other types of calcifications may be seen in the fibroglandular tissues at the surgical site. They may have the form of large globular calcifications, scattered smooth punctate calcifications, or large linear calcifications in the plane of the incision. Sutural calcification, which has a rod-shaped appearance, can occur. In addition, small, irregular clustered calcifications indistinguishable from malignant calcifications can develop in the surgical bed as the result of fat necrosis.

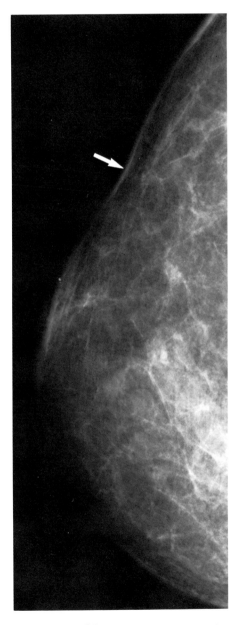

Fig. 15-6. Craniocaudal view in an asymptomatic 53-year-old woman with a history of a benign biopsy 1 year previously. A round area of lucency and a shell-like calcification is present medially. These changes are the result of surgically induced fat necrosis.

Fig. 15-7. Craniocaudal view in an asymptomatic 78-year-old woman with a history of a benign biopsy in the superolateral quadrant 5 years previously. Residual skin thickening and retraction is present at the surgical site *(arrow)*. Note the benign punctate calcification in the areola.

Skin calcifications can also develop in the area of incision. Large plaquelike calcifications have been described, but are observed infrequently. Occasionally, small punctate calcifications occur.

Skin thickening in the area of the biopsy is almost always seen. It rarely resolves completely. At times, there is associated retraction (Fig. 15-7).

Knowledge of a previous biopsy (e.g., quadrant, date, and any postsurgical complications) is critical for accurate interpretation of the mammogram. The radiologist must often examine the patient in order to correlate the physical findings with the mammogram.

REDUCTION MAMMOPLASTY

Reduction mammoplasty is performed for cosmetic and comfort reasons in women who have large breasts and for symmetry in the contralateral breast in women who have had breast conservation or who have a unilateral congenitally hypoplastic breast. Mammographic changes commonly occur postreduction and are dependent on the type of procedure.

Miller et al.[10] have described the mammographic findings in two of the more commonly used plastic procedures, nipple-areolar complex transposition and nipple-areolar complex transplantation. The procedures

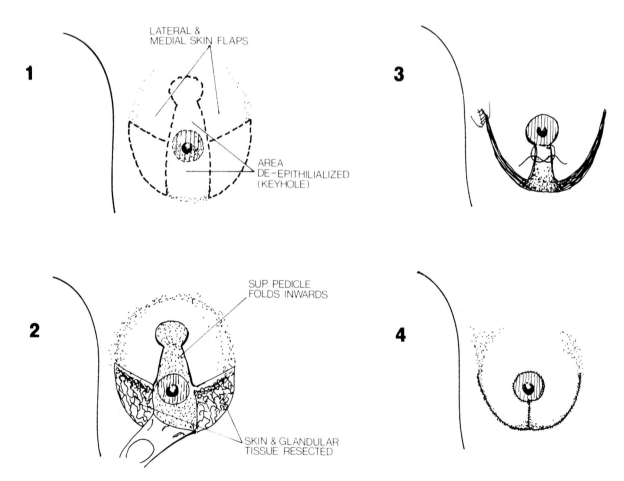

Fig. 15-8. Surgical technique commonly used in reduction mammoplasty. (Adapted from Miller et al.,[10] with permission.)

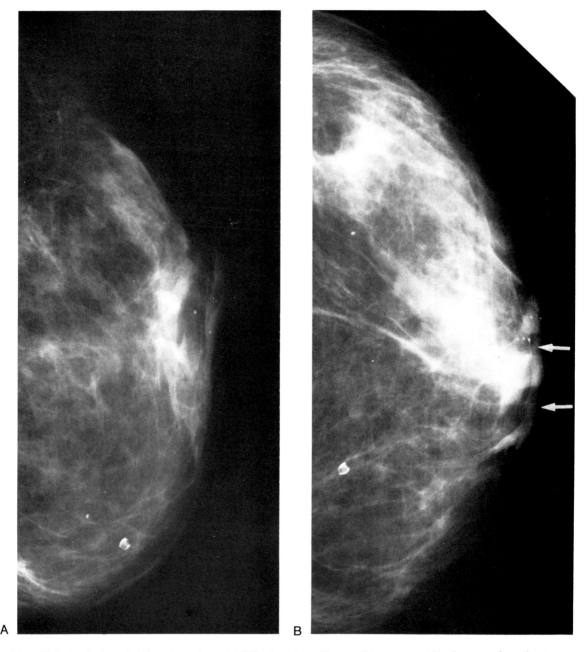

A   B

Fig. 15-9. Right lateral **(A)** and craniocaudal **(B)** views in a 40-year-old woman with a history of a reduction mammoplasty with transposition of the ducts. The lateral view demonstrates that the nipple is high. The areolar area is thickened, and several benign-appearing calcifications are present in the areola area, some of which can be definitely identified as within the skin. A retroareolar band *(arrows)* is seen on the craniocaudal view. The ducts connect to the nipple. Note the calcified oil cyst in the inferomedial quadrant.

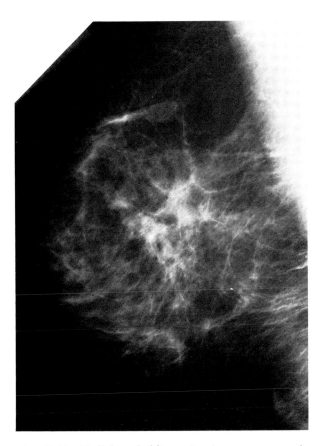

Fig. 15-10. Mediolateral oblique view in an asymptomatic 47-year-old woman with a history of a reduction mammoplasty. The fibroglandular tissues are distorted in appearance as the result of the mammoplasty.

are similar except the nipple-areolar complex remains connected to the ducts in the transposition procedure, and in the transplantation procedure the nipple-areolar complex is severed from the ducts. Beneath a "keyhole," which is drawn on the breast preoperatively, the area is de-epithelialized except for the areola. The skin, fat, and fibroglandular tissues medial and lateral to the inferior pedicle are resected. The nipple is displaced superiorly by suturing the medial and lateral skin flaps and infolding the superior pedicle (Fig. 15-8).

In their series, Miller et al.[10] found the mammographic findings similar in both procedures, except in the transposition procedure the ducts appear continuous; in the transplantation procedure they appeared discontinuous. In both procedures, findings that could be observed were displacement of fibroglandular tissues inferiorly, high nipple, superior tilt of the nipple, thickening of the skin inferiorly secondary to the linear

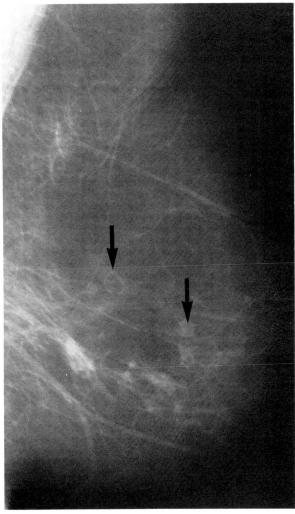

Fig. 15-11. Mediolateral oblique view in an asymptomatic 55-year-old woman with a history of a reduction mammoplasty 2 years previously. The study demonstrates round lucencies surrounded by a thin capsule *(arrows)*. These are oil cysts that developed secondary to fat necrosis.

scar, and skin retraction inferiorly. Other findings included areolar thickening, a retroareolar band, and areolar calcifications (Fig. 15-9).

Reduction mammoplasty can also cause the fibroglandular tissues to appear distorted as the result of fibrosis and fat necrosis (Fig. 15-10). Other manifestations of fat necrosis seen postmammoplasty are oil cysts, calcifications mimicking those seen in carcinoma, or a stellate mass with or without associated calcifications and skin retraction (Figs. 15-11 and 15-12).

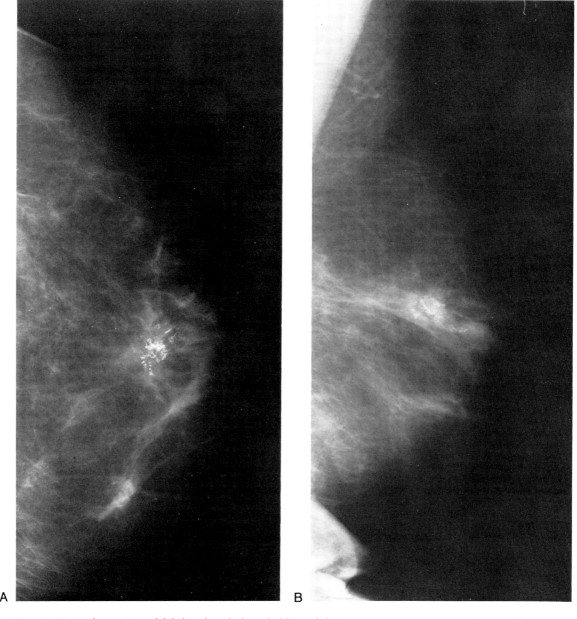

Fig. 15-12. Right craniocaudal **(A)** and mediolateral oblique **(B)** views in an asymptomatic 48-year-old woman, 1 year postreduction mammoplasty. The parenchyma is displaced inferiorly. A group of malignant-appearing microcalcifications is present. They were biopsied and proved to be the result of fat necrosis.

BREAST AUGMENTATION

Breast augmentation is performed by placing a Silastic envelope, which is filled with either silicone or saline, in the retromammary space or beneath the pectoralis muscle. Clinical examination of the fibroglandular tissues is easier with the prosthesis in the retromammary space, but the management of breast lesions is easier with the subpectoral location (Figs. 15-13 and 15-14). In either procedure, the prosthesis often precludes a satisfactory mammogram. Eklund et al.[4] have achieved better visualization of the breast parenchyma by displacing the prosthesis posteriorly and pulling the fibroglandular tissues forward during the examination.

Complications that can be observed radiographically include fractures, irregularities, and wrinkles of the prosthesis, leakage of silicone into the fibroglandular tissues, and findings associated with infection. If the prosthesis becomes encapsulated, it appears round and is hard on palpation. The encapsulated prosthesis is at risk for fracture during mammography if vigorous compression is used.

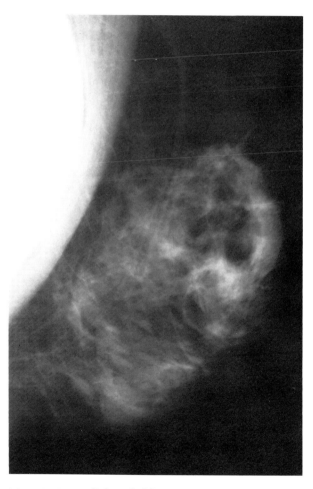

Fig. 15-13. Mediolateral oblique view in an asymptomatic 47-year-old woman with a history of an augmentation procedure. The prosthesis has been placed beneath the pectoralis muscle.

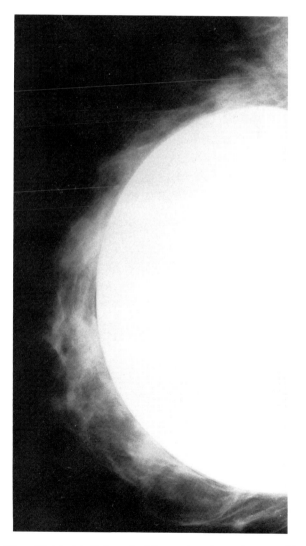

Fig. 15-14. Mediolateral oblique view in a 46-year-old woman with a prior augmentation. The prosthesis has been placed in the retromammary space.

SUGGESTED READINGS

1. Baber CE, Libshitz HI: Bilateral fat necrosis of the breast following reduction mammoplasties. AJR 128:508, 1977
2. Bassett LW, Gold RH, Cove HC: Mammographic spectrum of traumatic fat necrosis: the fallibility of "pathogomonic" signs of carcinoma. AJR 130:119, 1978
3. Bostwick J: Aesthetic and Reconstructive Breast Surgery. CV Mosby, St. Louis, 1981
4. Eklund GW, Busby RC, Miller SH, Job JS: Improved imaging of the breast. AJR 151:469, 1988
5. Heywang SH, Eiermann W, Basserman R, Fenzl G: Carcinoma of the breast behind a prosthesis — comparison of ultrasound, mammography and MRI (case report). Comput Radiol 9:283, 1985
6. Isaacs G, Rozner L, Tudball C: Breast lumps after reduction mammoplasty. Ann Plast Surg 15:394, 1985
7. Jensen SR, Mackey JK: Xeromammography after augmentation mammoplasty. AJR 144:629, 1985
8. Martin JE: Atlas of Mammography: Histologic and Mammography Correlations. Williams & Wilkins, Baltimore, 1982
9. Meyer JE, Silverman P, Ghandbir L: Fat necrosis of the breast. Arch Surg 113:801, 1978
10. Miller CL, Feig SA, Fox JW: Mammographic changes after reduction mammoplasty. AJR 149:35, 1987
11. Orson LW, Cigtay OS: Fat necrosis of the breast: characteristic xeromammographic appearance. Radiology 146:35, 1983
12. Robertson JL: A changed appearance of mammograms following breast reduction. Plast Reconstr Surg 59:347, 1977
13. Sickles EA: Breast calcifications: mammographic evaluation. Radiology 160:289, 1986
14. Sickles EA, Herzog KA: Intramammary scar tissue: a mimic of the mammographic appearance of carcinoma. AJR 135:349, 1980
15. Sickles EA, Herzog KA: Mammography of the postsurgical breast. AJR 136:585, 1981
16. Tabar L, Dean PB: Teaching Atlas of Mammography. Thieme-Stratton, New York, 1983
17. Wolfe JN: Xeroradiography of the Breast. 2nd Ed. Charles C Thomas, Springfield, IL, 1983

16

Mammographic Evaluation of the Postsurgical and Irradiated Breast*

Mary Ellen Peters

It is now commonplace for women to elect lumpectomy followed by radiation therapy for stages I and II breast carcinoma. Mammography is important in the preoperative assessment of these patients, in the detection of residual tumor postoperatively, and in the detection of recurrences and second primaries following radiation therapy.

PREOPERATIVE MAMMOGRAM

The limiting factors for breast conservation are the ability to obtain a satisfactory cosmetic result and the presence of only one dominant cancer. In the presence of two or more dominant cancers, mastectomy is advised. With a preoperative mammogram, the radiologist can evaluate the size of the tumor (mammography

is usually more accurate than physical examination), detect evidence of multicentric carcinomas, and assess the status of the contralateral breast (Fig. 16-1).

POSTLUMPECTOMY MAMMOGRAM

The postlumpectomy mammogram is used to detect any residual tumor and to establish a baseline for subsequent studies. The surgical procedure itself may take three forms: an excisional biopsy removing only a small border of normal-appearing tissue; a tylectomy, or wide local excision removing a 1 to 2 cm rim of normal parenchyma as well as an ellipse of the overlying skin; or a quadrectomy, resecting the one-fourth of the breast that encompasses the primary carcinoma. Most surgeons also perform an open axillary dissection removing all the level I and most of the level II nodes. Usually the apical nodes (level III) are not dissected, since level II will be positive if the apical nodes are involved with metastatic disease.

The postlumpectomy mammogram should be post-

---

* This chapter and Figures 16-1 through 16-16 are from Peters ME, Fagerholm MI, Scanlan KA et al: Mammographic evaluation of the postsurgical and irradiated breast. Radio-Graphics 8:873, 1988, with permission.

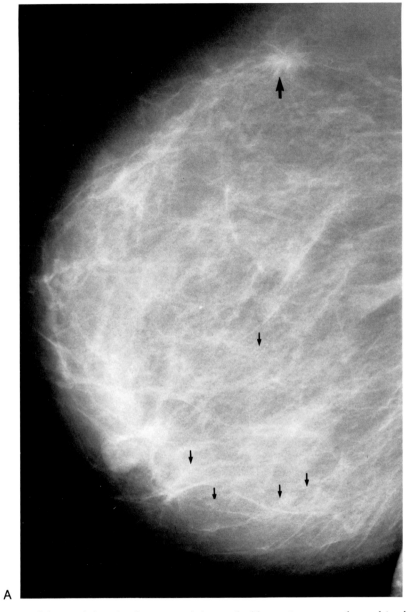

A

Fig. 16-1. Craniocaudal view **(A)** and enlargement **(B)**. A palpable carcinoma was located in the superolateral quadrant *(large arrow)*. The mammogram also demonstrated malignant calcifications *(small arrows)* in the inferomedial quadrant, which proved to be in multicentric, nonpalpable carcinomas. Because of the presence of more than one dominant cancer, the patient was ineligible for breast conservation. *(Figure continues.)*

poned for at least 2 weeks after the surgery. This gives time for the hematoma to resolve, yielding a more accurate radiographic interpretation, and for the incision to heal, permitting adequate compression of the breast during mammography. In evaluating a postlumpectomy mammogram, it is imperative to obtain the pre-

operative study. Critical information may be gained concerning the size, configuration, density, presence of associated microcalcifications, and exact location of the carcinoma.

Postoperative mammography is most effective in iden-

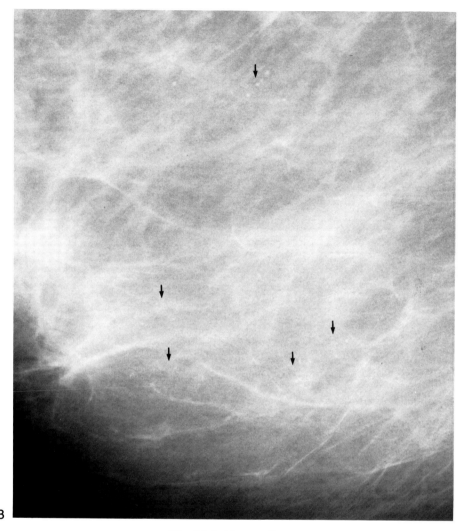

B

Fig. 16-1 *(Continued)*.

tifying residual tumors with associated calcifications (Fig. 16-2). In the fatty replaced breast, it can often be helpful even though the primary tumor did not contain calcifications. In the dense breast, however, it is usually not possible to recognize a residual tumor not associated with calcifications. In either case, the postoperative mammogram should be studied diligently for the presence of residual microcalcifications and/or masses (Fig. 16-3). Magnification views of the lumpectomy site may be useful in identifying residual tumor masses and calcifications.

The radiologist should be familiar with the mammographic findings caused by surgery, since some of the changes mimic the presence of carcinoma, while others can mask the presence of residual tumor. The immediate postoperative study invariably shows changes of edema of the fibroglandular tissues and skin. Typically, the edema is localized to the area of incision, but it can involve a much larger area. The edema of the fibroglandular tissues is manifested by a generalized increase in density and trabecular thickening (Fig. 16-3). These findings usually resolve within 4 weeks but may persist much longer. Commonly, however, the thickening of the skin in the area of the incision never completely resolves. Prominent periareolar edema is sometimes present as a result of surgical disruption of the lymphatics; this edema gradually resolves.

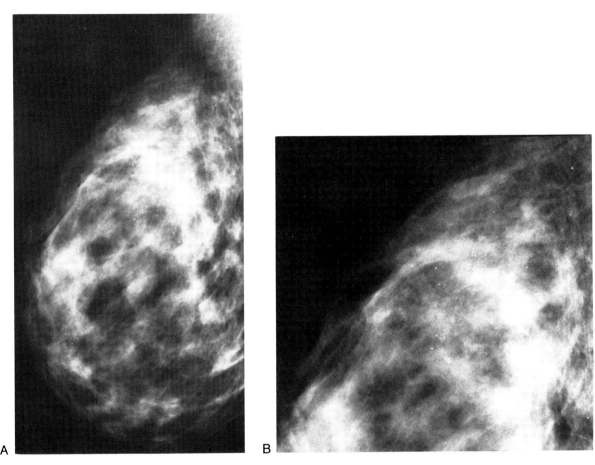

Fig. 16-2. Mediolateral oblique view **(A)** and enlargement **(B)** from the craniocaudal view. The patient was referred after resection of a superolateral quadrant infiltrating ductal carcinoma. Clinically, no residual mass was detected. However, diffuse, malignant calcifications at the lumpectomy site were evident on the mammogram. Residual carcinoma was confirmed at surgery.

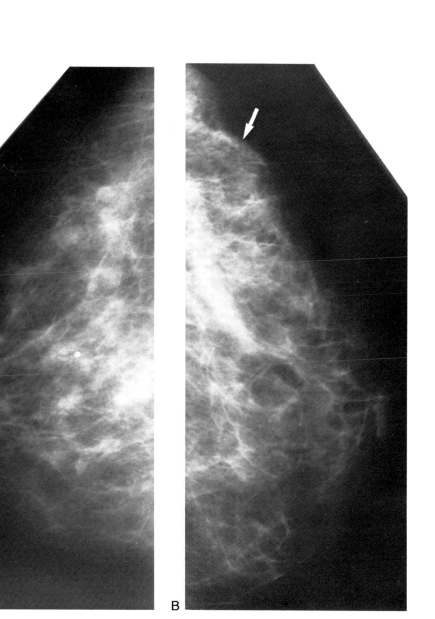

Fig. 16-3. Left and right craniocaudal **(A & B)** and mediolateral oblique **(C & D)** views. The patient was referred after resection of an infiltrating ductal carcinoma of the right superolateral quadrant. The mammogram was performed 2 days postoperatively, and a small, ill-defined mass *(large black arrow)* suggestive of carcinoma was seen at the lumpectomy site. Residual carcinoma was proven at surgery. This mammogram also demonstrated findings of postsurgical edema manifested by generalized increased density, trabecular thickening, and skin thickening *(white arrow). (Figure continues.)*

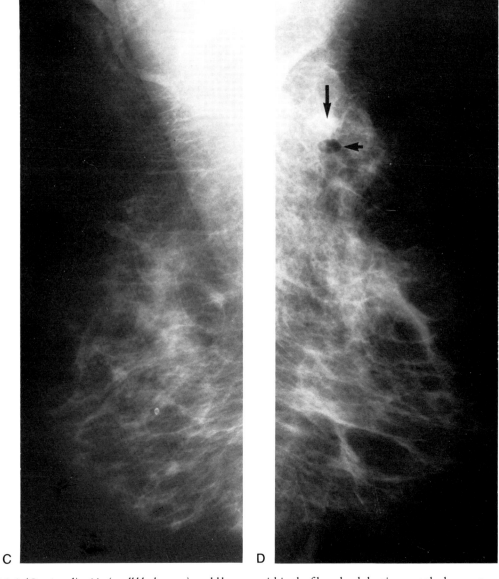

C   D

Fig. 16-3 *(Continued)*. Air *(small black arrow)* could be seen within the fibroglandular tissues at the lumpectomy site. No abnormalities were present on the left.

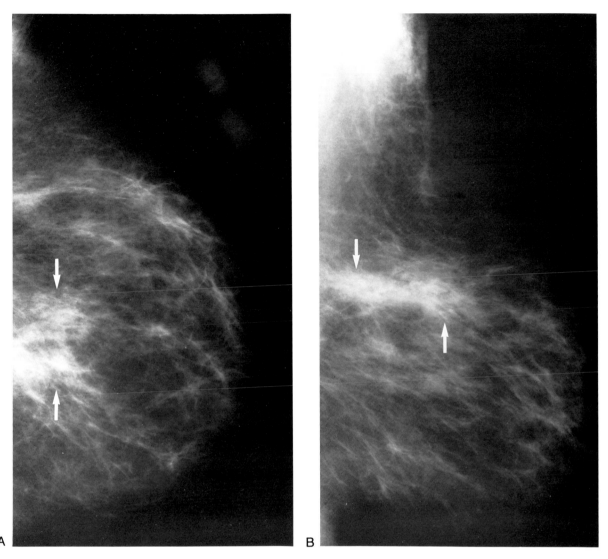

Fig. 16-4. Right craniocaudal **(A)** and mediolateral oblique **(B)** views and magnification of lumpectomy site **(C)**. Ill-defined areas of increased density were present in the area of the lumpectomy *(arrows)* on this study performed 2 weeks after surgery. The findings were probably secondary to edema and/or hematoma. No definite residual tumor was defined, but such a possibility could not be absolutely excluded. *(Figure continues.)*

The surgical bed can also contain air (Fig. 16-3) and hematoma. Radiographically, hematomas can present as fairly well-defined masses that can be so large as to preclude detecting residual tumor. They can also have the appearance of small, ill-defined densities that cannot be differentiated from islands of residual carcinoma or edema of the fibroglandular tissues (Fig. 16-4). Most hematomas resolve within 2 to 4 weeks, although they may persist as long as 8 weeks. Occasionally they form pseudocysts, mimicking the presence of carcinoma.

Lymphoceles (Fig. 16-5) and seromas can also develop

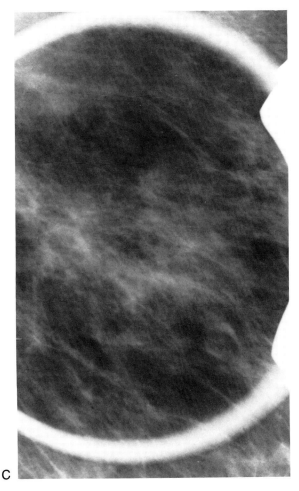

C

Fig. 16-4 *(Continued)*.

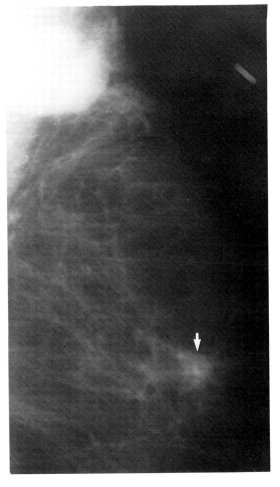

Fig. 16-5. Mediolateral oblique view. The study was performed 17 days postlumpectomy and demonstrated a large, round, palpable mass in the lower axilla. Chylous fluid was aspirated, proving that it was a lymphocele. A well-defined mass *(arrow)* that did not conform to the original carcinoma was present at the lumpectomy site; the findings were consistent with a residual hematoma.

after axillary dissection and lumpectomy. Radiographically, they present as fairly well-defined masses. Although demonstrable with mammography, they are infrequent and usually clinically evident.

POSTRADIATION MAMMOGRAM

In postmenopausal women, radiation therapy is begun 2 to 3 weeks after lumpectomy if the axillary nodes are negative. If the nodes are positive, four to five cycles of adjuvant chemotherapy are administered prior to radiation therapy at the University of Wisconsin. Adjuvant chemotherapy is also given to premenopausal women with negative nodes and positive estrogen receptor tumors prior to radiation therapy. The timing of the adjuvant chemotherapy is controversial, and it varies in different institutions. The typical radiation dose is 50 Gy to the entire breast, boosting to 60 Gy at the lumpectomy site. The first postradiation mammograms should be obtained at 6 and 12 months after the initiation of therapy, followed by annual studies unless suspicious findings warrant earlier examinations.

The most pronounced mammographic changes evident after radiation therapy are the result of edema

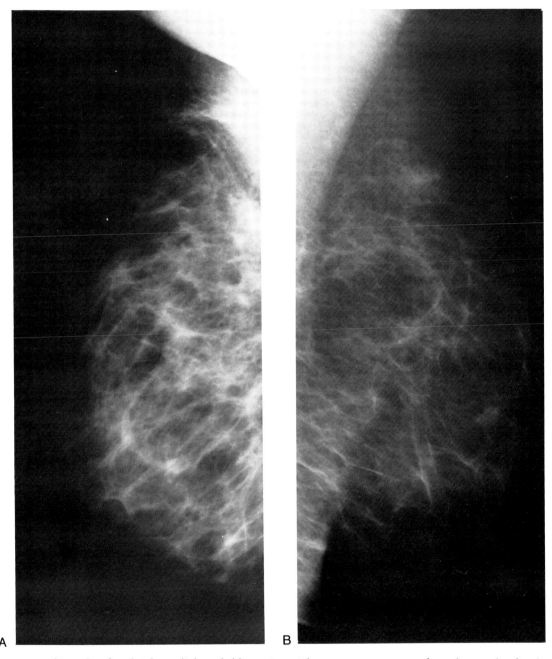

Fig. 16-6. (A & B) Left and right mediolateral oblique views. The mammogram was performed 6 months after the initiation of radiotherapy to the left breast. It demonstrated findings of edema manifested by generalized increased density of the fibroglandular tissues and associated trabecular thickening on the left. The right was normal.

affecting the fibroglandular tissues, subcutaneous tissues, and skin. The findings of edema following radiation are more dramatic, compared with the postsurgical changes. In addition, the edema always involves the entire breast and persists much longer. As in the postsurgical breast, there is an overall increase in density of the fibroglandular tissues and thickening of the trabeculae (Figs. 16-6 to 16-8). These changes are most prominent 6 months after the initiation of therapy. The generalized increased density of the fibroglandular tissues usually resolves within 1 year. The trabecular thickening clears more slowly and may never completely resolve.

The edema of the subcutaneous tissues is seen on mammograms as small, linear opacities resulting from dilated lymphatics and blood vessels and as irregularity of the inner surface of the skin (Fig. 16-9). These findings are most pronounced at 6 months and will usually resolve within 24 months.

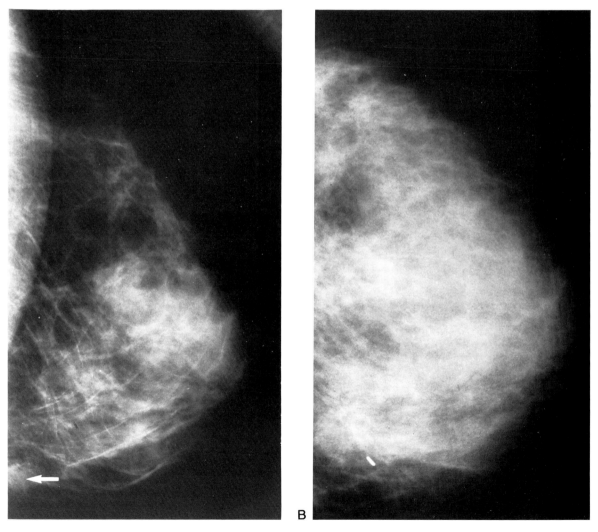

A

B

Fig. 16-7. (A) Craniocaudial view. A carcinoma was present in the inferomedial quadrant *(arrow)*. A lumpectomy was performed. **(B)** Craniocaudial view. The 6-month study after initiation of radiation therapy demonstrated a marked increase in density. The breast was very firm as the result of the therapy, and adequate compression during mammography could not be achieved. The inability to obtain good compression of the irradiated breast contributes to the overall appearance of increased density.

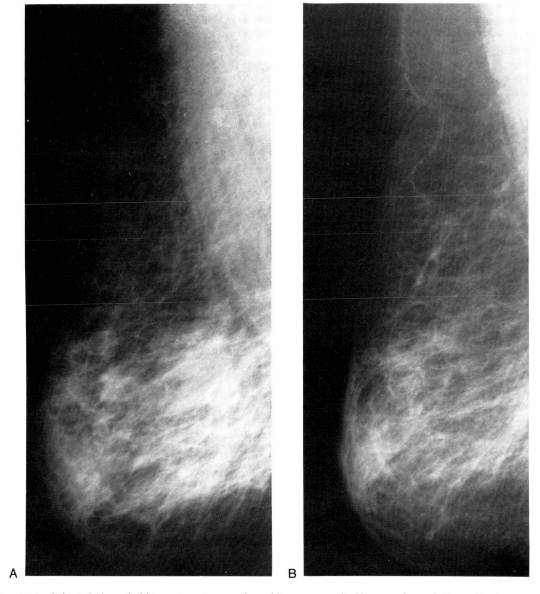

Fig. 16-8. **(A)** Mediolateral oblique view. A superolateral lumpectomy had been performed. Generalized increased density of the fibroglandular tissues and trabecular and skin thickening were evident on the 6-month study after initiation of radiation therapy. **(B)** Mediolateral oblique view. The 12-month study demonstrated an overall decrease in density, but the trabecular and skin thickening persisted. The breast was smaller as the result of fibrosis.

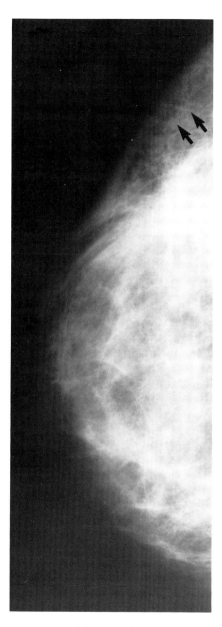

Fig. 16-9. Craniocaudal view. The patient had a superolateral lumpectomy. Subcutaneous edema was evident on this 6-month study after initiation of radiation therapy. The inner surface of the skin lacked its normal clear definition, and linear opacities could be observed in the subcutaneous area *(arrows)*. Note also the associated skin thickening.

Skin edema, which is most prominent at the incision site and periareolar area, is greatest at 6 months and gradually decreases (Fig. 16-10). In the majority of cases treated to 50 Gy, the skin thickness returns to near normal, except for the area of incision.

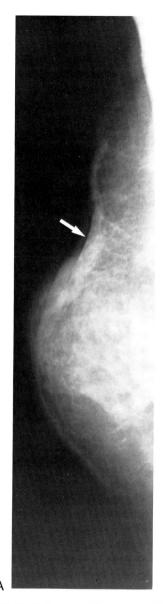

A

Fig. 16-10. (A) Mediolateral oblique view. This 6-month study after initiation of radiation therapy demonstrated generalized skin thickening, which was greatest at the surgical site *(arrow)* and periareolar area. *(Figure continues.)*

CALCIFICATIONS FOLLOWING SURGERY AND RADIATION THERAPY

Calcification in the wall of an oil cyst is the most characteristic type observed in the postsurgical breast,

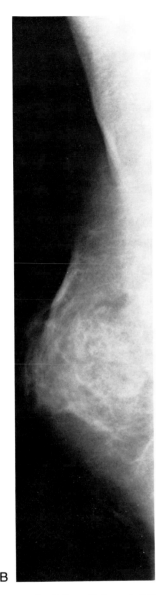

B

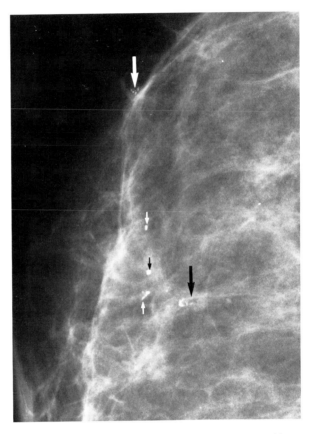

Fig. 16-10 *(Continued)*. **(B)** Mediolateral oblique view. Partial resolution of the skin thickening had occurred by 12 months.

Fig. 16-11. Enlargement from a craniocaudal view of lumpectomy site. This 2-year study demonstrated development of benign-appearing calcifications in the area of the lumpectomy. Coarse linear calcifications *(large black arrow)* in the plane of the incision, a calcified oil cyst *(small black arrow)*, large linear and globular calcifications *(small white arrows)*, and a group of smooth, relatively large calcifications *(large white arrow)* were present.

as has been previously discussed. An area of low density or lucency can be present as early as the postlumpectomy mammogram. The capsular calcification may be observed on the initial 6-month study, or it may not be visible for years. Oil cysts can also occur outside the surgical site in the conservatively treated breast, probably as the result of radiation-induced fat necrosis. Less

frequently, calcifications of varying size, shape, and density, mimicking those seen in malignancy, develop secondary to fat necrosis at the lumpectomy site.

Other types of calcifications can develop in the area of

the lumpectomy: smooth, round calcifications, which can be grouped or scattered; large linear calcifications oriented in the plane of the incision; large globular calcifications; sutural calcifications, which are rod-shaped; and dermal calcifications, which can be either plaquelike or punctate (Figs. 16-11 to 16-13). Development of secretorylike calcifications has been described in the irradiated breast, but this is uncommon. All of these calcifications may develop by 6 months, but their occurrence is quite variable.

ARCHITECTURAL DISTORTION AND PARENCHYMAL SCAR

The most difficult problem in mammography of the conservatively treated breast is to differentiate recurrent carcinoma from architectural distortion resulting from fibrosis and fat necrosis. The discussion of parenchymal scar versus carcinoma that was presented in

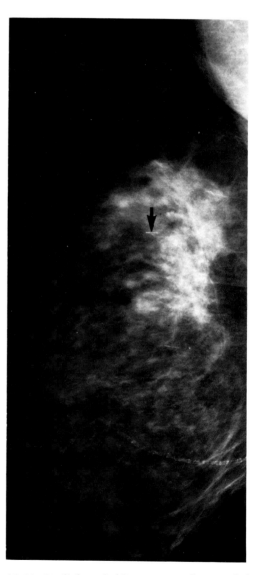

Fig. 16-12. Enlargement from a mediolateral oblique view of lumpectomy site. Malignant-appearing calcifications, not evident on previous studies, were seen at the lumpectomy site on this 4-year study. The histopathology of the biopsied specimen showed sclerosis.

Fig. 16-13. Mediolateral oblique view. A large, rod-shaped calcification, compatible with a sutural calcification, developed *(arrow)* in the area of the lumpectomy. (Areas of vascular calcification were also present.)

Chapter 15 on the benign postsurgical breast applies here as well. Careful follow-up mammography of these patients is mandatory, since it can often be beneficial in differentiating scars from recurrent carcinoma.

MAMMOGRAPHIC CHANGES OF RECURRENCES

The recurrence rate of carcinoma in the conservatively treated breast has been found to be 2 percent/year during the first 14 years. The mammographic signs of recurrence are an increase in size of a pre-existing density (Fig. 16-14), development of a new mass, development of malignant-appearing calcifications (Fig. 16-15), and an inappropriate increase in edema.

In the series of Stomper et al.,[14] 35 percent of recurrences were detected by mammography alone, and 61 percent of all recurrences were seen on mammography. They found that recurrences detected by mammogra-

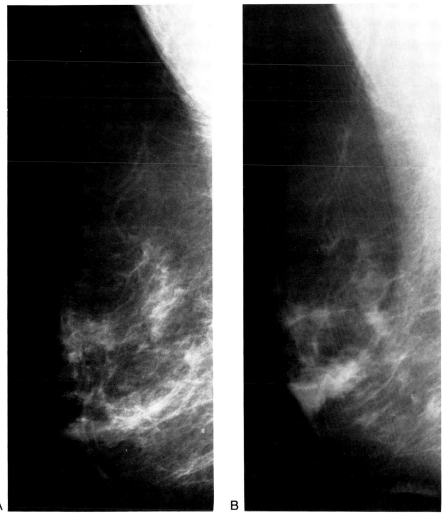

Fig. 16-14. (A) Mediolateral oblique view. The study was performed 3 years after initiation of radiation therapy and was stable, compared with previous studies. **(B)** Mediolateral oblique view. The study 1 year later demonstrated greater opacity in the lumpectomy site located in the retroareolar area, nipple retraction, and an increase in skin thickening. These findings indicated recurrence of the carcinoma. Clinically, no mass was detected. A biopsy confirmed the presence of a recurrence.

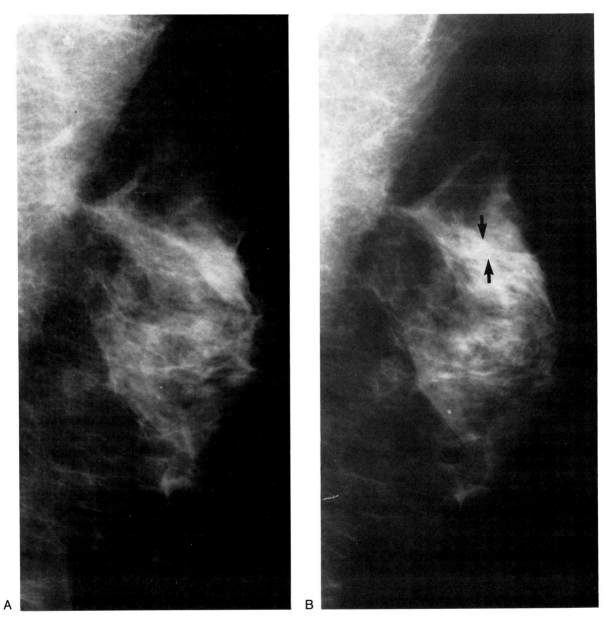

A

B

Fig. 16-15. **(A)** Mediolateral oblique view. The patient had a superolateral lumpectomy. The 12-month study after initiation of therapy demonstrated no evidence of recurrence. **(B)** Mediolateral oblique view and **(C)** enlargement. The 2-year study showed the development of microcalcifications *(arrows)* in the area of the lumpectomy. No mass was palpated. Recurrence was proven on biopsy. *(Figure continues.)*

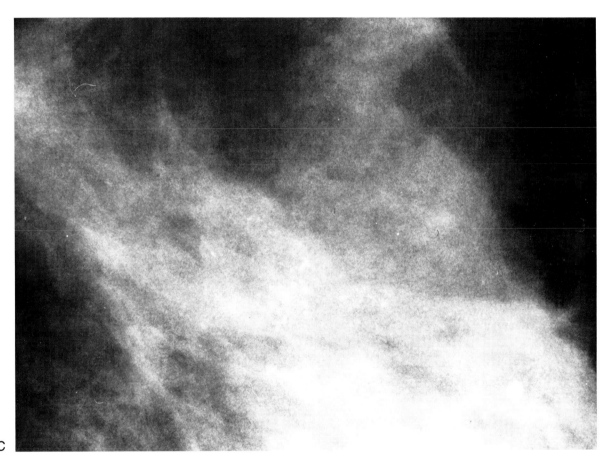

C

Fig. 16-15 *(Continued).*

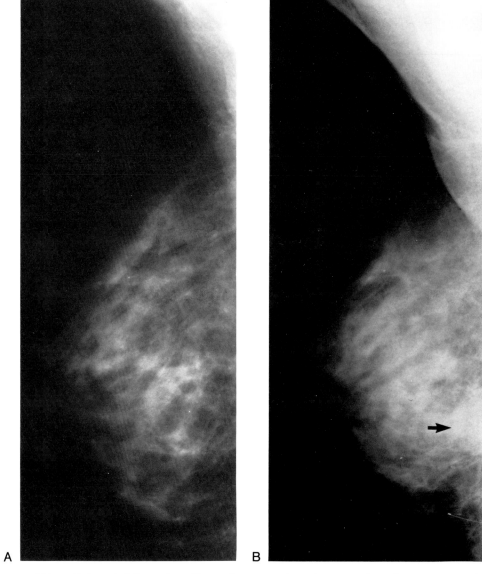

Fig. 16-16. (A) Mediolateral oblique view. The study was performed 5 years after a lumpectomy and radiation therapy for a superolateral quadrant medullary carcinoma. No recurrence was evident on this study. **(B)** Mediolateral oblique view. The 6-year study demonstrated a new mass *(arrow)* in the conservatively treated breast that was not detected clinically. Histopathology showed an infiltrating ductal carcinoma indicating the presence of a second primary.

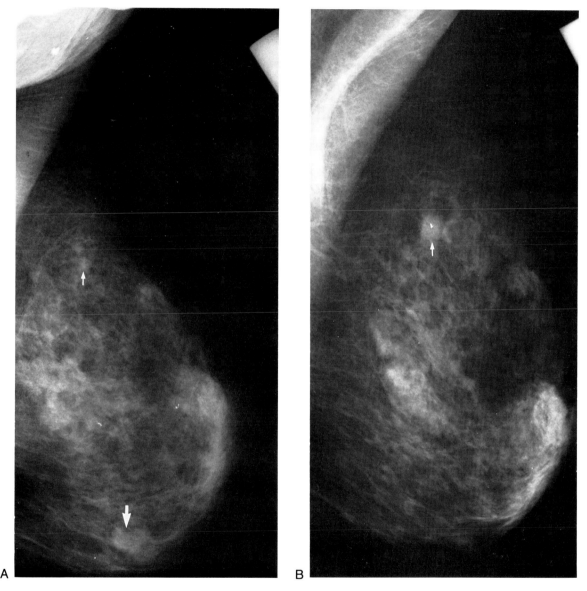

Fig. 16-17. (A) Mediolateral oblique view. An infiltrating ductal carcinoma *(large arrow)* was resected in this 81-year-old woman. **(B)** Mediolateral oblique view 3 years later. The size of the previous density *(small arrow)* has increased; it proved to be an infiltrating ductal carcinoma. It is not known if it is a second primary or metastasis, since it is the same cell type.

phy alone were more apt to be noninvasive, compared with those found on physical examination. Sixty-five percent of the recurrences in their series developed at the lumpectomy site, 22 percent occurred at other sites, and 13 percent were multifocal.

The conservatively treated breast is at a higher risk for developing a second primary. However, this diagnosis can only be made if the second primary is of a different histopathologic cell type (Figs. 16-16 and 16-17). Remember that the contralateral breast is also at a higher risk for developing carcinoma.

SUGGESTED READINGS

1. Bassett LW, Gold RH, Mirra JM: Nonneoplastic breast calcifications in lipid cysts: development after excision and primary irradiation. AJR 138:335, 1982
2. Bosworth JL, Ghossein NA: Limited surgery and radiotherapy in the treatment of localized breast cancer: an overview. Surg Clin North Am 64:1115, 1984
3. Buckley JH, Roebuck EJ: Mammographic changes following radiotherapy. Br J Radiol 59:337, 1986
4. Fisher B, Bauer M, Margolese R et al: Five-year results of a randomized clinical trial comparing total mastectomy and segmental mastectomy with or without radiation in the treatment of breast cancer. N Engl J Med 312:665, 1985
5. Gefter WB, Friedman AK, Goodman RL: The role of mammography in evaluating patients with early carcinoma of the breast for tylectomy and radiation therapy. Radiology 142:77, 1982
6. Libshitz HI, Montague ED, Paulus DD: Calcifications and the therapeutically irradiated breast. AJR 128:1021, 1977
7. Libshitz HI, Montague ED, Paulus DD: Skin thickness in the therapeutically irradiated breast. AJR 130:345, 1978
8. Montague ED, Paulus D, Schell S: Selection and follow-up of patients for conservation surgery and irradiation. Front Radiat Ther Onc 17:124, 1983
9. Paulus DD: Conservative treatment of breast cancer: Mammography in patient selection and follow-up. AJR 143:483, 1984
10. Recht A, Connolly JL, Schnitt SJ et al: Conservative surgery and radiation therapy for early breast cancer: results, controversies, and unsolved problems. Semin Oncol 113:434, 1986
11. Sickles EA: Breast calcifications; mammographic evaluation. Radiology 160:289, 1986
12. Sickles EA, Herzog KA: Intramammary scar tissue: a mimic of the mammographic appearance of carcinoma. AJR 135:349, 1980
13. Sickles EA, Herzog KA: Mammography of the postsurgical breast. AJR 136:585, 1981
14. Stomper PC, Recht A, Berenberg AL, Jochelson MS, Harris JR: Mammographic detection of recurrent cancer in the irradiated breast. AJR 148:39, 1987
15. Tabar L, Dean PB: Teaching Atlas of Mammography. Thieme-Stratton, New York, 1983
16. Tinker M, Wise L: Breast-preserving operations. p. 225. In Ariel IM, Cleary JB (eds): Breast Cancer Diagnosis. McGraw-Hill, New York, 1986
17. Wolfe JN: Xerography of the Breast. 2nd Ed. p. 399. Charles C Thomas, Springfield, IL, 1983

17

The Male Breast

Kathleen A. Scanlan

The male breast is a site of frequent benign pathology and infrequent but life-threatening malignancy. Mammography plays a role in the evaluation of male breast abnormalities.

EMBRYOLOGY AND STRUCTURE

The breasts of male and female children are quite similar structurally. Both are composed of 15 to 25 lobar units, each centered around a lactiferous duct. At puberty sexual dimorphism takes place. Estrogen/progesterone-dependent development does not, of course, take place in the male. Only remnants of a ductal system with atrophic epithelium can be seen histologically in the normal adult male breast. In the female breast, however, estrogen is responsible for growth, division, and elongation of the duct system. The synergistic action of progesterone is required for alveolar (acinar) development.

MAMMOGRAPHIC APPEARANCE OF THE MALE BREAST

The normal male breast is composed predominantly of fat, with no parenchymal density and only rudimentary ducts. It appears on mammographic images as a small, lucent structure with a few radiopaque strands coursing posteriorly from the nipple (Fig. 17-1). Obesity may increase the size and adipose content of the male breast, mimicking gynecomastia clinically (Fig. 17-2).

GYNECOMASTIA

The most common male breast abnormality seen clinically is gynecomastia, a benign enlargement of one or both breasts. Tenderness is frequently present, and a localized nodule may be palpable. Although gynecomastia can coexist with male breast cancer, this occurrence is extremely rare. In most series the only true association of gynecomastia and breast cancer occurs with Klinefelter's syndrome.

Etiology

Gynecomastia is not in itself a pathologic entity. It is a histologic manifestation of an underlying disturbance in steroid hormone physiology, specifically an abnormal androgen/estrogen ratio. The causative factors are many and include physiologic, genetic, and enzymatic abnormalities. Gynecomastia occurs most commonly in adolescent boys and in men over 50. Virtually all boys have some gynecomastia during pubescence. This variant may occur in adolescent boys because plasma estradiol reaches an adult level prior to that of testosterone.

Gynecomastia is relatively common in the elderly, due in part to drug therapy and in part to endocrine changes

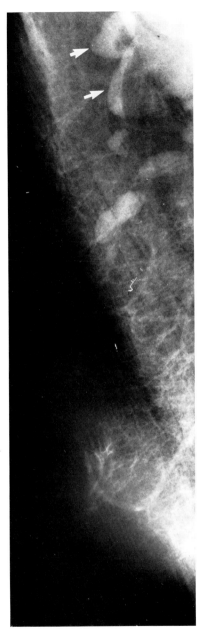

Fig. 17-1. Mediolateral oblique view of a normal male breast. A few radiopaque strands extend posteriorly from the nipple in the radiolucent fatty breast tissue. Normal axillary lymph nodes with fat-replaced hila are visualized *(arrows)*.

that occur in many aging men. Usually after age 70 plasma testosterone binding globulin increases so that the level of free testosterone falls, accompanied by an increase in the rate of conversion of androgens to estro-

gens in the peripheral tissues. Obesity can further contribute to the rate of peripheral conversion of androgens to estrogens.

Pathologic gynecomastia occurs in certain disease states that alter normal steroid hormone metabolism. The two major categories include diseases that involve deficient production or action of testosterone and those that result in increased estrogen production. Examples of the first category include Klinefelter's syndrome and secondary testicular failure. Increased estrogen production may occur with some testicular tumors, in liver disease, and with adrenal disease.

Multiple drugs may cause gynecomastia via several modes, including those that inhibit testosterone synthesis or action, those that are estrogenic, and those that act as gonadotropins. Certain drugs cause gynecomastia via an as yet unknown mechanism. Several drugs known to cause gynecomastia are listed below.

DRUGS THAT INDUCE GYNECOMASTIA

Inhibitors of Testosterone Synthesis or Action

    Spironolactone
    Cyproterone
    Flutamide
    Cimetidine

Estrogenic Drugs

    Diethylstilbesterol
    Digitalis
    Marihuana (tetrahydrocannabinol)
    Gonadotropins

Unknown Mechanism

    Methyldopa
    Busulfan
    Isoniazid
    Ethionamide
    Tricyclic antidepressants

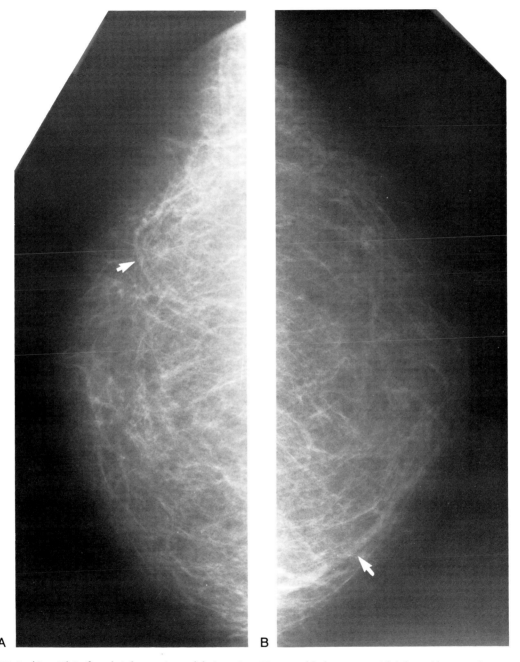

Fig. 17-2. (A & B) Left and right craniocaudal views in a 43-year-old obese man with bilateral breast enlargement demonstrate increased adipose tissue enlarging both breasts. No glandular tissue is identified. Veins *(arrows)* and minimal connective tissue strands are seen.

Histology

The histologic changes of gynecomastia tend to correlate with the duration of the abnormal hormone balance. In early stages, proliferation of both the fibroblastic stroma and the duct system occurs. The duct system undergoes elongation, budding, and duplication. If gynecomastia persists with continued hormonal alteration, progressive fibrosis and hyalinization develop as the epithelial proliferation regresses. Ultimately a mononuclear cell infiltration can be seen. Resolution of the process may occur if the fibrosis has not become too extensive. When marked fibrosis has occurred, complete resolution of gynecomastia will not occur, even when the hormonal imbalance has been corrected.

Gynecomastia is commonly quite asymmetric. Initially gynecomastia may present as a unilateral process, which may ultimately progress to the development of bilateral gynecomastia.

Clinical Assessment

The evaluation of the patient with gynecomastia should include a drug history, testicular examination to assess for small or asymmetrical testes, and an assessment of liver function. If necessary, a limited endocrine evaluation to assess urinary ketosteroid levels, plasma luteinizing hormone, and plasma testosterone levels is obtained. When the possibility of breast carcinoma is a clinical consideration, mammography can be a useful adjunct to clinical examination and chemical screening. Typically, in the smaller male breast, only mediolateral oblique views are obtained. Craniocaudal views are attempted when warranted.

Mammographic Appearance

The radiologic appearance of gynecomastia can vary (Figs. 17-3 to 17-5). The findings may be unilateral or bilateral and when bilateral are most frequently asymmetric (Fig. 17-6). Typically the radiographic appearance of gynecomastia consists of a triangular or flare-shaped increase in glandular density extending from the nipple posteriorly into the fatty tissue of the breast. In the majority of cases the density is symmetrically positioned behind the nipple. Nipple retraction has been reported with benign gynecomastia resulting

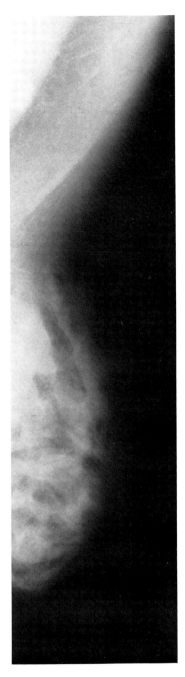

Fig. 17-3. Mediolateral oblique view in a 26-year-old man with right breast enlargement shows dense tissue replacing and enlarging the entire breast. The left breast was normal. No etiology for the unilateral gynecomastia was known.

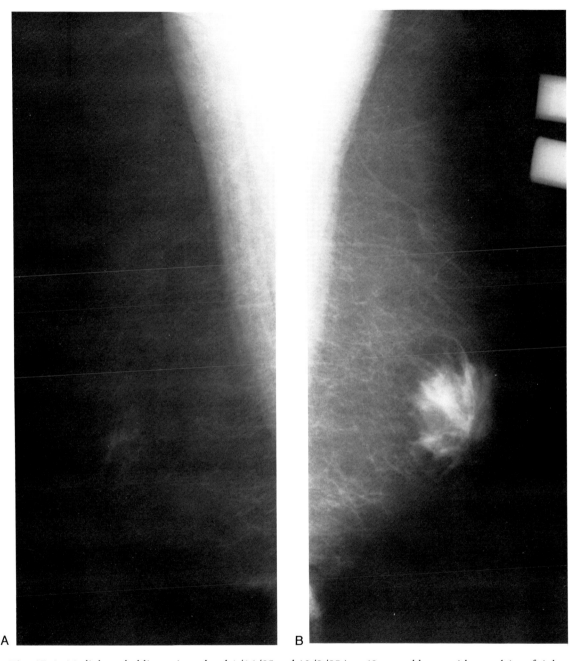

Fig. 17-4. Mediolateral oblique views dated 1/16/85 and 10/9/85 in a 69-year-old man with complaint of right breast tenderness and mass. The left breast **(A & B)** shows progression from normal breast tissue to a dense retroareolar nodule on the follow-up examination. The right breast **(C & D)** demonstrates gynecomastia, which has regressed slightly in the interval. *(Figure continues.)*

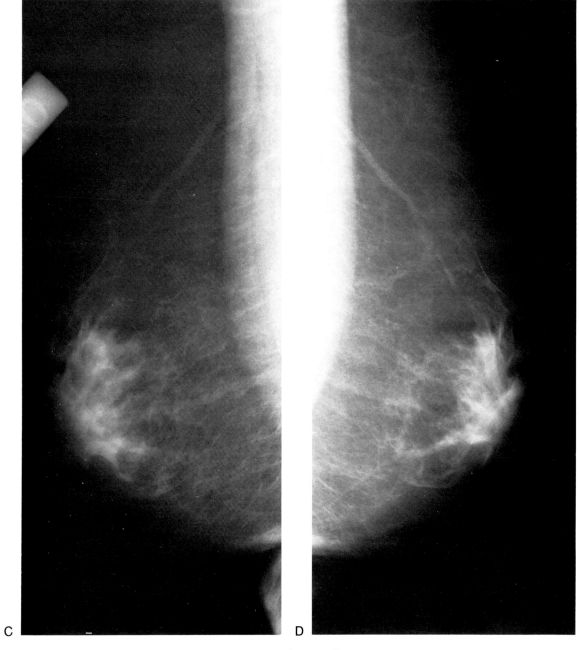

Fig. 17-4. *(Continued).*

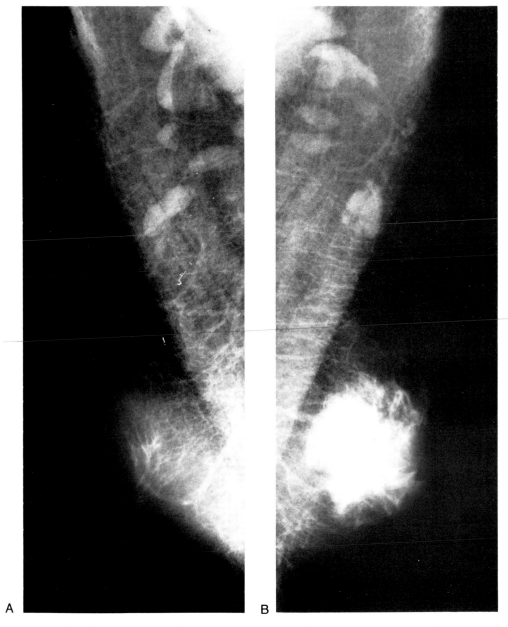

A

B

Fig. 17-5. Left and right mediolateral oblique views in a 66-year-old man with a complaint of right tender breast enlargement demonstrate increased right retroareolar density with extensions radiating into the fat. The left breast is normal.

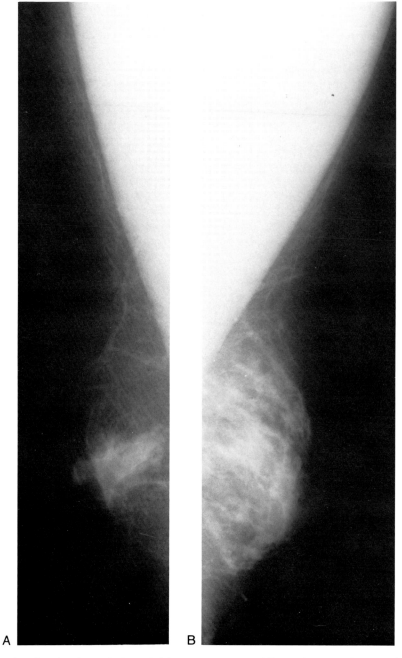

A   B

Fig. 17-6. (A & B) Left and right mediolateral oblique views in a middle-aged man with a complaint of bilateral breast enlargement and tenderness show an increased amount of dense glandular tissue in the retroareolar areas bilaterally. The changes are much more pronounced in the right breast. The patient's medications included spironolactone.

from the development of fibrosis. Some authors divide the mammographic findings into two types, the early florid and the later dendritic or fibrous variant. The florid gynecomastia is of shorter duration, usually less than 6 months. Histologically, there are an increased number of ducts, with proliferation of the ductal epithelium. Periductal edema with a highly cellular fibroblastic stroma mixed with adipose tissue can be seen. Mammographically, this type is manifest as a triangular retroareolar soft tissue density with very few posteriorly radiating extensions (Fig. 17-7). Pubertal gynecomastia usually demonstrates the florid variant. The dendritic or fibrous variant histologically involves less epithelial proliferation, edema, and cellular stroma. Hyalinization and fibrosis are the predominant histologic findings. This type corresponds mammographically to a pattern of retroareolar density with extensions that radiate posteriorly into the deeper adipose tissue (Fig. 17-8).

Sonography has been used in an attempt to evaluate gynecomastia. Described patterns include retroareolar hypoechogenicity or a more diffuse pattern of increased echoes. No evidence exists to suggest that sonography can differentiate gynecomastia from breast carcinoma.

MALE BREAST CARCINOMA

Carcinoma is a relatively unusual lesion with a frequency of only 0.9 percent of the occurrence of female breast cancer and comprising only 0.2 percent of malignancies in men. Breast cancer in men is most common after the age of 60, with a reported mean age of 71. The prognosis is approximately the same as that of female breast cancer when similar disease stages are compared. In the smaller male breast the primary lesion tends to be nearer the chest wall, leading to earlier invasion. Earlier detection of lesions could theoretically improve survival. The only known potentially predisposing factors for male breast carcinoma are breast irradiation and Klinefelter's syndrome. Factors that influence survival rates for males are the same as those for females. The malignant mass itself may be well delineated or may have a stellate appearance similar to that of a scirrhous carcinoma in the female breast. A well-defined nodule in the male breast is more likely to represent carcinoma than in the female, and in such a situation biopsy is indicated (Fig. 17-9). Male breast

carcinoma may be centrally or eccentrically located; however, an eccentric lesion is more likely to be malignant than a central lesion. The frequency of microcalcifications in malignant male breast masses varies widely depending on the reported series, ranging from 0 to 30 percent. As in the female breast, lymphatic obstruction may occur, whether from benign or malignant adenopathy (Fig. 17-10).

Histology

Male breast cancer duplicates most of the features of female breast carcinoma except for the in situ lobular and highly metaplastic types found in the female breast. There is an increased tendency toward the eosinophilic (sweat gland) variety of breast carcinoma in the male. This tumor is composed of acidophilic cells with granular cytoplasm. The pattern is similar to that of the cutaneous sweat gland carcinoma and the rarer apocrine gland cancer of the axilla.

MISCELLANEOUS BENIGN CONDITIONS

Papillomatosis of the male breast has been reported. The pattern of papillomas may be solitary or may involve the entire breast. These papillomas are similar to those described in the female breast and may calcify in a similar fashion. Papillomatosis can cause bloody nipple discharge and has been associated with florid gynecomastia.

Fat necrosis may occur in the male breast just as in the female. A history of trauma can often be elicited. Similar patterns, including both a stellate mass (Fig. 17-11) and eggshell-type calcification surrounding liquifactive necrosis (oil cysts) can be seen.

Cellulitis of the male breast occurs and may present as in the female with redness, induration, and skin thickening. Frank abscess formation may develop. Chronic inflammation may be associated with the development of fibrosis and accompanying nipple retraction. A spiculated mass composed of fibrotic tissue may develop.

Assorted benign lesions occasionally found in the male breast include cysts, lipomas (Fig. 17-12), hematomas,

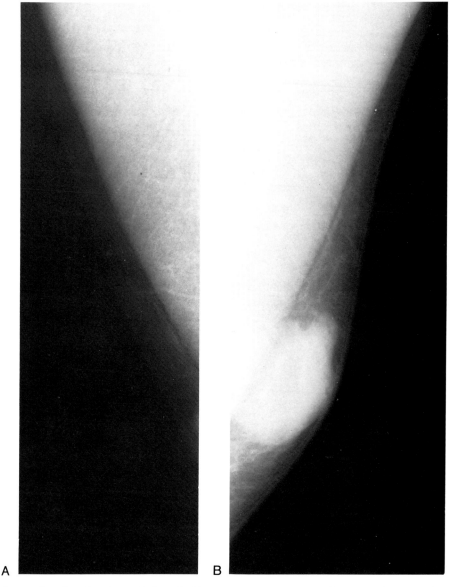

A   B

Fig. 17-7. (A & B) Left and right mediolateral oblique views in a 51-year-old man with a complaint of recent painful right breast enlargement demonstrate a uniform area of increased density with no radiating extensions in the right retroareolar area. This mammographic pattern corresponds to the florid variant. The left breast is normal.

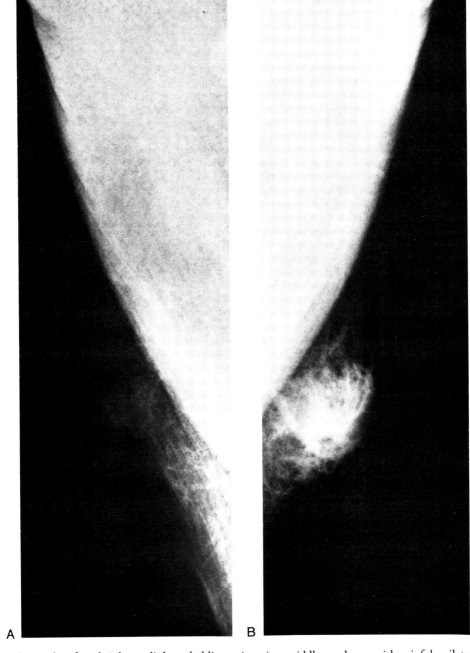

Fig. 17-8. (A & B) Left and right mediolateral oblique views in a middle-aged man with painful unilateral breast enlargement show increased right retroareolar density with extensions radiating into the fat. This mammographic type corresponds to the dendritic or fibrous variant.

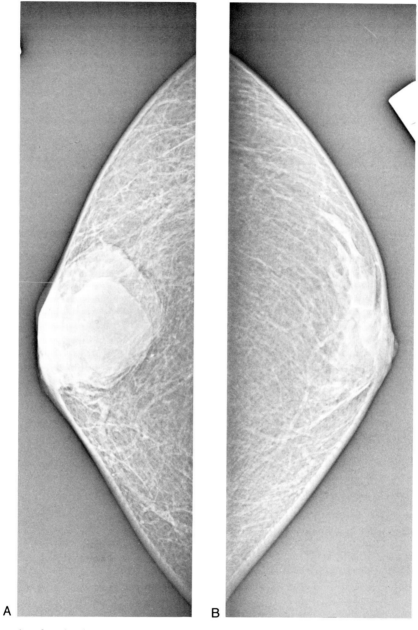

Fig. 17-9. **(A & B)** Left and right craniocaudal xeromammograms demonstrate a centrally located, fairly well-circumscribed mass on the left in a 60-year-old man with a 1-year history of a palpable, lobulated left breast mass. Nipple retraction was present. The right breast shows minimal gynecomastia. No calcifications are seen. Biopsy of the left breast revealed mucinous adenocarcinoma.

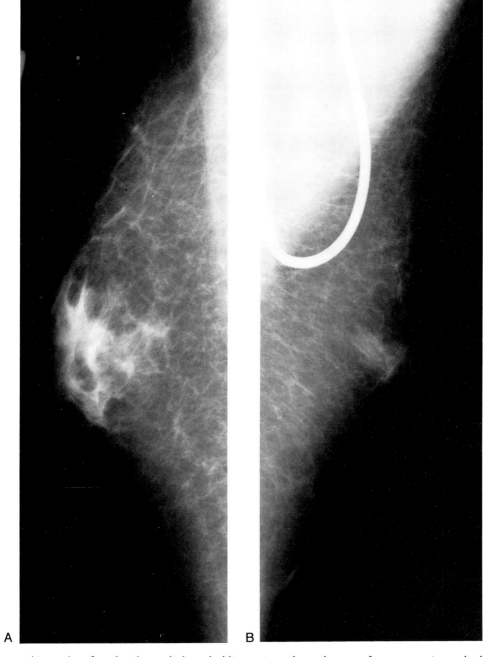

Fig. 17-10. (A & B) Left and right mediolateral oblique views show changes of gynecomastia on the left in a 64-year-old man undergoing therapy for Hodgkin's disease with a complaint of tender left breast enlargement. There is diffuse increased reticular density bilaterally from a degree of lymphatic obstruction. A central venous catheter overlies the upper portion of the right breast.

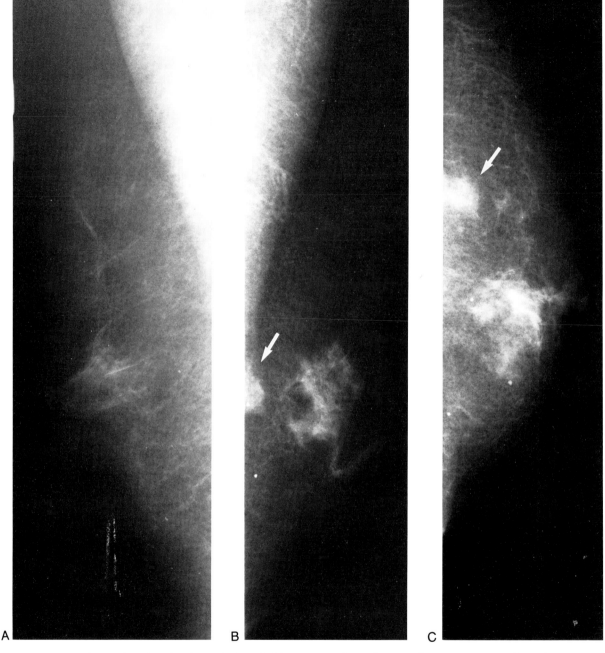

A   B   C

Fig. 17-11. (A & B) Left and right mediolateral oblique views show changes of gynecomastia on the right in a 71-year-old man with a complaint of right breast tenderness. A previous biopsy had been performed on the right. Physical examination showed tender right breast enlargement as well as a hard mass in the upper-outer quadrant. A small spiculated mass is also seen in the upper-outer quadrant *(arrow)*. The appearance of the mass is suggestive of malignancy. A needle aspiration of the mass showed fat necrosis. **(C)** Craniocaudal view of the right breast demonstrates the small posterior mass *(arrow)*.

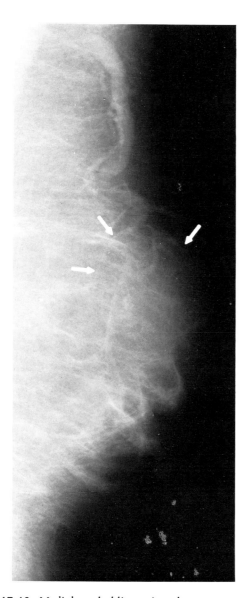

Fig. 17-12. Mediolateral oblique view shows a mass of fat density surrounded by a very thin capsule *(arrows)* in a 63-year-old man with a complaint of painless, soft left breast mass of uncertain duration. Histologic examination showed adipose tissue consistent with lipoma.

lymphoid hyperplasia, intramammary lymph nodes, and chronic granulomatous disease. Clinical findings, history, and mammography and/or ultrasound examination, combined when necessary with fine-needle aspiration, will usually differentiate the process involved.

SUGGESTED READINGS

1. Cohen R, Schauer PK: Male breast cancer following repeated fluoroscopy. Am J Med 76:929, 1984
2. Dershaw DD: Male mammography. AJR 146:127, 1986
3. Detraux P, Benmussa M, Tristant H, Garel L: Breast disease in the male: galactographic evaluation. Radiology 154:605, 1985
4. Jackson VP, Gilmor RL: Male breast carcinoma and gynecomastia: comparison of mammography with sonography. Radiology 149:533, 1983
5. Kapdi CC, Parekh NJ: The Male Breast. Radiol Clin North Am 21:137, 1983
6. McDivitt RW, Stewart FW, Berg JW: Tumors of the breast. 2nd Series. Armed Forces Institute of Pathology, Washington, DC, 1967
7. Michels LG, Gold RH, Arndt RD: Radiography of gynecomastia and other disorders of the male breast. Radiology 122:117, 1977
8. Moore DC, Schlaepfer LV, Paunier L, Sizonenko PC: Hormonal changes during puberty. V. Transient pubertal gynecomastia: abnormal androgen-estrogen ratios. J Clin Endocrinol Metab 58:492, 1984
9. Ouimet-Oliva D, Hebert G, Ladouceur J: Radiology of breast tumors in the male. J Can Assoc Radiol 28:249, 1977
10. Ouimet-Oliva D, Herbert G, Ladouceur J: Radiographic characteristics of male breast cancer. Radiology 129:37, 1978
11. Weshler Z, Sulkes A: Contrast mammography and the diagnosis of male breast cysts. Clin Radiol 31:341, 1980
12. Wigley KD, Thomas JL, Bernardino ME, Rosenbaum JL: Sonography of gynecomastia. AJR 136:927, 1981
13. Wilson JD, Aiman J, MacDonald PC: The Pathogenesis of Gynecomastia. p. 1. Year Book Medical Publishers, Chicago, 1980

18

Galactography

Dawn R. Voegeli

Galactography is the injection of radiopaque contrast material into the mammary ducts. It is performed to identify the source of abnormal nipple discharge and is particularly helpful when there is no palpable or mammographically detectable abnormality. Accurately localizing the source of abnormal discharge can result in a less radical surgical procedure and may demonstrate that surgery is unnecessary. It may also be performed to evaluate a solitary dilated duct in an asymptomatic patient. Prior to galactography, cytologic examination of the discharged material should be done, although it has been reported that negative results are unreliable.

The procedure is performed with the patient sitting or supine. An attempt to express secretions is made in order to identify the duct of origin. The nipple is prepped in sterile fashion, and the specific duct is cannulated with a blunt needle (pediatric sialogram set). The abnormal discharge often causes enlargement of the affected duct orifice, which makes it easier to cannulate. A head-mounted magnifying glass may be used for better visualization.

Approximately 0.1 to 2 cc of sterile water-soluble contrast is slowly injected, while compressing the tip of the nipple to improve the seal around the needle. Care is taken to exclude air bubbles from the contrast. Injection is stopped when the patient reports a sensation of pressure, and films in the craniocaudal and mediolateral projections are immediately performed. Magnification views may also be helpful. Only minimal breast compression is used, as vigorous compression could cause

the contrast material to be expelled. Compression on the nipple by the patient may help to keep the contrast media within the ducts.

It is possible to perforate the duct and cause extravasation of contrast material, especially if the needle is inserted too deeply (greater than a few millimeters) or if the contrast material is injected too rapidly (Fig. 18-1). The patient will complain of a burning sensation or sharp pain, and the injection should be stopped immediately.

Infection and abscess formation were complications associated with the use of oil-based contrast for galactography, but they have not been reported with the use of water-soluble media. However, pre-existing mastitis or breast abscess can be exacerbated by galactography and are contraindications to the procedure.

Abnormalities causing abnormal nipple discharge include ductal ectasia, fibrocystic changes, papilloma, papillomatosis, and intraductal carcinoma. Ductal ectasia is manifested by dilated ducts of varying caliber (Figs. 18-2 and 18-3). Inspissated material within the ducts may be difficult to distinguish from true masses (Fig. 18-4). Galactography in the presence of fibrocystic changes often demonstrates filling of small cysts.

Papillomas present as smooth filling defects within the ducts and can be round or serpiginous in shape. Often the duct is completely obstructed by the mass (Fig. 18-5). Multiple filling defects are demonstrated in papillomatosis (Fig. 18-6). Intraductal carcinoma classi-

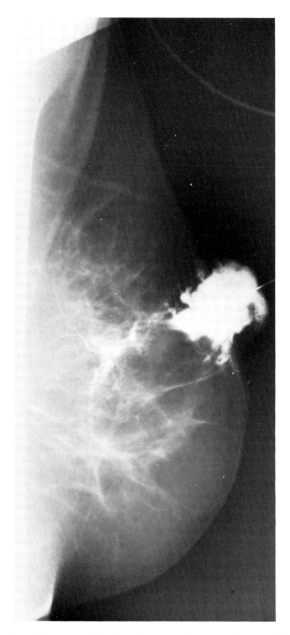

Fig. 18-1. Rapid injection of contrast during galactography
may result in ductal perforation and extravasation of contrast.

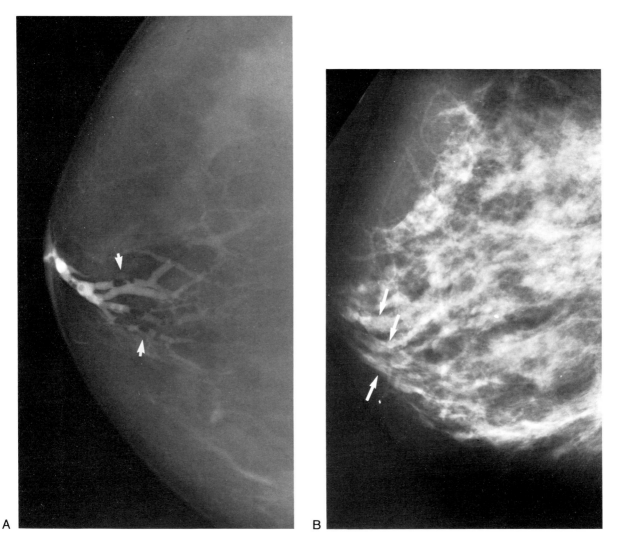

A   B

Fig. 18-2. **(A)** Galactogram in a 50-year-old woman with nipple discharge demonstrates diffuse ductal ectasia. Filling defects within the ducts are due to inadvertent injection of air *(arrows)*. **(B)** Mediolateral oblique view in the same patient shows multiple retroareolar dilated ducts *(arrows)*.

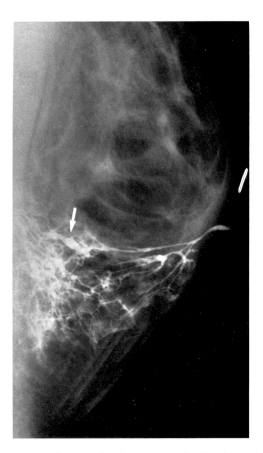

Fig. 18-3. Galactography demonstrates localized ductal ectasia *(arrow)* in this 33-year-old woman with unilateral nipple discharge. No filling defects are present.

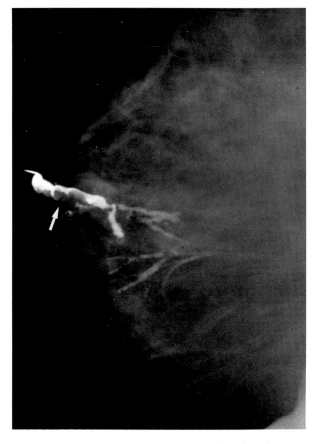

Fig. 18-4. Galactogram shows retroareolar ductal ectasia and filling defects *(arrow)* in this 54-year-old woman with nipple discharge. No cellular atypia was noted on cytologic examination of the discharge. Histology: dilated ducts containing debris, with chronic periductal inflammation and no evidence of malignancy.

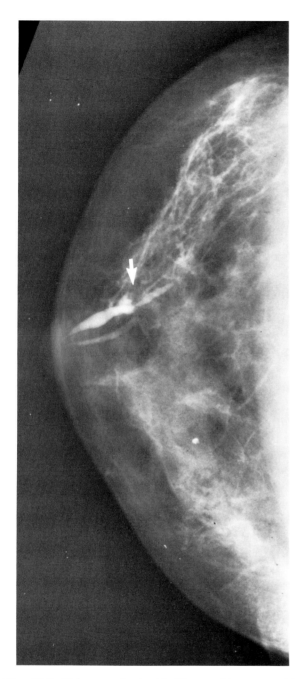

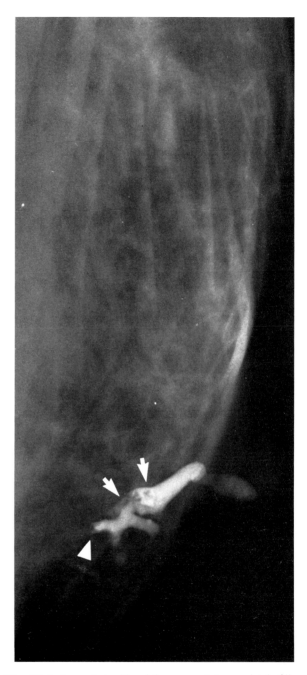

Fig. 18-5. Galactography in this 60-year-old woman with nipple discharge reveals abrupt termination of a duct by a smooth but lobulated intraductal mass *(arrow)*. Histology: intraductal papilloma.

Fig. 18-6. Irregularly dilated ducts containing multiple filling defects *(arrows)* are present in this patient with papillomatosis. Note complete obstruction of some ducts by the intraluminal masses *(arrowhead)*. The patient presented with bloody nipple discharge.

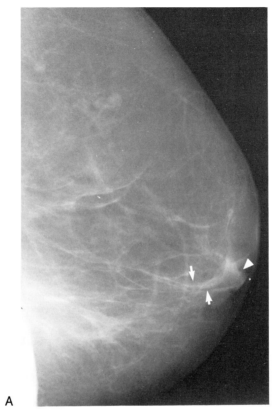

A

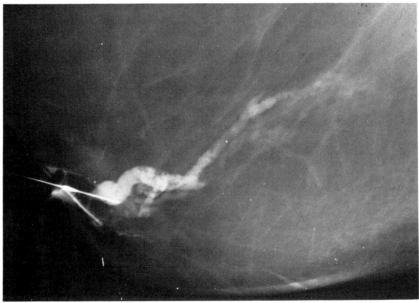

B

Fig. 18-7. (A) Mediolateral oblique view in a 46-year-old woman with unilateral blood-streaked nipple discharge. A single dilated retroareolar duct is present *(arrows)*. The round density anteriorly is the nipple, which is not in profile *(arrowhead)*. **(B)** Galactography demonstrates tiny filling defects in multiple dilated ducts. Histology: intraductal carcinoma and premalignant papillomas.

cally presents as single or multiple ill-defined masses within the ducts, and the ducts may have irregular contours (Fig. 18-7). In reality, the appearance of benign and malignant lesions within the ducts overlaps significantly. Galactography is performed to localize the abnormality, not to make a histologic diagnosis.

Galactography with the injection of methylene blue dye rather than radiopaque contrast can be repeated just prior to surgical resection, specifically localizing the area to be excised.

SUGGESTED READINGS

1. Bjorn-Hansen R: Contrast-mammography. Br J Radiol 38:947, 1965
2. DiPietro S, Coopmans De Yoldi G, Bergonzi S, et al: Nipple discharge as a sign of preneoplastic lesion and occult carcinoma of the breast. Clinical and galactographic study in 103 consecutive patients. Tumori 65:317, 1979
3. Gregl A: Color Atlas of Galactography. Schattauer, Stuttgart, 1980
4. Hicken NF: Mammography. The roentgenographic diagnosis of breast tumors by means of contrast media. Surg Gynecol Obstet 64:593, 1937
5. Hoeffken W, Lányi M: Mammography. WB Saunders, Philadelphia, 1977
6. Ries E: Diagnostic lipiodol injection into milk-ducts followed by abscess formation. Am J Obstet Gynecol 20:414, 1980
7. Tabár L, Dean PB, Péntek Z: Galactography: the diagnostic procedure of choice for nipple discharge. Radiology 149:31, 1983
8. Threatt B, Appleman HD: Mammary duct injection. Radiology 108:71, 1973

19

Preoperative Localization of Nonpalpable Breast Lesions

Dawn R. Voegeli

Preoperative localization has become an important technique for the removal or biopsy of nonpalpable breast lesions. In the past, these lesions were biopsied "blindly" by estimating their location from previous mammograms. Since the shape of the breast during upright compression mammography is quite different from the shape of the supine breast during surgery, this triangulation method was not very precise and often resulted in large biopsy specimens. Preoperative placement of a needle or self-retaining wire with its tip at or adjacent to the abnormality results in more precise localization and in a smaller biopsy specimen. Resection of a smaller volume of breast tissue causes less mammary distortion and scarring, which is especially desirable if the lesion turns out to be a minimal carcinoma or a benign lesion.

These localization techniques have simplified breast biopsy to the extent that many centers are now performing the majority of biopsies on an outpatient basis, which decreases the morbidity associated with general anesthesia and can be highly cost-effective.

LOCALIZATION DEVICES

Several needles and self-retaining wires have been devised to aid in preoperative localization of nonpalpable breast lesions. One commonly used device is a wire with a hook on its end, which is introduced through a needle. Upon needle withdrawal, the barbed end expands, anchoring the wire in the desired location in the breast (Fig. 19-1). Once the wire is anchored, it can no longer be withdrawn into the needle, and it is very difficult to remove without surgery.

Another device available is a curved-end retractable wire. When the wire is advanced through a needle into the breast, its curved end anchors the tip in the desired location (Fig. 19-2). The wire is composed of a nitinol alloy that possesses some elastic quality, so it can be advanced into the breast and withdrawn into the needle repeatedly, allowing for repositioning without having to place a second wire. This wire is also strong enough to eliminate inadvertent transection during surgery, a complication that has been reported with the hooked wire.

Preoperative placement of a needle through which dye can be injected (Evans blue or methylene blue) is another technique that has been used (Fig. 19-3). The surgeon then excises the volume of breast tissue that has been stained. One drawback of this technique is that the tip of the needle is not anchored, and there is potential for movement in the time span from needle placement to surgery, especially with changes in the shape of the breast as the patient changes position. Also, the dye can diffuse rather rapidly and result in a large biopsy specimen.

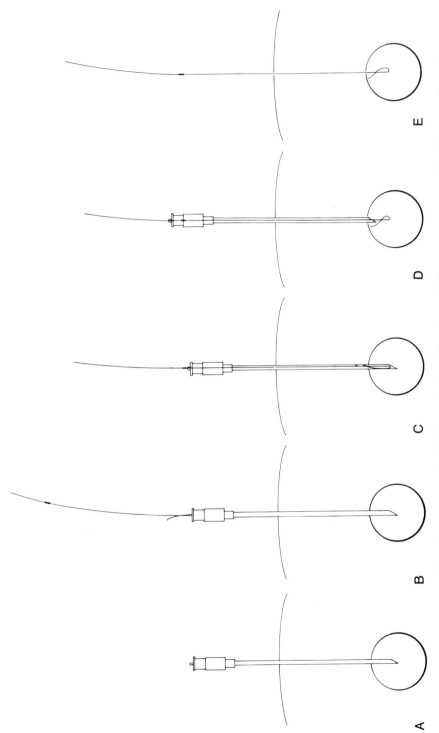

Fig. 19-1. Method of localization using a hooked wire. **(A)** Needle in lesion. **(B)** Insert wire into needle. **(C)** Wire advanced so that burnished area is at hub. **(D)** Needle pulled back, and wire springs open. **(E)** Needle removed.

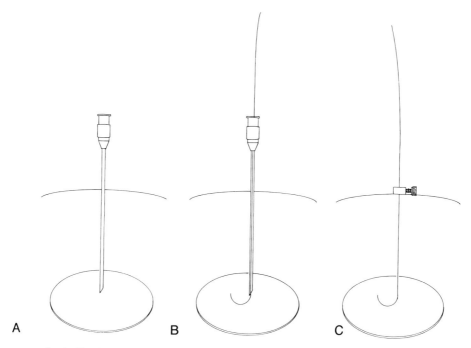

Fig. 19-2. Method of localization using the curved-end retractable wire. A stabilizer device is attached to the wire at the end of the procedure to keep the wire from advancing into the breast. **(A)** Needle in lesion. **(B)** Wire through needle. **(C)** Needle removed, and stabilizer in place.

TECHNIQUE

Preprocedural planning is important for successful localization. Previous mammograms are studied to determine the exact position of the suspicious lesion in two views and to plan the approach for needle placement (from the medial, lateral, or superior aspect of the breast). The safest approach is to place the needle parallel to the chest wall. Localization with the needle directed toward the chest wall often lacks accuracy, and there is a potential risk of pneumothorax and actually advancing the wire into the thorax. An exception is with very superficial lesions, which can be approached tangentially. Preprocedural determination of the best position for the patient (sitting or lying on her side) and optimum needle length (depending on the depth of the lesion) is also important.

Lesions located in the lateral half of the breast can be approached from the lateral aspect, with the patient lying on her side and the nonaffected breast dependent. The breast is compressed in the lateromedial position.

Lesions in the superiolateral quadrant can also be localized from the superior aspect, with the patient in the sitting position and the breast compressed in the craniocaudal projection. The approach offering the shortest distance to the lesion is usually the best.

Lesions in the medial half of the breast are usually localized from the superior or medial aspect. Lesions in the superiomedial quadrant can be approached from the superior aspect, with the breast compressed in the craniocaudal position. Lesions in either the superiomedial or inferomedial quadrants can be localized from the medial aspect of the breast, with the patient in the sitting position and the breast compressed in the mediolateral or mediolateral oblique position. It is nearly impossible to localize these lesions with the patient lying on her side and the affected breast dependent. In this position, it is extremely difficult to pull the breast under the compression paddle, and the other breast is usually in the way.

A method of localizing lesions in the lower half of the breast with needle entry from below has been de-

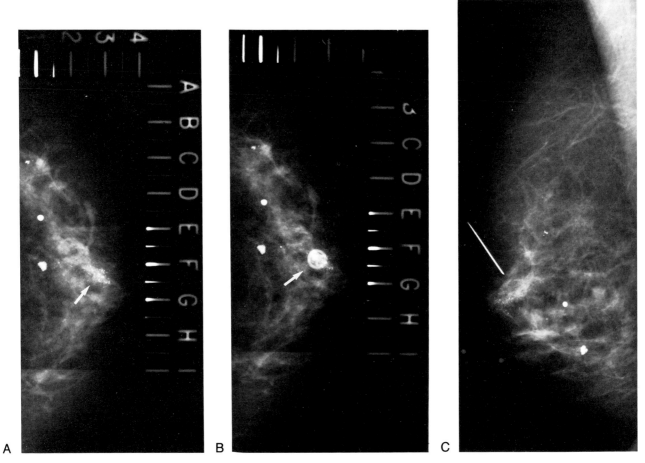

Fig. 19-3. (A) Craniocaudal localizer view demonstrates cluster of suspicious calcifications in the retroareolar area *(arrow)*. **(B)** A 25-gauge needle (seen on end) has been placed into the suspicious area through the opening in the compression paddle *(arrow)*. **(C)** A view perpendicular to the first demonstrates that the needle tip is within 2 cm of the suspicious calcifications. At surgery, methylene blue was injected through the needle, and the stained area was excised. Histology: intraductal carcinoma.

scribed. A small metallic marker is taped on the undersurface of the breast so that it projects over the abnormality in the craniocaudal projection. The marker indicates the site of eventual needle entry. A lateral view is then performed, and the distance of the lesion from the metallic marker and the angle of needle insertion is determined. The patient is then placed in the supine position. The physician simulates the geometry of lateral compression with one hand, and advances the needle into the breast at the proper angle and to the needed depth with the other hand. The needle is thus placed essentially parallel to the chest wall, with minimal angulation.

With any breast localization, selecting a needle of the proper length may be difficult initially but becomes easier with experience. A common mistake is to overestimate the depth of the lesion. An example is given in Figure 19-4. On the craniocaudal views, one would expect a needle 10 cm in length to be the correct length for localization of both lesions A and B. However, the lateral views show that lesion A is higher in the breast and is therefore more superficial than lesion B. This is because the breast is orb-shaped and is not as wide superiorly or inferiorly as it is in its midportion. A somewhat shorter needle is needed for lesion A.

The measured depth of a lesion in the breast also changes when the breast is compressed differently (Fig. 19-5). You must take this into account when choosing your needle length. If in doubt, use the longer needle, as it is better to pass through the lesion than to fall short of it.

If the suspicious lesion can only be identified in one mammographic view, it is difficult to determine the correct depth for needle placement. Several methods to overcome this difficulty have been described, including the use of alternate orthogonal projections and parallax, computed tomography, and sonography.

Localization is performed within several hours of biopsy, and patients are often very anxious when they enter the mammography suite. Explaining the procedure to the patient prior to beginning may alleviate some of this anxiety. As it is usually necessary for the patient to sit or stand during the localization procedure, it is important that no premedication be given.

Following procedural planning, the patient is positioned, and a scout radiograph is performed. Modified compression paddles are often used to facilitate needle placement. One compression paddle commonly used has a large fenestration or "window," which is marked on the sides with lead markers in gridlike fashion (Fig. 19-6). With the breast positioned so that the lesion will be within the "window," a scout radiograph is obtained. It is important to work quickly at this point, as the compression on the breast is uncomfortable, and it is important that the patient remain immobile. The developed film demonstrates the lesion and its coordinates, which are used to guide needle placement (Fig. 19-7A – C).

Another modified compression paddle contains multiple perforations that are visible on the radiographs (Fig. 19-8). The localization needle will be placed through the perforation most closely overlying the lesion.

The hooked wire technique will be described first. The skin is cleansed in sterile fashion. Lidocaine can be given intradermally and is recommended if the lesion is deep and multiple attempts could be required. A needle of the required length is advanced into the breast at the chosen coordinates, at right angles to the compression device. If the skin has been anesthetized, patients usually have only a brief feeling of pressure or mild pain.

Another radiograph is exposed in the same projection to ensure proper needle placement (Fig. 19-7D). If repositioning of the needle is necessary, that is done, and another radiograph is performed. The compression is released while supporting the breast and allowing it to expand up around the needle, while the tip stays in place. The needle can be anchored loosely in place with steri-strips if desired.

A film is then obtained at 90 degrees to the first, to confirm proper placement in this projection (Fig. 19-7E). If necessary, the needle can be withdrawn slightly and another film obtained to confirm its location.

At this point, a wire can be placed through the needle and the needle removed while leaving the wire in place. The wire is anchored in place with tape or a stabilizer

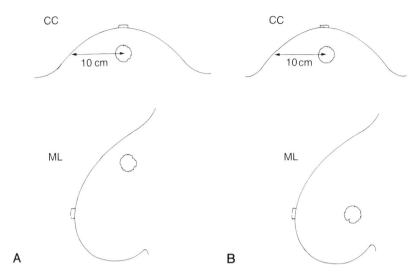

Fig. 19-4. Lesions A and B will both be localized from a lateral approach, with the breast compressed in the mediolateral position. Craniocaudal views used to estimate needle length suggest that 10-cm-long needles should be used in each case. Comparison with the mediolateral views demonstrates that lesion A is actually more superficial than lesion B (the orb-shaped breast is thinner superiorly and inferiorly than it is in its midportion). A needle somewhat shorter than 10 cm should be used for lesion A. CC, craniocaudal view; ML, mediolateral view.

device to prevent migration into the breast, and another radiograph with the projection perpendicular to the initial film is performed to confirm wire tip location (Fig. 19-7F). If this film demonstrates that the tip of the wire is greater than 2 cm from the lesion, a second wire should be placed with its tip closer to the abnormality.

It is important to directly communicate the position of the wire to the surgeon and to send the carefully labeled films to the operating room for reference purposes. Lack of communication between the radiologist and surgeon is a potential cause for failure.

If the curved-end retractable wire is being used, it may be advanced into the breast following initial needle placement to help in anchoring the needle in place. If repositioning is necessary, the wire can be retracted and then readvanced. The curved-end retractable wire sys-

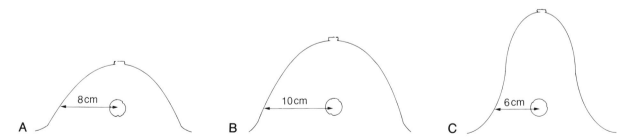

Fig. 19-5. The actual depth of a lesion within the breast must be estimated from both the craniocaudal and mediolateral views. Viewing the uncompressed breast from the superior aspect **(A)** demonstrates the mass to be 8 cm from the skin. Craniocaudal compression spreads the breast out **(B)**, and the lesion is now 10 cm from the skin. Mediolateral compression **(C)** causes the lesion to be only 6 cm from the skin.

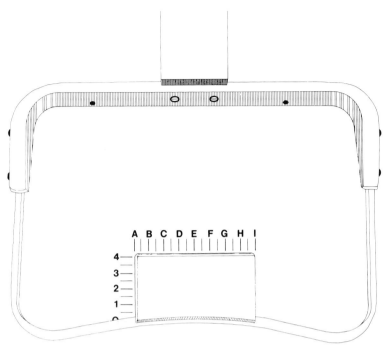

Fig. 19-6. Fenestrated compression paddle for needle localization. Lead markers along the sides of the "window" guide needle placement.

tem also has a fixation device that attaches to the wire at the skin and holds the wire in place.

The most common surgical approach is to dissect along the wire until the lesion is reached. If a circumareolar approach is desired, a needle can be replaced over the localizing wire in the operating room, as this is more easily palpable to the surgeon. It is preferable not to leave the needle in the breast for the time between mammographic localization and surgery, as this would be uncomfortable for the patient.

If the abnormality being localized is actually a cyst, and if the tip of the localization needle is placed directly within it, fluid will squirt out of the needle. If this occurs, a film of the breast will usually confirm that the mass has disappeared. If the localizing needle does not go directly through the cyst, the surgeon will usually report "popping" of the cyst at surgery. In either case, follow-up films in 3 to 6 months are necessary to detect any recurrence of the abnormality, which could indi-

cate the presence of a rare intracystic carcinoma (Fig. 19-9).

SPECIMEN RADIOGRAPHY

Specimen radiography is imperative to confirm removal of the lesion. The specimen is brought from the operating room, and a radiograph is obtained. If the lesion is identified within the specimen, the procedure is ended (Fig. 19-7G). If not, another specimen is obtained and radiographed. It is helpful for the surgeon to resect the initial specimen with the localization wire within it, as this may give some clue as to where to take the second specimen. Usually no more than one or two attempts are required. If the lesion has not been identified within three or four specimens, it is advisable to terminate the procedure and have the patient return for a repeat mammogram after the surgical changes have resolved (at least 6 weeks). If the lesion is still present, a repeat needle localization and biopsy can be performed.

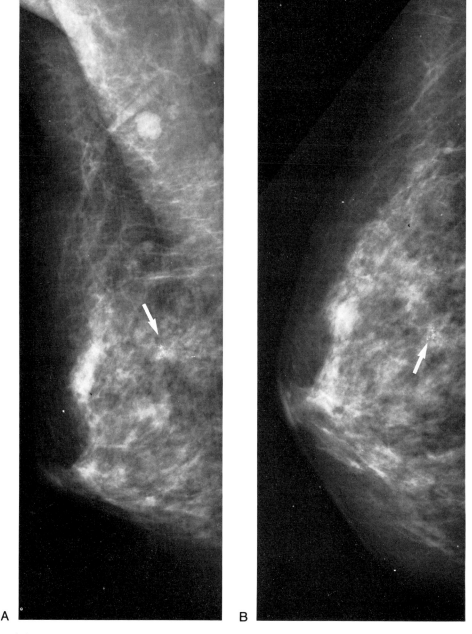

Fig. 19-7. (A) Mediolateral oblique screening view in a 52-year-old woman reveals a cluster of suspicious calcifications deep in the breast *(arrow).* **(B)** Craniocaudal view shows calcifications just lateral to the nipple *(arrow).* These views are used to plan the approach for biopsy and estimate needle length. *(Figure continues.)*

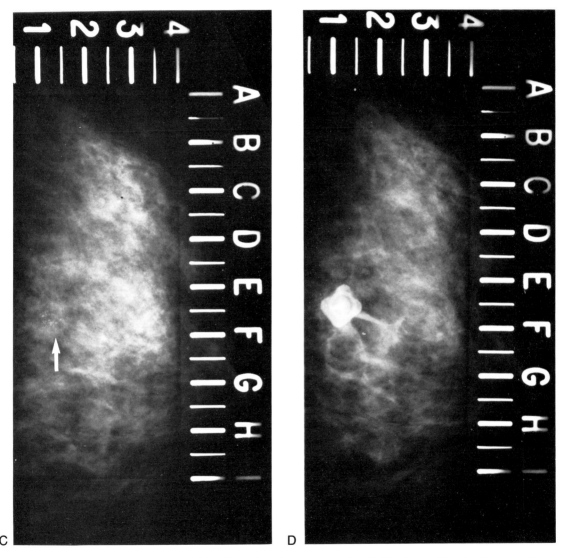

Fig. 19-7 *(Continued).* **(C)** Craniocaudal localizer view demonstrates the calcifications within the fenestrated area of the paddle at the coordinates "1" and "half-way between E and F" *(arrow).* **(D)** Repeat craniocaudal view after needle placement shows satisfactory position in this projection. *(Figure continues.)*

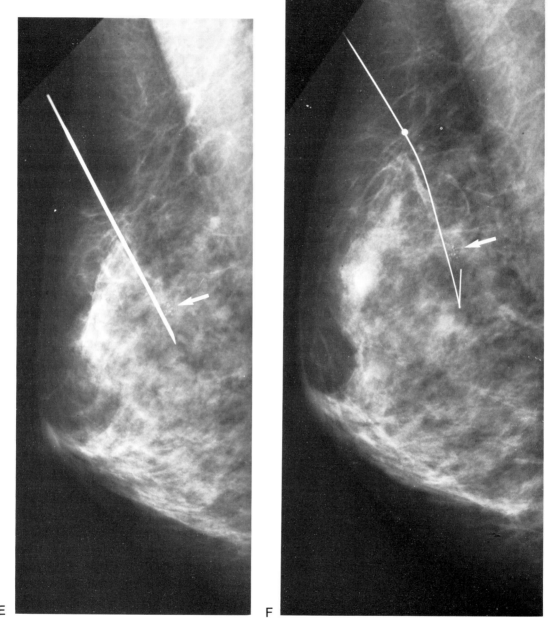

E

F

Fig. 19-7 *(Continued).* **(E)** Film obtained perpendicular to the first demonstrates the needle tip is just beyond the calcifications *(arrow).* **(F)** Repeat view following wire placement and removal of the needle reveals good position of the wire *(arrow* demonstrates calcifications). *(Figure continues.)*

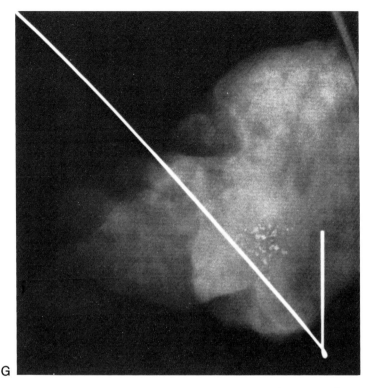

Fig. 19-7 *(Continued).* **(G)** Specimen radiography performed at the time of biopsy confirms removal of the calcifications. The wire is intact within the specimen. Histology: early infiltrating carcinoma.

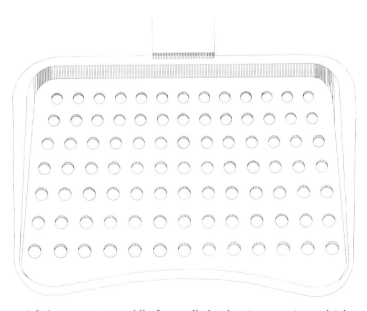

Fig. 19-8. Modified compression paddle for needle localization contains multiple perforations.

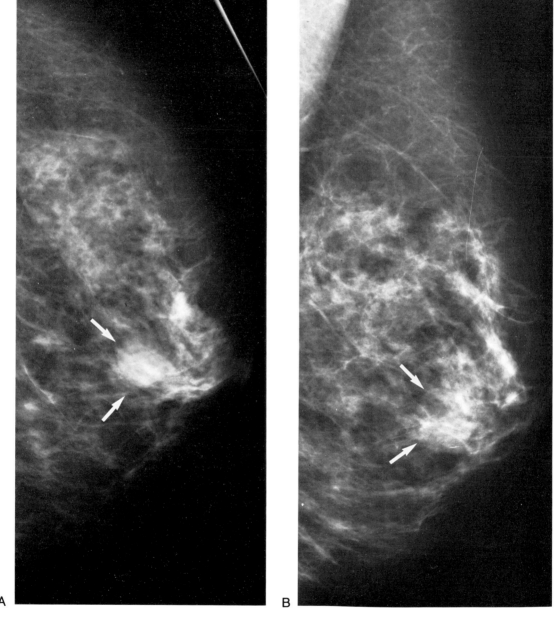

A

B

Fig. 19-9. **(A)** Craniocaudal screening view in this 42-year-old woman shows a poorly defined nonpalpable mass in the breast *(arrows)*. **(B)** Mediolateral oblique view also demonstrates mass *(arrows)*. *(Figure continues.)*

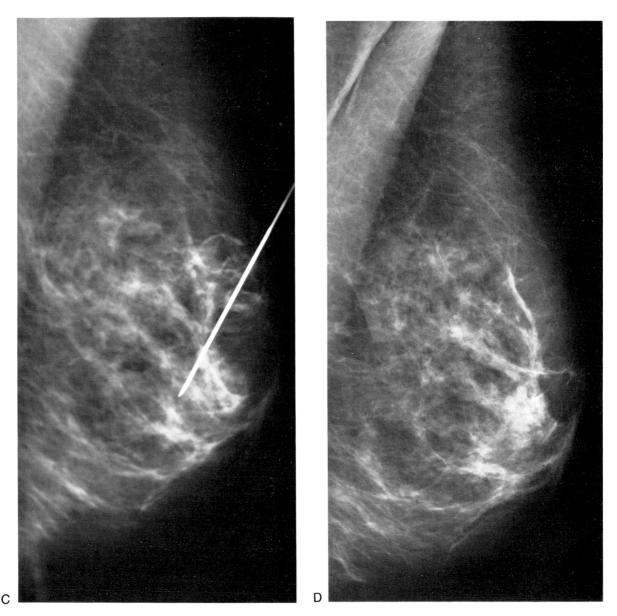

C

D

Fig. 19-9 *(Continued).* **(C)** During localizing needle placement, clear yellow fluid squirted out of the needle. A film demonstrates disappearance of the mass, confirming that it was a cyst. Presumably its borders were poorly defined due to overlying fibroglandular tissue. **(D)** Mediolateral oblique view 6 months later shows no recurrence of the cyst.

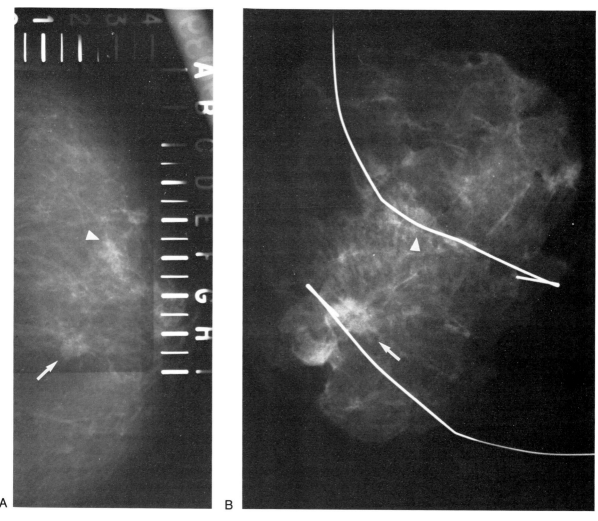

Fig. 19-10. (A) Localizer view demonstrates a spiculated mass *(arrow)* and a second, less defined mass *(arrowhead)*, which was seen better on the other view. Both lesions were localized with hooked wires. **(B)** Specimen radiograph confirms removal of the spiculated mass *(arrow)*. The less defined mass is more difficult to identify *(arrowhead)*. Histology: two foci of infiltrating ductal carcinoma.

Calcifications are easily identified within a specimen, but solid masses can sometimes be extremely difficult to identify, especially if they are not very dense (Fig. 19-10). Occasionally a lesion not identified on the initial specimen radiograph will be seen on a film obtained at an angle 90 degrees to the first one. Some radiologists feel that they can better identify soft tissue lesions if the specimen is submerged in water. Magnified compression views may also be helpful.

Once the lesion has been identified within the speci-

men, a 25-gauge needle can be advanced into the abnormal area to guide histologic sampling (Fig. 19-11).

COMPLICATIONS OF NEEDLE LOCALIZATION

Complications of localization are few. An occasional patient will experience a vasovagal reaction, which can be treated by supportive measures and medication if necessary. Minimal bleeding rarely occurs and can result in a small and clinically insignificant hematoma.

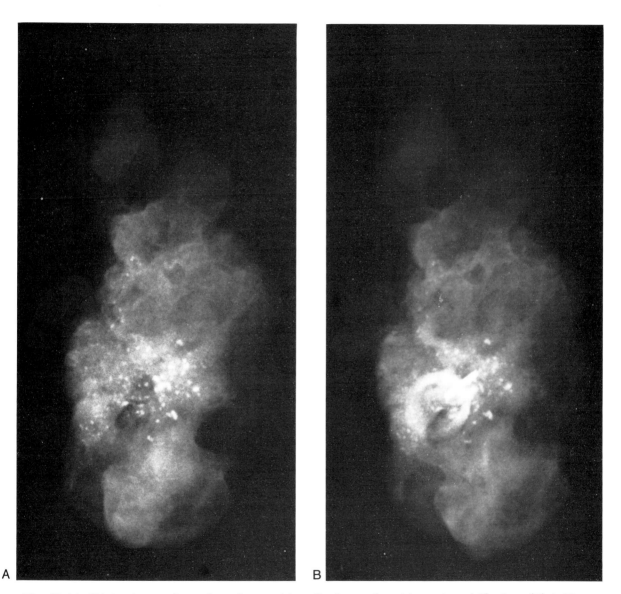

Fig. 19-11. (A) Specimen radiograph confirms excision of a cluster of suspicious microcalcifications. **(B)** A 25-gauge needle placed into the specimen localizes the main area of interest for the pathologist.

The localizing wire can retract into the breast, especially with fatty breasts. In one reported case, the wire actually migrated into the pleural space, necessitating thoracotomy. These problems can be avoided by placing needles parallel to the chest wall and anchoring the wire at the skin.

Some wires can be inadvertently transected intraoperatively. The surgeon must be cautioned about this possibility and urged to dissect with a scalpel rather than scissors.

Failure to remove the suspicious lesion is a complication that occurs approximately 3 to 5 percent of the time. These patients are managed by repeat localization and biopsy.

SUGGESTED READINGS

1. Bristol JB, Jones PA: Transgression of localizing wire into the pleural cavity prior to mammography. Br J Roentgenol 54:139, 1981
2. Budge JC, Knight RM: Dye localization of small breast lesion. Rocky Mt Med J 75:322, 1978
3. Dixon GD: Preoperative computed-tomographic localization of breast calcifications. Radiology 146:836, 1983
4. Frank HA, Hall FM, Steer ML: Preoperative localization of nonpalpable breast lesions demonstrated by mammography. N Engl J Med 295:259, 1976
5. Gisvold JJ, Martin JK, Jr: Prebiopsy localization of nonpalpable breast lesions. AJR 143:477, 1984
6. Goldberg RP, Hall FM, Simon M: Preoperative localization of nonpalpable breast lesions using a wire marker and perforated mammographic grid. Radiology 146:833, 1983
7. Homer MJ: Transection of the localization hooked wire during breast biopsy. AJR 141:929, 1983
8. Homer MJ: Nonpalpable breast lesion localization using a curved-end retractable wire. Radiology 157:259, 1985
9. Homer MJ: Preoperative needle localization of lesions in the lower half of the breast: needle entry from below. AJR 149:43, 1987
10. Homer MJ, Pile-Spellman ER: Needle localization of occult breast lesions with a curved-end retractable wire: technique and pitfalls. Radiology 161:547, 1986
11. Homer MJ, Smith TJ, Marchant DJ: Outpatient needle localization and biopsy for nonpalpable breast lesions. JAMA 252:2452, 1984
12. Kalisher L: An improved needle for localization of nonpalpable breast lesions. Radiology 128:815, 1978
13. Kopans DB, Lindfors K, McCarthy KA, Meyer JE: Spring hookwire breast lesion localizer: use with rigid compression mammographic systems. Radiology 157:537, 1985
14. Kopans DB, Meyer JE: Computed tomography guided localization of clinically occult breast carcinoma—the "N" skin guide. Radiology 145:211, 1982
15. Kopans DB, Meyer JE: Versatile spring hookwire breast lesion localizer. AJR 138:586, 1982
16. Kopans DB, Meyer JE, Lindfors KK, Bucchianeri SS: Breast sonography to guide cyst aspiration and wire localization of occult solid lesions. AJR 143:489, 1984
17. Kopans DB, Waitzkin ED, Linetsky L, Swann CA, Hall DA, White G: Localization of breast lesions identified on only one mammographic view. AJR 149:39, 1987
18. Laing FC, Jeffrey RB, Minagi H: Ultrasound localization of occult breast lesions. Radiology 151:795, 1984
19. Loh CK, Perlman H, Harris JH, Jr, Rotz CT, Jr, Royal DR: An improved method for localization of nonpalpable breast lesions. Radiology 130:244, 1979
20. Lou MA, Mandal AK, Alexander JL: The pros and cons of outpatient breast biopsy. Arch Surg 111:668, 1976
21. Parekh NJ, Wolfe JN: Localization device for occult breast lesions: use in 75 patients. AJR 148:699, 1987
22. Rebner M, Pennes DR, Baker DE, Adler DD, Boyd P: Two-view specimen radiography in surgical biopsy of nonpalpable breast masses. AJR 149:283, 1987
23. Sitzman SB: A new needle for pre-operative localizations of nonpalpable breast lesions. Radiology 131:533, 1979
24. Stephenson TF: Chiba needle-barbed wire technique for breast biopsy localization. AJR 135:184, 1980
25. Swann CA, Kopans DB, McCarthy KA, White G, Hall DA: Localization of occult breast lesions: practical solutions to problems of triangulation. Radiology 163:577, 1987
26. Vyborny CJ, Merrill TN, Geurkink RE: Difficult mammographic needle localizations: use of alternate orthogonal projections. Radiology 161:839, 1986
27. Walker GM, II, Foster RS, Jr, McKegney CP, McKegney FP: Breast biopsy. A comparison of outpatient and inpatient experience. Arch Surg 113:942, 1978

20

Ultrasound of the Breast

Kathleen A. Scanlan

The major purpose of breast imaging is to achieve an early and accurate diagnosis of malignant changes. Characterization of benign lesions using noninterventional modalities will avoid unnecessary surgery. Breast ultrasound has become an accepted adjunct method for evaluation of breast pathology. Its chief role is in the differentiation of cystic from solid masses that have been identified either by mammography or physical examination. While the diagnosis of palpable lesions can often be confirmed with fine-needle aspiration alone, ultrasound is frequently used to characterize the internal structure of a mass. In some series, ultrasound mammography has proven useful in the evaluation of the radiographically dense breast, a situation in which screen-film mammography has its lowest sensitivity. There is universal agreement that ultrasound cannot be substituted for mammography as a screening test for malignancy. Effective use of ultrasound requires both an understanding of basic ultrasound interaction with breast tissue and familiarity with normal breast anatomy.

INSTRUMENTATION AND PHYSICS

Instrumentation

There are two techniques of breast ultrasound, the dedicated whole breast scanner and the hand-held transducer. Dedicated whole breast units offer the advantage of computerization to ensure an orderly, sequential, and reproducible examination of the entire breast. With many automated units, transverse, longitudinal and rotational sections are possible. The entire examination can be videotaped and reviewed at a later time. Additionally, the same location and plane in each breast can be reviewed simultaneously to assess symmetry. Sonic coupling is achieved with a water path in prone automated units and a step-off device in supine scanners.

Disadvantages of automated units include the additional cost of operating an ultrasound unit dedicated solely to breast imaging and a relatively long examination time. The images are often of lower resolution than that of a hand-held unit, as dedicated scanners tend to use transducers of a frequency less than 5 MHz. Patient discomfort is often encountered due to positioning and prolonged examination times. Another disadvantage, particularly with prone water path scanning, is that it is not possible to localize precisely a lesion site for surgical biopsy. There is disagreement concerning the utility of whole breast scanners. Some investigators believe that their use is unnecessary and may in fact lead to false-positive and -negative results. Changes of carcinoma can sometimes be mimicked by scars and focal fibrosis, while false-negative examinations may occur if the acoustic properties of a carcinoma are not significantly different from the surrounding tissue. In our experience, dedicated breast ultrasound has not offered sufficient additional diagnostic information over mammography to warrant its cost and time expenditure. Most diagnostic problems can be adequately solved with a combination of mammography and, when indicated, a hand-held ultrasound examination.

When using a hand-held transducer, the frequency should be 5 MHz or greater, as axial resolution improves with higher frequencies. A water path or solid gel step-off device can be useful in combination with the hand-held transducer and coupling gel to allow improved superficial imaging by bringing the skin into the focal zone of the transducer. The hand-held transducer is suited to the evaluation of a specific breast area such as a localized mass identified on mammography or a mass identified on physical examination. Unlike the dedicated imaging unit, it is not possible to obtain a reproducible survey of the entire breast with a hand-held transducer. Superficial changes such as skin thickening or thickening of Cooper's ligaments will be more difficult to see with a hand-held examination, compared with a prone water path examination.

Physics

A full explanation of ultrasound physics is beyond the scope of this book, and the reader is referred to texts on this topic for more detailed information. The operator

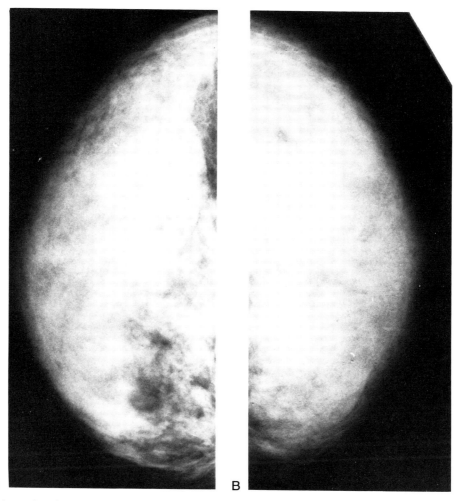

A   B

Fig. 20-1. (A & B) Left and right craniocaudal views demonstrating extremely dense breast tissue. Mammography is less sensitive with this type of tissue. *(Figure continues.)*

must have a familiarity with certain aspects of ultrasound physics for a diagnostic and artifact-free examination. An important factor is transducer frequency, which determines to a large degree the resolution of the image. For hand-held examinations a transducer frequency of 5 MHz or greater should be used. Water path units generally use transducers somewhat lower in frequency. In addition to frequency-dependent resolution, care must be taken to ensure that the area of interest is within the focal zone of the transducer. In mechanical transducers this is an inherent characteristic of the instrument, while in electronically focused units the focal zone can be adjusted to a specific level. If necessary an ultrasonic offset pad can be used to place the area of interest in the breast within the focal zone of the transducer.

It is also important that penetration be adequate to see the entire thickness of the breast, to avoid missing lesions near the chest wall. On occasion this may require switching to a lower frequency transducer for improved penetration or compressing the breast to reduce its thickness. Such a situation may be encountered in the large or very dense sound-attenuating breast (Fig. 20-1).

Acoustic power setting, over-all gain, and time gain compensation curves also require attention for optimal

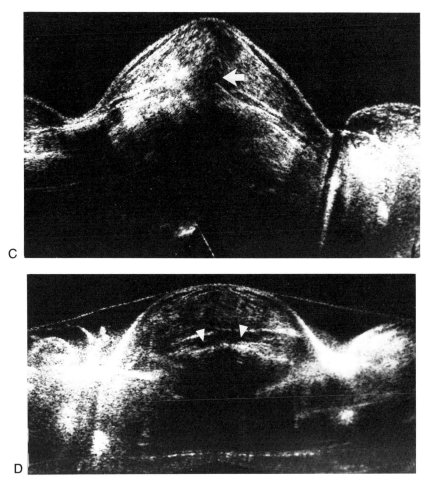

Fig. 20-1 *(Continued).* **(C)** Water path ultrasound examination of the right breast. The central posterior portion of the breast is difficult to image *(arrow).* **(D)** Compression of the breast facilitates ultrasound imaging by decreasing breast thickness and placing the breast tissue more perpendicular to the ultrasound beam. The pectoralis muscle can now be seen *(arrowheads).*

image quality. These factors may need to be adjusted during the examination to enhance specific aspects of the lesion, such as internal echo characteristics and through transmission. With these technical factors in mind the best quality image can be obtained and the unintentional generation of artifacts reduced.

ULTRASOUND ANATOMY OF THE NORMAL BREAST

The ability to distinguish between the various types of tissue in the breast is based on differences in acoustic impedance. The skin is seen superficially as an echogenic line. The nipple, because of its shape and thickness, causes an area of sonic attenuation posteriorly. Deep to the skin the subcutaneous fat is seen as a relatively hypoechoic layer, with scattered echogenic bands representing Cooper's ligaments. All fatty tissue in the breast is relatively hypoechoic, in contradistinction to the adipose tissue found elsewhere in the body, which is generally hyperechoic. Centrally a cone of breast parenchyma is seen and is somewhat more echogenic than the subcutaneous fat. Hypoechoic adipose lobules may be distributed throughout the cone of breast parenchyma. The volume of the central parenchymal cone will vary depending on the degree of fatty replacement of the breast. The echogenicity of the parenchyma will be dependent on its relative composition of fibrous, glandular, and fatty tissues.

Mammary ducts course through the central cone of parenchyma in a radial orientation toward the nipple. A focal dilatation (the ampulla) of each duct is seen immediately beneath the nipple. The lactiferous ducts are frequently not visualized if they are of normal caliber. Posterior to the cone of parenchyma lies the retromammary fat layer. It is relatively hypoechoic and similar in echogenicity to the subcutaneous fat. The deepest layer is the pectoralis muscle, in which echogenic connective tissue bands can be identified (Fig. 20-2). Behind the pectoralis muscle lie the ribs and intercostal muscles. The ribs and costochondral cartilages are seen in cross section as ovoid hypoechoic structures with posterior acoustic attenuation (Fig. 20-3).

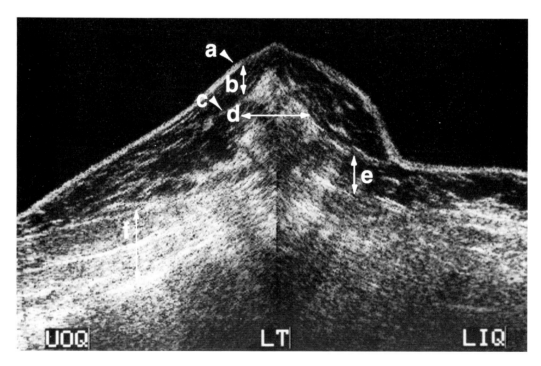

Fig. 20-2. Automated water path breast ultrasound of an asymptomatic 40-year-old woman. The following structures can be identified: *a,* skin; *b,* subcutaneous fat; *c,* Cooper's ligament; *d,* central breast parenchyma; *e,* retromammary fat layer; and *f,* pectoralis muscle.

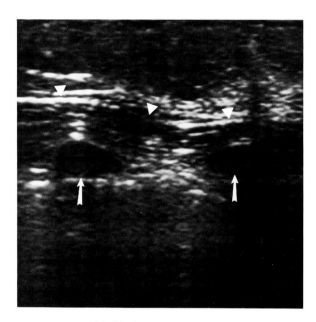

Fig. 20-3. Hand-held ultrasound examination of the breast demonstrating the costochondral cartilages in cross section *(arrows)*. They are ovoid with low-level internal echoes and some posterior attenuation. They should not be mistaken for a breast mass. Anterior to the cartilages lie the pectoralis muscles and pectoralis fascia *(arrowheads)*.

INDICATIONS

The major indication for breast ultrasound is to characterize a mass found on mammography or physical examination as cystic or solid in nature. The ultrasonic differentiation between benign and malignant solid masses, however, is not reliable. Ultrasound is most helpful in evaluating the solitary mass seen on mammography. When there are several lesions to evaluate within one breast, it becomes difficult to assure that the lesion seen on ultrasound correlates with a given mass on mammography. Ultrasound can be useful in conjunction with mammography in the evaluation of nipple discharge associated with ductal ectasia or occasionally the bloody discharge associated with an intraductal papilloma. Localizing a dilated duct may be simplified by ultrasound, because either hand-held or automated transducers can be oriented radially in the plane of the ducts (Fig. 20-4). Occasionally a solid intraductal papilloma may be identified in a fluid-distended duct. Al-

though dilated ducts can be localized, normal-caliber ducts cannot be consistently identified on ultrasound.

Ultrasound can also be used in the elevation of mastitis. In this circumstance film mammography is frequently not helpful due to generally increased tissue density. Its use may also be precluded by pain. Ultrasound can serve to identify any localized fluid collections in a relatively pain-free fashion.

In some series, ultrasound has proven useful for identifying masses in the radiographically dense breast. If such an examination is to be performed, an automated unit should be used to generate a reproducible ultrasound mammogram of the entire breast (Fig. 20-5). Even in women with known dense breast tissue, however, ultrasound examination is not a substitute for mammography. Alterations in breast architecture identified on a mammogram may be missed on ultrasound examination, and microcalcifications are rarely seen with ultrasound.

In the patient with a breast prosthesis, normal tissue is compressed, and the density of the prosthesis masks the tissue, limiting the mammogram's usefulness. Automated ultrasound examination may provide adjunctive information under this circumstance, and hand-held examination can be performed if a specific area is in question.

Finally, hand-held ultrasonography can be useful to guide aspiration biopsy of those nonpalpable lesions that have been previously identified by ultrasound examination. Some authors have also used ultrasound to guide aspiration of masses identified previously via mammography.

EVALUATION OF
BREAST LESIONS

The ultrasound characteristics of a mass include its margins and shape, as well as the size and homogeneity of any internal echoes. The attenuation characteristics of the lesion must also be evaluated. These range from the nonattenuating cyst with strong posterior enhancement to the highly attenuating desmoplastic lesions.

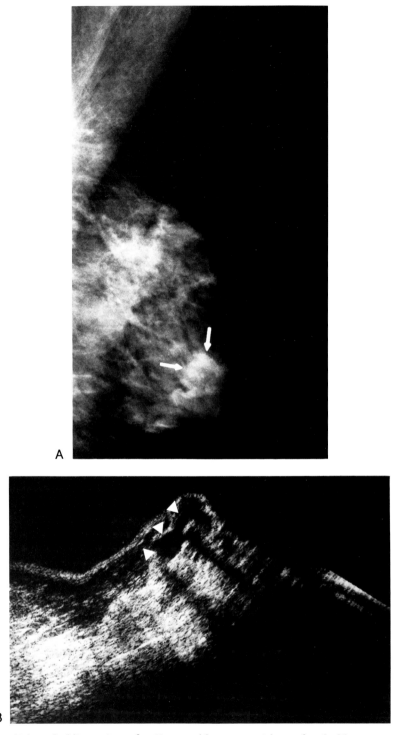

Fig. 20-4. (A) Mediolateral oblique view of a 48-year-old woman with a soft palpable retroareolar mass. The mammogram demonstrates a lobulated retroareolar mass *(arrows).* **(B)** An automated water path ultrasound study of the same breast. A dilated duct extending to the nipple is evident *(arrowheads).*

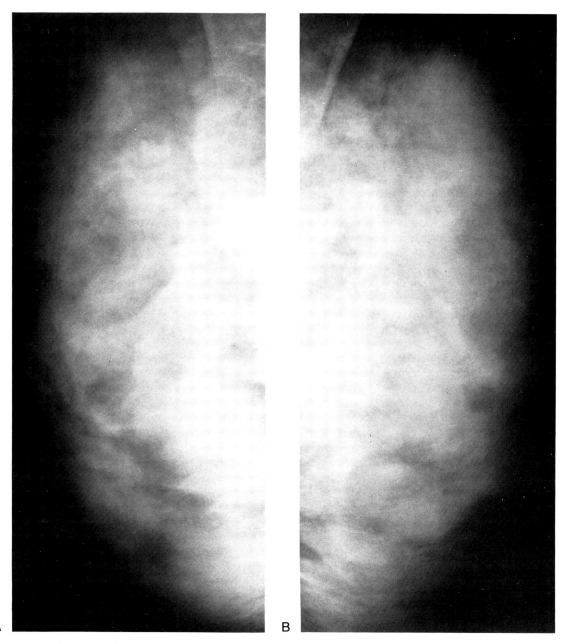

A   B

Fig. 20-5. (A & B) Left and right mediolateral oblique views of a 27-year-old woman with a palpable right breast mass and a positive family history of breast cancer. Very dense breast tissue is seen bilaterally. No masses are identified. *(Figure continues.)*

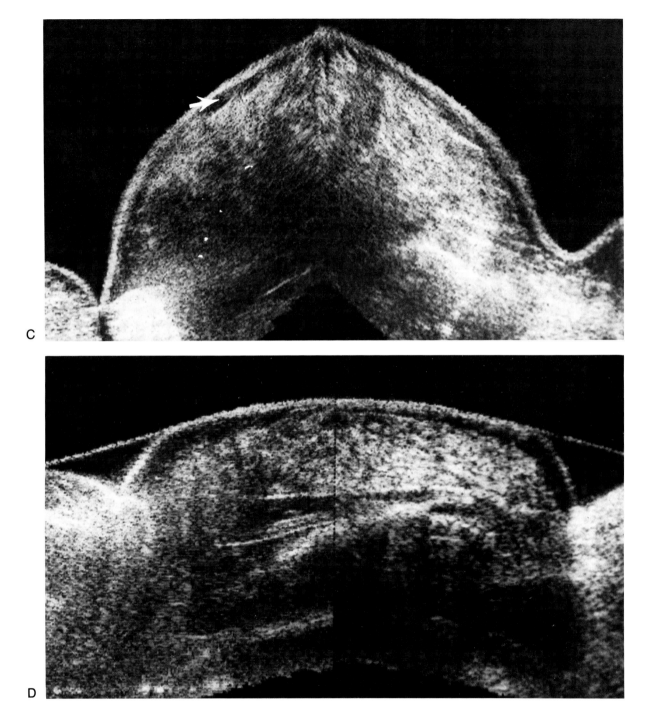

Fig. 20-5 *(Continued)*. **(C)** Automated water path ultrasound of the right breast. Echogenic central glandular tissue is seen. There is a very thin layer of subcutaneous fat *(arrow)*. No mass is identified. The posterior midportion of the breast is difficult to image, because the tissue is highly attenuating. **(D)** The study was repeated with compression, allowing penetration to the posterior aspect of the breast. No masses were identified on compression examination.

Cysts

Most cysts arise at the level of the lobule as a result of an imbalance in the production and absorption of lobular fluid generated by the epithelial lining cells. Cyst formation can be encouraged by obstructive fibrosis at the outlet of the lobule. Occasionally obstruction of a duct or lobule by a mass lesion may result in formation of a cyst. The characteristics of a simple breast cyst include sharp margins, the absence of internal echoes, and strong posterior enhancement (Fig. 20-6). Microcysts, those measuring less than 3 mm in diameter, occur as a result of dilated, fluid-filled lobules. These are considered a normal finding. It is more difficult to demonstrate posterior enhancement in smaller cysts. With larger cysts, some lobulation can be noted (Fig. 20-7), and several cysts may lie in close proximity, producing the appearance of a single mass on mammography. Occasionally blood or proteinaceous debris within a cyst may create fine uniform internal echoes, causing confusion with a solid mass. Mechanical compressibility of the mass, if demonstrable, may help to confirm that it is fluid-filled.

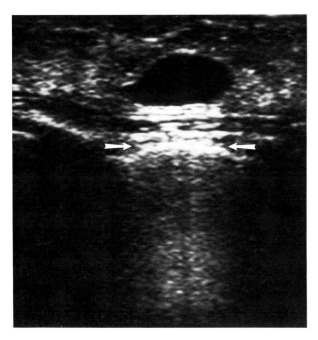

Fig. 20-6. Hand-held ultrasound examination in a 50-year-old woman with a palpable breast mass demonstrates a classic simple cyst. It has smooth margins, marked through transmission *(arrows)*, and no internal echoes.

Galactoceles

Galactoceles appear much like a simple cyst; however, they may have a few internal echoes from the presence of inspissated milk. Sonic absorption by the internal contents will diminish through transmission when compared with a simple cyst. Although the origin of the galactocele is in the lactating breast, it is most often identified sometime after the conclusion of breast feeding.

Inflammatory Disease

Cellulitis of the breast may occur in association with nursing or as a result of leakage of lipoid material into the parenchyma from dilated ducts. It may also occur as a complication of trauma. In the absence of frank fluid collections, skin thickening and diffuse hypoechoic change from edema may be noted in the area of inflammation.

Fluid collections in the inflamed breast may be the result of either frank purulent material, as in the classic bacterial mastitis of the lactating breast, or as a result of sterile inflammation, as in plasma cell mastitis (ductal ectasia). The latter condition is the result of leakage of fatty material from the ducts into the breast parenchyma, inciting a sterile lipoid inflammation. Ductal enlargement may be identified on ultrasound (Fig. 20-8) together with irregular fluid collections that may contain a few internal echoes (Fig. 20-9). Ultimately fibrotic tissue may be formed as the result of the chronic inflammatory process.

The purulent abscess is identified as a fluid-filled cavity that may be irregular and have a thick, ragged wall. Most often internal echoes and septations are identified from the presence of internal debris and partial organization of the contents (Fig. 20-10).

Hematoma/Fat Necrosis

Trauma to the breast may result in hematoma formation and ultimately fat necrosis. The acute hematoma can be seen on ultrasound as an irregular, fluid-containing area with moderate through transmission and usually a few internal echoes. Liquefaction of the hematoma causes clearing of the internal structure, and finally organization will occur, showing echogenic

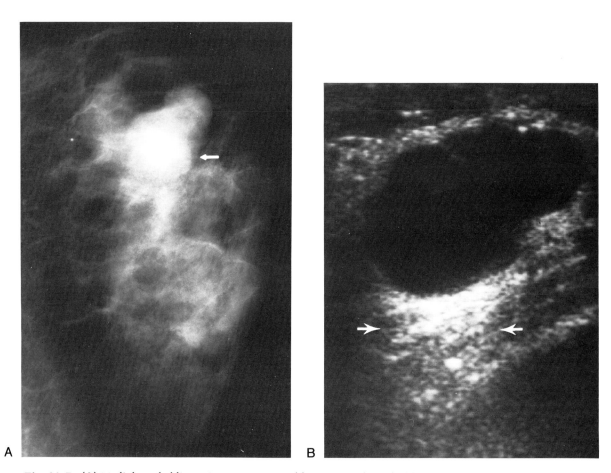

Fig. 20-7. **(A)** Mediolateral oblique view in a 45-year-old woman with a palpable right breast mass demonstrates a bilobed structure with partially well-defined borders. Sections of the margin show a halo sign *(arrow)*. **(B)** Hand-held ultrasound examination of the palpable mass demonstrates a completely clear bilobed cystic structure that correlates with the lesion identified on the mammogram. Strong posterior enhancement is seen *(arrows)*.

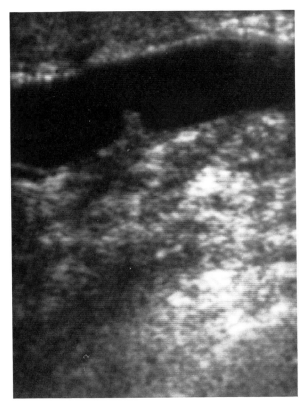

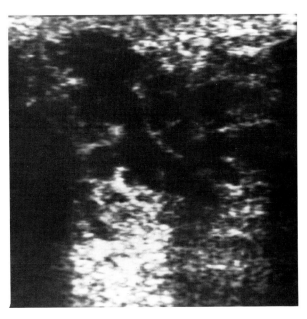

Fig. 20-8. Real-time ultrasound examination with the transducer oriented radially demonstrates enlarged ducts in a 48-year-old woman complaining of intermittent breast pain and redness. The duct measures approximately 1 cm in diameter. The papillary projection is of uncertain significance.

Fig. 20-9. Hand-held ultrasound examination demonstrates several fluid collections, some of which communicate with the ductal system in a 27-year-old woman with a clinical history of mammary duct ectasia and serous nipple discharge. There was increased fullness to palpation superior and lateral to the nipple.

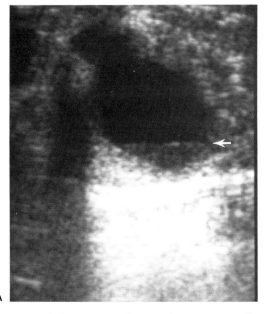

A

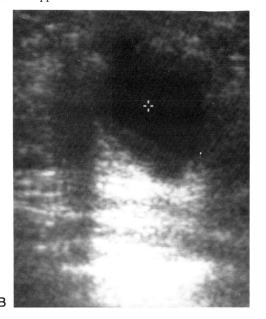

B

Fig. 20-10. (A) Real-time ultrasound examination of a 45-year-old woman complaining of a warm, red, painful breast demonstrates a thick-walled, slightly irregular cystic structure with marked through transmission and a sediment level *(arrow)*. **(B)** The contents of the cavity show gravity-dependent shift when the patient is placed in a decubitus position. Aspiration of the contents produced purulent material.

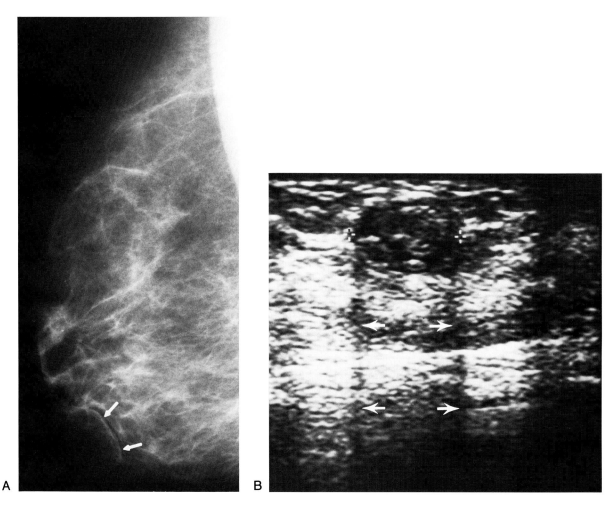

A B

Fig. 20-11. **(A)** Craniocaudal view shows an ovoid lucent mass with a very thin calcific rim *(arrows)* in a 37-year-old woman with palpable left breast mass. There was a history of subacute trauma. The mammographic findings are those of circumscribed fat necrosis. **(B)** Ultrasound examination of the palpable abnormality demonstrates a well-marginated mixed echogenicity mass with no visible posterior attenuation. Hypoechoic posterior bands *(arrows)* at the poles of the mass are caused by refraction at the curved surface.

septae extending through the fluid collection. Fibrotic tissue may ultimately form in the area of tissue trauma.

Fat necrosis may also occur following trauma, including surgery. Fat necrosis takes two forms, that of the calcified oil cyst and a solid stellate form. In the first instance a small focal area of adipose tissue becomes liquefied and at this early stage appears as a focal fluid collection. Later irritation from the fatty acids causes deposition of calcium at the periphery of the focus, appearing as a spherical, shell-shaped calcification surrounding a fluid or mixed fluid/solid center. Sonographically this appears as a curvilinear echogenic line with posterior attenuation of the sound from the presence of a calcific shell. If calcification is minimal, posterior attenuation will not be present (Fig. 20-11).

When fat necrosis results in a stellate lesion, the ultrasound appearance is not characteristic and may mimic malignancy. The presence of a focal fibrotic scar can result in the ultrasound appearance of an irregular, hypoechoic mass with posterior attenuation.

Solid Benign Lesions

The prototype of the solid, benign lesion is the fibroadenoma. It is characterized by smooth margins, low-level internal echoes, and posterior characteristics ranging from minimal sonic attenuation to moderate posterior enhancement (Figs. 20-12 to 20-14). The lesion is usually round or ovoid in configuration. If macrocalcifications are present within the fibroadenoma,

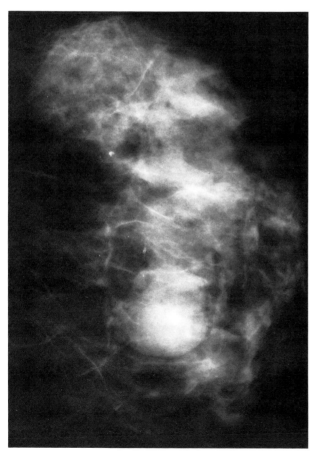

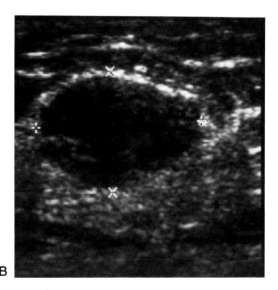

A   **B**

Fig. 20-12. (A) Craniocaudal oblique view in a 66-year-old woman with a palpable mass demonstrates a smooth ovoid mass with sharp margination at most of the periphery. **(B)** Hand-held ultrasound examination of the area shows a smoothly demarcated mass with low-level internal echoes and no posterior enhancement or attenuation. Histology: fibroadenoma.

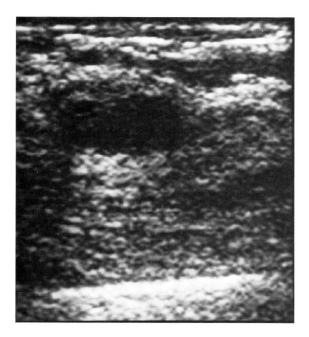

Fig. 20-13. Hand-held ultrasound examination of a 28-year-old woman with a mobile palpable breast mass shows a circumscribed ovoid mass with low-level internal echoes and slight posterior enhancement. Diagnosis: fibroadenoma

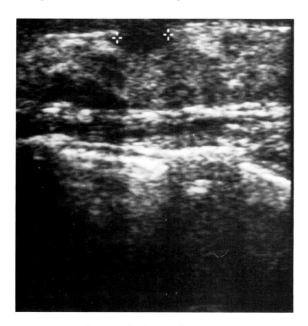

Fig. 20-14. Ultrasound of the left breast demonstrates an ovoid, well-circumscribed mass, with low-level internal echoes and moderate posterior enhancement in a 30-year-old woman with bilateral palpable breast masses. Two fibroadenomas had been previously excised on the right. The ultrasound findings in a patient of this age are most consistent with fibroadenoma.

they appear on ultrasound as echogenic foci with sharply defined posterior attenuation.

Intramammary lymph nodes may occasionally be encountered on breast ultrasound and are usually located in the axillary tail. They are smoothly demarcated, ovoid, and hypoechoic, with a few low-level internal echoes. Posterior enhancement is usually seen.

Although a smoothly defined ovoid mass seen on ultrasound usually indicates a benign lesion, any solid mass must be viewed with suspicion because certain malignant tumors, particularly the medullary and colloid carcinomas, may have characteristics virtually identical to those of the fibroadenoma. Occasionally a hyperechoic or mixed echogenicity lesion is identified on ultrasound. The findings are nonspecific, however, and virtually all solid masses will require surgical excision (Fig. 20-15).

"Fibrocystic" Masses

A focus of sclerosing adenosis occasionally manifests clinically as a palpable isolated breast mass. This type of histologic change is usually seen on ultrasound as an area of high-level homogeneous echoes containing a few hypoechoic lobules of fat. A focus of dense fibrotic tissue may cause posterior attenuation. Most authors agree that the degree of posterior echo attenuation is proportional to the amount of fibrous connective tissue present. This can cause confusion with the infiltrating ductal carcinoma, which often contains a large amount of desmoplastic fibrosis. Fibrocystic changes involving only epithelial hyperplasia are not identifiable on ultrasound examination. Cysts can usually be readily identified.

Malignant Lesions

The classic stellate scirrhous ductal carcinoma is demonstrated on ultrasound as a solid mass with irregular margins and heterogeneous internal echoes (Fig. 20-16). Attenuation properties of malignancies are proportional to the degree of associated desmoplasia. Posterior attenuation may be so strong that the entire breast mass cannot be visualized because the posterior wall cannot be imaged.

Certain malignant lesions may be difficult to differentiate from benign lesions, and ultrasound findings must

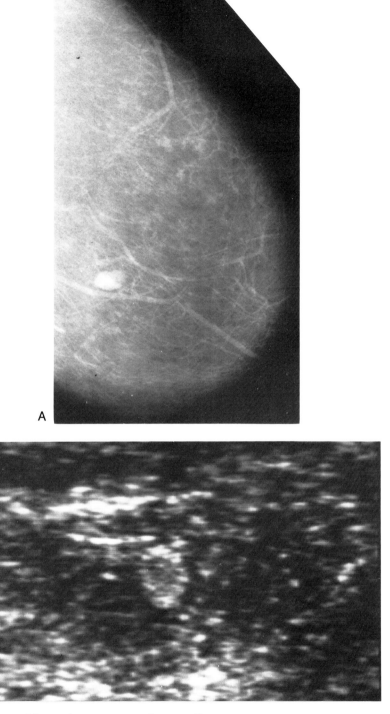

Fig. 20-15. (A) Craniocaudal view demonstrates a solitary, well-circumscribed mass in a 61-year-old asymptomatic woman. **(B)** Real-time ultrasound examination revealed a hyperechoic well-circumscribed mass with a relatively hypoechoic central area. No posterior attenuation or posterior enhancement was identified. Excisional biopsy showed a benign adenoma. The histologic characteristics were similar to a lactating adenoma, although the patient was postmenopausal.

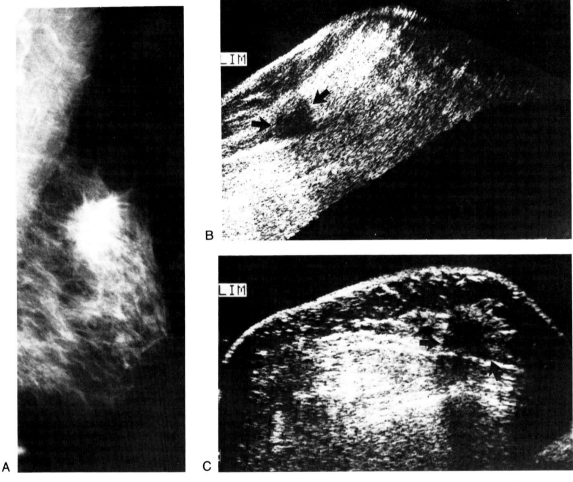

Fig. 20-16. (A) Mediolateral oblique view demonstrates a spiculated dense mass in the upper right breast in a 54-year-old woman with a palpable breast mass. **(B & C)** Automated water path ultrasound examination of the area shows an irregular hypoechoic mass *(arrows)* with a few internal echoes. Moderate posterior acoustic attenuation is noted. Pathology: infiltrating ductal carcinoma.

therefore be correlated with the clinical history and age of the patient.

Both the medullary and the colloid carcinomas are characteristically well circumscribed and show fine, low-level internal echoes with a mild degree of posterior enhancement, similar to the ultrasound appearance of a fibroadenoma.

The cystic papillary carcinoma is a relatively rare lesion that may have well-defined margins on mammography. Ultrasound demonstrates a cystic structure with a variable amount of solid tumor projecting into it (Fig. 20-17).

Histologically, infiltrating lobular carcinoma is frequently a poorly marginated mass that blends imperceptibly into the normal breast stroma, a characteristic that can make this entity difficult to identify on both mammography and ultrasound. In addition, this type of carcinoma may be multicentric. Reports of its appearance with ultrasound imaging vary from an ill-defined area of architectural distortion to an area of decreased echogenicity relative to normal breast tissue.

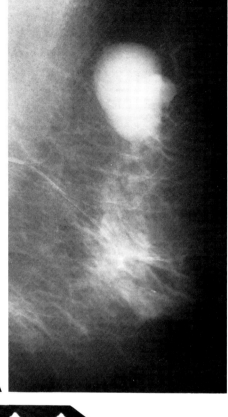

A

Fig. 20-17. (A) Mediolateral oblique view in a 75-year-old woman with a palpable mass. A sharply marginated mass with two components is present. **(B)** Hand-held ultrasound examination of the same breast demonstrates a cystic component with an accompanying solid portion extending partially into the cyst. The mass was removed. Diagnosis: Intracystic papillary carcinoma.

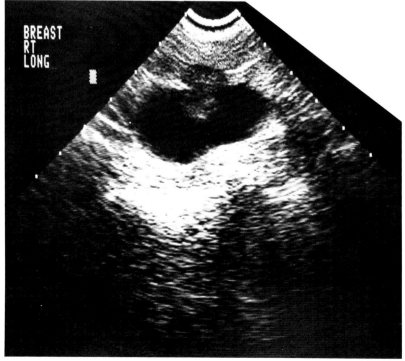

B

Metastatic lesions to the breasts, although rather rare, are occasionally reported. They are usually rounded, well circumscribed, and have weak internal echoes. Attenuation has been reported as minimal to intermediate. Melanoma is the most common source of hematogenous metastasis to the breast.

THE FUTURE OF BREAST ULTRASOUND

There is hope that ultrasound techniques for breast examination can be further refined to contribute additional information. Use of higher frequency transducers has been investigated in the identification of microcalcifications. Doppler ultrasound holds some promise for differentiating benign from malignant lesions. Research to date has shown an increased Doppler frequency shift in malignant lesions as a result of the high velocity of blood flow from the neovascularity of malignant lesions. Tissue characterization via measurement of transmitted or back-scattered waves may also be used in the future to better define breast pathology. Frequency-dependent attenuation characteristics of both benign and malignant breast tissues is also being investigated.

SUMMARY

Breast ultrasound is a useful adjunct to mammography, primarily in the differentiation of a solid from a cystic mass, whether found on mammography or as a palpable mass on physical examination. Ultrasound cannot be used as a primary method of breast carcinoma screening for several reasons. Ultrasound is of limited usefulness in the fatty breast due to poor resolution from increased refraction of the ultrasound beam. Depending on the breast type and operator, there is inconsistent identification of solid masses measuring less than 1 cm in diameter. Additionally, minimal carcinoma cannot be identified because microcalcifications are not demonstrable by currently available ultrasound techniques. Doppler examination of breast masses and ultrasonic tissue characterization may provide useful information in future applications.

SUGGESTED READINGS

1. Bassett LW, Gold RH, Kimme-Smith C: Hand Held and Automated Breast Ultrasound. Slack Inc., Thorofare, NJ, 1986
2. Bloomberg TJ, Chivers RC, Price JL: Real-time ultrasonic characteristics of the breast. Clin Radiol 35:21, 1984
3. Cole-Beuglet C, Soriano RZ, Kurtz AB, Goldberg BB: Ultrasound analysis of 104 primary breast carcinomas classified according to histopathologic type. Radiology 147:191, 1983
4. Cole-Beuglet C, Schwartz G, Kurtz AB et al: Ultrasound mammography for the augmented breast. Radiology 146:737, 1983
5. Davros WJ, Madsen EL, Zagzebski JA: Breast mass detection by ultrasound: a phantom study. Radiology 156:773, 1985
6. Derchi LE, Rizzatto G, Giuseppetti GM et al: Metastatic tumors in the breast: sonographic findings. J Ultrasound Med 4:69, 1985
7. Fleischer AC, Thieme GA, Winfield AC et al: Breast sonotomography and high-frequency, hand-held, real-time sonography: a clinical comparison. J Ultrasound Med 4:577, 1985
8. Foster FS, Strban M, Austin G: The ultrasound macroscope: initial studies of breast tissue. Ultrasonic Imaging 6:243, 1984
9. Guyer PB, Dewbury KC: Ultrasound of the breast in the symptomatic and x-ray dense breast. Clin Radiol 36:69, 1985
10. Guyer PB, Dewbury KC, Warwick D et al: Direct contact b-scan ultrasound in the diagnosis of solid breast masses. Clin Radiol 37:451, 1986
11. Harper P: Ultrasound Mammography. University Park Press, Baltimore, 1985
12. Harper AP, Kelly-Fry E, Noe JS et al: Ultrasound in the evaluation of solid breast masses. Radiology 146:731, 1983
13. Hayashi N, Tamaki N, Yonekura Y et al: Real-time sonography of palpable breast masses. Br J Radiol 58:611, 1985
14. Heywang SH, Lipsit ER, Glassman LM, Thomas MA: Specificity of ultrasonography in the diagnosis of benign breast masses. J Ultrasound Med 3:453, 1984
15. Hilton S, Leopold GR, Olson LK, Willson SA: Real-time breast sonography: application in 300 consecutive patients. AJR 147:479, 1986
16. Jackson VA, Kelly-Fry E, Rothschild PA et al: Automated breast sonography using a 7.5-MHz PVDF transducer: preliminary clinical evaluation. Radiology 159:679, 1986

17. Jackson VA, Rothschild PA, Kreipke DI et al: The spectrum of sonographic findings of fibroadenoma of the breast. Invest Radiol 21:34, 1986
18. Kobayashi T, Hayashi M, Arai M: Current status of ultrasonic tissue characterization in breast cancer. J Univ Occupational Environ Health (Jpn) 6:397, 1984
19. Kobayashi T, Hayashi M, Arai M: Echographic characteristics and ultrasonic tissue characterization in breast tumor. J Univ Occupational Environ Health (Jpn) 7:419, 1985
20. Kopans DB, Meyer JE, Lindfors KK: Whole-breast US imaging: four-year follow-up. Radiology 157:505, 1985
21. Kremkau FW: Diagnostic Ultrasound: Principles, Instrumentation, and Exercises. 2nd Ed. Grune & Stratton, Orlando, FL, 1984
22. Landini L, Sarnelli R: Evaluation of the attenuation coefficients in normal and pathological breast tissue. Med Biol Eng Comput 24:243, 1986
23. Marques BJ, Perez MR, Alvarado G: The value of image post-processing in sonomammography: a preliminary report. Bol Asoc Med PR 77:138, 1985
24. Maturo VG, Zusmer NR, Gilson AJ, Bear B: Ultrasonic appearance of mammary carcinoma with a dedicated whole-breast scanner. Radiology 142:713, 1982
25. McSweeney MB, Murphy CH: Whole-breast sonography. Radiol Clin North Am 23:157, 1985
26. Muller JW: Diagnosis of breast cysts with mammography, ultrasound and puncture. Diagn Imaging Clin Med 54:170, 1985
27. Pluygers E, Burion J: Work presented at the third international congress on the ultrasonic examination of the breast. J Belge Radiol 67:253, 1984
28. Pluygers E, Burion J, Takehara Y, Takamizawa K: C-mode ultrasonography in breast disease. J Belge Radiol 67:235, 1984
29. Rosner D, Blaird D: What ultrasonography can tell in breast masses that mammography and physical examination cannot. J Surg Oncol 28:308, 1985
30. Rubin E, Koehler RE, Urist MM: Ultrasound of the breast; what are the indications? Ala J Med Sci 23:192, 1986
31. Rubin E, Miller VE, Berland LL et al: Hand-held real-time breast sonography. AJR 144:623, 1985
32. Sarnelli R, Landini L, Martini L, Squartini F: A comparative ultrasonic-histologic study in breast cancer tissue characterization. J Nucl Med Allied Sci 29:253, 1985
33. Walsh P, Baddeley H, Timms H, Furnival CM: An assessment of ultrasound mammography as an additional investigation for the diagnosis of breast disease. Br J Radiol 58:115, 1985
34. Weber WN, Sickles EA, Cullen PW, Filly RA: Nonpalpable breast lesion localization: limited efficacy of sonography. Radiology 155:783, 1985
35. Zusmer NR, Goddard J, Maturo VG et al: Automated sonomammographic - xeromammographic - pathologic correlations in the assessment of carcinoma of the breast. J Ultrasound Med 1:19, 1982

21

The Mammography Report

Dawn R. Voegeli

The mammography report should be concise and directive, and should address any specific questions raised by the referring clinician. There are several issues unique to mammography that must also be addressed within the report.

FALSE-NEGATIVE MAMMOGRAMS

Mammography has at least a 10 percent false-negative rate in the detection of carcinoma, which may be due to errors in interpretation, poor radiographic technique, absence of radiographic criteria of malignancy, or inability to identify a mass within a dense breast. Some radiologists include a disclaimer to this effect in every mammography report. Although routine disclaimers are not recommended, it is important to educate referring physicians with regard to the limitations of mammography. When there is a clinical abnormality without a corresponding mammographic finding, an additional statement, such as "lack of radiographic findings should not delay further investigation of a palpable mass," should be included in the report.

Abnormalities within fatty breasts are often more easily recognized than those within very dense breasts. This difference in the radiologist's confidence level should be conveyed to the clinician with a statement such as

"the breasts are very dense, which makes interpretation difficult." If there is a clinical abnormality without corresponding mammographic findings in a patient with very dense breasts, a statement such as "the breasts are very dense and a mass could be hidden" may be added to the report.

USE OF THE WORD "BIOPSY"

Many surgeons object to radiologists recommending a biopsy within a written report, stating that it forces their hand. In these situations, the radiologist can substitute other strong language that conveys the same meaning, such as "the mass is very suspicious for carcinoma." The discovery of a suspicious lesion should be personally conveyed to the referring clinician, either in person or by telephone.

USE OF THE WORD "DYSPLASIA"

Radiologists often use the word "dysplasia" to describe mammographically dense breasts. This use is erroneous for two reasons. First, dense breasts may be a normal finding in many patients. Second, dysplasia is a specific pathologic condition, which cannot be identified mammographically, and should not be mentioned

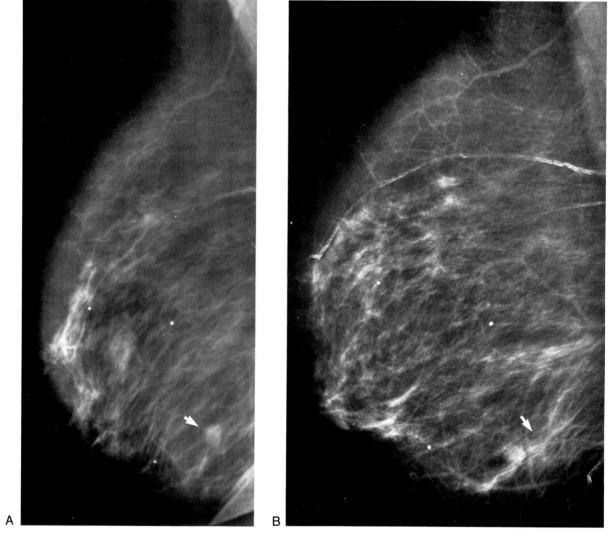

A   B

Fig. 21-1. (A) Mediolateral oblique view in a 54-year-old woman who underwent contralateral mastectomy for malignancy. A well-defined round mass is present inferiorly *(arrow)*. **(B)** Yearly follow-up showed no change in the mass, although this mammogram performed 3 years later suggests slight architectural distortion posteriorly *(arrow)*. *(Figure continues.)*

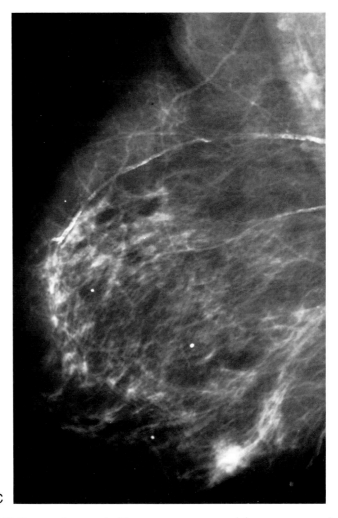

C

Fig. 21-1 *(Continued)*. **(C)** One year later a palpable mass was present, and the mammogram demonstrates increased architectural distortion and size of the mass. Histology: infiltrating ductal carcinoma.

within a mammographic report. Patients may have difficulty in obtaining health insurance because the word "dysplasia" has been used on their mammogram reports.

TIMING OF FOLLOW-UP STUDIES

Many mammographically detected abnormalities will not undergo biopsy. For example, a patient may have multiple, bilateral, well-defined masses, none of which is more suspicious than any of the others. Rather than undergo biopsy of all of these lesions, it is likely

that the patient will be followed with repeat mammography. Mammography often demonstrates areas of asymmetric density that are of questionable significance or are only identified on one view. Most of these areas of asymmetry represent normal glandular tissue, but some may be the only sign of breast cancer. It is important to follow these lesions with repeat mammography to rule out a developing cancer (Fig. 21-1). In other cases, the surgeon or patient may prefer follow-up to biopsy, regardless of the radiologist's opinion.

The first follow-up study is usually performed within 3 to 6 months, depending on the degree of suspicion.

Interval studies are then performed yearly for a minimum of 2 to 3 years. If the lesion remains unchanged after this time, it is assumed to be benign in nature, although there are reports of lesions changing up to 7 years after they were first detected.

SUGGESTED READINGS

1. Homer MJ: Analysis of patients undergoing breast biopsy. The role of mammography. JAMA 243:677, 1980
2. Homer MJ: Nonpalpable mammographic abnormalities: timing the follow-up studies. AJR 136:923, 1981
3. Homer MJ: The mammography report. AJR 142:643, 1984
4. Martin JE, Moskowitz M, Milbrath JR: Breast cancer missed by mammography. AJR 132:737, 1979
5. Newsome JF: A word of caution concerning mammography. JAMA 255:528, 1986
6. Page DL, Winfield AC: The dense mammogram. AJR 147:487, 1986
7. Wolfe JN: Xeroradiography: Uncalcified Breast Masses. Charles C Thomas, Springfield, IL, 1977
8. Wolfe JN: Xeroradiography: Breast Calcifications. Charles C Thomas, Springfield, IL, 1977
9. Wolfe JN: Mammography reporting. AJR 143:924, 1984

Index

Page numbers followed by *f* indicate figures; those followed by *t* indicate tables.

339